# INDIVIDUAL DIFFERENCES
# IN MOVEMENT

# INDIVIDUAL
# DIFFERENCES
# IN MOVEMENT

Editor

## BRUCE D. KIRKCALDY

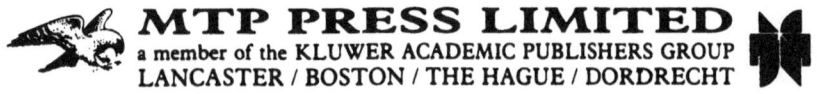
**MTP PRESS LIMITED**
a member of the KLUWER ACADEMIC PUBLISHERS GROUP
LANCASTER / BOSTON / THE HAGUE / DORDRECHT

Published in the UK and Europe by
MTP Press Limited
Falcon House
Lancaster, England

**British Library Cataloguing in Publication Data**

Individual differences in movement.
1. Human mechanics   2. Man – Attitude and
movement
I. Kirkcaldy, Bruce D.
612'.76      QP301

ISBN 0-85200-896-1

Published in the USA by
MTP Press
A division of Kluwer Boston Inc
190 Old Derby Street
Hingham, MA 02043, USA

**Library of Congress Cataloging in Publication Data**

Individual differences in movement

Bibliography: p.
Includes index.
1. Movement, Psychology of   2. Individuality.
3. Difference (Psychology)   4. Personality.
5. Psychology, Physiological. I. Kirkcaldy, Bruce D.
(Bruce David), 1952-
   BF295.I52      1985     152.3      85-18098

ISBN-13: 978-94-010-8676-9      e-ISBN-13: 978-94-009-4912-6
DOI: 10.1007/978-94-009-4912-6

Typesetting by Blackpool Typesetting Services Ltd., Blackpool.

# Contents

# Introduction

This book is an attempt to bridge the gap between differential psychology and human movement. It is curious that each discipline has received considerable attention in its own right but little effort has been made to cross-fertilize them. Some experimentalists view this union as the equivalent of committing academic adultery; they have tended to concentrate on general theories and models of motor control and movement, viewing individual differences as awkward and best assigned to the error variance component of an analysis. By neglecting person variables, valuable information is discarded: people do differ in terms of ability, attitude, motivation and temperament and it is hardly surprising that such differences interact with a variety of experimental and situational paradigms. The causes and determinants of individual differences must be examined at an interdisciplinary level, incorporating studies from experimental, physiological, clinical and educational psychology. This synthesis could not have been actualized by any single contributor. For this reason, a multi-authored approach has been adopted, in which 17 specialists have been assembled to present the current position of individual difference research in their respective disciplines.

The authors were granted maximum freedom in their selection and presentation of material. What emerges is, hopefully, a novel and informative collection of articles addressed to a wide audience and providing an impulse for further research. The plurifacultative approach combined with an appropriate level of communication should assure its appeal amongst students, practitioners and researchers in clinical and educational psychology, as well as psychiatrists, counsellors and physical educators.

The book is organized more or less into three sections covering various aspects of the spectrum of human movement ranging from an examination of primarily laboratory-oriented studies (experimental and developmental) involving behavioural measures of motor skills and performance, to the more macroscopic events (social and applied studies) including non-verbal communication, expressive styles, sport and playful behaviour. An intermediate section is devoted to the neurophysiological bases underlying such behavioural variation.

The opening chapter on individual differences in voluntary movement (Sheridan) considers, as its central theme, sources of variation in skill and ability underlying individual differences in motor performance, and a distinction is made between the kinematics or form of a movement, and the outcome of a movement. Attention is also given to consistencies in motor behaviour, since these can illustrate the constraints operating on human motor behaviour at a number of different levels. Intra- and interindividual movement variation are discussed at a number of levels, and it is argued that there are individual differences in initial potential, in practice and in experience, which at one level affect movement production, and at another level affect action, by influencing the knowledge that the organism has about itself and its world.

In Chapter 2, a novel amalgamated theory of extraversion is presented drawing on theories from Pavlov and Eysenck. Eysenck's theoretical standpoint (reactive inhibition and arousal theory) is examined at different stages of development. Brebner suggests that central mechanisms can either be in a state of excitation or inhibition, dependent on the demands imposed by stimulus-analysis or response-organization (both S-analysis and R-organization occur prior to the execution of the response). Extraverts ought to make frequent and faster motor responses than introverts due to their ability to generate excitation from R-organization and inhibition from S-analysis. Introverts should prefer a strategy in which excitation is derived from frequent stimulus analysis and the feedback stimulation from discrete responses. Brebner attempts a selective review of currect literature on movement and personality to gain empirical support for this revitalized model of extraversion.

Runeson's contribution presents a recently developed principle – Kinematic Specification of Dynamics (KSD) – based on concepts from physics, biomechanics, robotics and recent advances in motor control theory. The principle asserts that the kinematic pattern of a person in action is, by necessity, specific to the movement relevant properties of the person. These properties include, for example, anatomical proportions, intentions and expectations. It could also be extended to psychological states and properties such as emotions and personality when these are construed as transient and stable conditions of readiness of the motor system. He goes on to review studies exploring the consequences of the KSD principle for visual perception of persons and action. In particular, the review considers studies of gender and identity perception from displays of human kinematic patterns as published by Cutting and colleagues as well as Runeson and Frykholm. Emphasis is laid on the possibility of faking one's movements so as to give observers false impressions of oneself or what one is doing. The discussion concludes by stressing the richness of unfakeable information about person and action available in human movements, their role in social interaction and consequences in social psychology.

Eysenck's contribution on the role of reminiscence in the acquisition of skilled movements focuses on theories studied within the laboratory context (a microscopic analysis). The phenomenon of reminiscence is described – the observation that performance tends to improve after a period of rest – an event which is easily characterized but is difficult to define adequately. The two major theories of reminiscence are examined (inhibition and consolidation);

particular attention is given to Ammon's concept of inhibition theory which has been supported by large scale experimental studies, as well as to Kimble's two-factor theory of inhibition (in which drive serves as a motivational basis for habit development). Eysenck offers an array of empirical studies primarily involving the pursuit rotor task in which the effects of motivation and personality variables on reminiscence are considered. The chapter culminates in the presentation of the Eysenck and Frith revised version of consolidation theory which, in addition to taking account of previous criticisms, is open to empirical testing. Reminiscence emerges as a very important factor in the acquisition of motor skills, both practically and even more theoretically.

Glanzmann examines the theories and empirical evidence concerning the relationship between trait anxiety, state anxiety and performance in different stress situations on the basis of drive theoretical concepts. In addition to outlining basic drive theory constructs, the trait–state distinction of anxiety and problems related to the assessment of state anxiety by means of self-reports are considered, as well as examination of the worry–emotionality distinction and the issues of generality of anxiety traits. Revisions of drive theory are suggested pertaining to the effects of task difficulty on learning performance, the integration of coping behaviour in the drive theory model and the anxiety–performance relationship in ego threatening and pain threatening situations. He concludes with a brief overview of current theory and research on anxiety.

Campbell's first chapter provides a review of the various methods used in the measurement of the timing and duration of information processing activities (mental chronometry). He expresses scepticism of the reliance occasionally placed on using the behavioural index, mean or median reaction time, since it is laden with methodological problems. An assumption of serial model information processing is that the reaction process entails a linear sequence of discrete stages. Group differences in mean reaction time are therefore difficult to interpret because they can arise for a variety of reasons. Reaction time is also susceptible to an individual's bias towards speed or accuracy in responding strategy. Campbell describes the advantages of using a physiological measure, the average evoked potential, which can be divided into components in much the same manner as the information processing stages of behavioural studies. The late positive wave, P300, seems to be primarily affected by stimulus evaluation processes, whereas reaction time involves stimulus evaluation and response production. The difference between P3 and reaction time latency may thus serve as an indication of the contribution of response bias to the overall reaction time.

The second chapter by Campbell, co-authored with Noldy-Cullum, is devoted to studies on group differences in the 'speed of decision-making'. Five typical areas reflecting individual differences in reaction time have been sampled in this review: (1) intelligence, (2) extraversion, (3) hyperactivity, (4) brain trauma and (5) ageing. The possibility that individual differences in response bias could influence group differences is discussed. In many cases, group differences in mean reaction time are impossible to interpret. Alternative methods of analysis that employ a sophisticated trial-by-trial analysis of reaction time, taking error into consideration, are recommended. Examples of how the use of the latency of the P3 component can dramatically alter interpretation of group reaction time differences are also provided since it (P3) is determined by processes leading to stimulus evaluation and is relatively independent of response bias. By combining both reaction time and P3 latencies, it can be demonstrated that at least in some cases, group differences in mean reaction time may be due to variation in response bias and not to processes leading to stimulus evaluation.

Bechtereva and Kambarova describe details of studies performed at the Soviet Academy of Sciences in Leningrad using long-term intracerebral electrode implantation for diagnostic and therapeutic purposes in neurological patients. By directly registering neurophysiological dynamics of brain states, valuable information is gained concerning the interrelationship between anatomical structure and function. This is achieved by a combination of local electrostimulative techniques together with infra-slow physiological processes (ISPP). Such psychophysiological correlates of behaviour enabled the identification of spatial cerebral patterns related to normal and pathological emotional states. A central area of investigation was the dynamic character of rearrangement of brain processes during emotional responses (evoked and spontaneous) and movement processes, including speech-motor behaviour.

Stelmack's paper examines individual differences in motor behaviour from a psychophysiological perspective. He commences with a review of studies relating personality factors (focusing on Eysenck's concept of extraversion for ease of exposition) with responsivity to sensory stimulation. He proceeds to examine the relationship between the personality variables, extraversion and anxiety, and the physiological measure, contingent negative variation (an electrocortical measure assumed to assess motor preparedness). In addition, the differential effects of cortically excitatory and inhibitory drugs such as chlordiazepoxide, caffeine, nicotine and cannabis are considered. Cardiovascular activity, which together with electrocortical activity is functionally related to motor activity, is examined in relation to the dimensions of type A, sensation-seeking and extraversion (personality dimensions with common descriptive characteristics). Furthermore, the differential effects of incentives and rewards on heart rate in various personality groups are examined.

Castell and Blumenthal begin their contribution with a series of definitions pertinent to the area of research in physical exercise and mood, paying particular attention to the health-related aspects (psychological and physical benefits) of aerobic exercise. A distinction is made between the acute and chronic effects of such exercise on anxiety and depression in clinical as well as normal populations. They review much of the contemporary research of clinical and laboratory studies with emphasis on methodological limitations, e.g. need for random experimental designs, more adequate descriptions of subject characteristics involved and less reliance on self-report methods of assessment. They conclude their chapter by providing possible directions for future research.

Bull's chapter is concerned with individual differences in both the encoding and decoding of non-verbal cues in the context of the social skills model. With regard to encoding, people may vary in their ability to express themselves non-verbally, while non-verbal cues may also provide encoded information concerning what sort of individual they are. Individuals vary as well in their ability to decode non-verbal cues, although there may be different types of skill, such that the person who is good at decoding intentional or posed communications may not necessarily be good at decoding spontaneous or unintentional communications. These theoretical issues of decoding and encoding non-verbal cues are discussed in terms of differences in age, culture, sex, personality and psychopathology.

Conley's chapter on movement and personal styles is hypothetical in character; the theoretical linkages which are suggested are important and revealing. He examines the work of Allport and Vernon on expressive styles as an example of an exciting and promising attempt at relating personality theory with movement studies. He considers it a lost opportunity that this approach was never actively pursued by researchers. The chapter describes the original work of Allport and Vernon on expressive movement and elaborates the theory of personal styles as integrative heuristic for the study of human movement and other forms of expressive behaviour.

An unusual situation has emerged in sport psychology: trait psychology has fallen into disrepute, as its value has been questioned as a result of the many inconsistencies in the literature. Even in those instances where statistically significant findings have been reported they have generally been of low explanatory and predictive value, leading some to refer to 'experimenter suicide' for those who choose to employ traditional trait strategies. This controversial area is characterized by many deficiencies arising from methodological and statistical weaknesses. Kirkcaldy's contribution examines critically the value of implementation of personality studies in sport settings, discussing the need for a control of response distortion, assessment of the magnitude of effect, secondary source errors, moderator variables and the importance of theoretical enquiry.

The article by Nias, on recreational behaviour and personality, commences with a review of a series of large-scale factor analyses aimed at providing an appropriate classification of interests. Personality and demographic factors are amongst the determinants of lifestyle preference and recreational pursuits which are considered. Furthermore, Nias goes on to examine the influence of family and peers in the selection of activities: for example, husband–wife and parent–child similarities as well as the relationship between marital satisfaction and type of leisure preference. The motivational aspects of participating in particular pursuits are also examined. The needs for preferring certain activities are assumed to be partially attributable to genetic factors. Finally, the possible beneficial effects of recreation (in terms of improved well-being and mental health) as well as the effect of competition are raised.

Liss examines children's play with toys and relates such play to skilled learning. She reviews literature on sex differences in playing behaviour in children, particularly the manner in which boys and girls differ in their toy play in terms of factors of high and low activity level and gross and fine motor skills. The issue is raised as to whether children acquire identical skills from male- or female-traditional toys, as well as the degree of transference of such skills to other toys. She considers the possibility of incorporating intervention procedures such as modelling and reinforcement, for changing sex-typed play.

Teacher influences and clothing, group size and type of play are amongst the variables considered which determine sex differences in playful behaviour.

It is inevitable that some of the articles have been somewhat arbitrarily assigned to a particular section. Furthermore, the task of integrating technical and substantive findings from a wealth of psychological material was enormous and there are obviously some areas which were neglected in the process. I realize that as editor I am ultimately responsible for the structure and content of the product, which to some extent reflects my personal interests. The problem inherent in most multi-authored books in which there is a certain degree of overlap between contributions has been generally viewed positively, since authors were frequently interested in finding out how others perceived similar topics. Furthermore, this led to clarification of several earlier conceptual inadequacies as well as promoting good informal contacts amongst the contributors which has, in my case, made the task of editing that much more enjoyable.

It remains for me to perform the pleasurable task of expressing my deep gratitude to all those contributors who considered this a sufficiently worthwhile venture in which to participate. The execution of such a comprehensive and exploratory text owes much to the co-operative effort and enthusiasm of its authors. I am also appreciative of the assistance offered by several in reviewing various sections of the book; special thanks go to Gunther Barrie (Senior Psychologist at the IBA), Maurice Yaffe (York Clinic, Guy's Hospital, London), Michael Eysenck (Birkbeck College, University of London), Patrick Chauvel (Institut National de la Santé et de la Recherche Médicale, Paris) and Marvin Zuckerman (University of Delaware). They provided valuable criticisms and suggestions for improvement. I am particularly grateful for the encouragement and continued support offered by MTP Press UK who did significantly more than provide editorial guidance throughout, thanks going to David Bloomer, Managing Director and Lesley Cassar, Editorial Liaison Officer. I should like to take the opportunity of extending my appreciation to Kurt Alphons Jochheim, Director of the Rehabilitation Clinic, University of Cologne for his support and Hans J. Eysenck, Institute of Psychiatry, University of London whose work has influenced much of my own research in movement studies. Finally, Elisabeth Thomé (Fachschule für Sozial Pädagogik, Düsseldorf) has been a patient and comforting friend during the incubation phase of this venture and her optimism did much to reassure me.

# List of Contributors

N. P. BECHTEREVA
Department of Human Neurophysiology
Institute of Experimental Medicine
USSR Academy of Medical Sciences
12 Pavlov's Street, Leningrad 197022
USSR

J. A. BLUMENTHAL
Department of Psychiatry
Behavioural Physiology Laboratory
Box 3926
Duke University Medical Center
Durham, North Carolina 27710
USA

J. BREBNER
Psychology Department
University of Adelaide
Box 498, Adelaide 5001
Australia

P. E. BULL
Department of Psychology
University of York
Heslington, York YO1 5DD
UK

K. B. CAMPBELL
School of Psychology
University of Ottawa
Ottawa KIN 6N5
Canada

P. J. CASTELL
Research Training Program Center for
  the Study of Aging and Human
  Development
Box 2969
Duke University Medical Center
Durham, North Carolina 27710
USA

J. J. CONLEY
Stonington Institute
North Stonington
Connecticut 06359
USA

H. J. EYSENCK
Institute of Psychiatry
Department of Psychology
De Crespigny Park
University of London
London SE5 8AF
UK

P. GLANZMANN
Psychological Institute
University of Mainz
6500 Mainz, Saarstrasse 21
Jacob-Welder-Weg 18, Postfach 3980
West Germany

D. K. KAMBAROVA
Institute of Experimental Medicine
USSR Academy of Medical Sciences
12 Pavlov's Street, Leningrad 197022
USSR

B. D. KIRKCALDY
Rehabilitation Clinic of the
   University of Cologne
Lindenburger Allee 44
5000 Cologne, 41-Lindenthal
West Germany

M. B. LISS
Department of Psychology
California State University
San Bernardino
5500 University Parkway
California 92407
USA

D. K. B. NIAS
Institute of Psychiatry
Department of Psychology
De Crespigny Park
University of London
London SE5 8AF
UK

N. NOLDY-CULLUM
School of Psychology
University of Ottawa
Ottawa KIN 6N5
Canada

S. RUNESON
Department of Psychology
University of Uppsala
Box 227, S-75104 Uppsala
Sweden

M. R. SHERIDAN
Department of Psychology
University of Hull
Hull HU6 7RX
UK

R. M. STELMACK
School of Psychology
University of Ottawa
Ottawa KIN 6N5
Canada

# SECTION 1

# EXPERIMENTAL AND DEVELOPMENTAL STUDIES

# 1
## Individual differences in voluntary movement

*Martin R. Sheridan*

---

## INTRODUCTION

Over 50 years ago Bartlett[1] illustrated the complexity of motor behaviour by reference to the high level skill of an experienced tennis player. As with Bartlett we can all marvel at people possessed of high level skills, the professional golfer, the gymnast, the pilot, the musician, and this leads us to speculate what accounts for the success achieved by some individuals while others remain relative novices. Variation in human performance occurs not only in what may be termed skilled behaviour, but also in more general performance. For example, of the 18 647 runners in the 1984 London Marathon, the first competitor completed the course in a time of somewhat over 2 hours, while the last recorded competitor, a sufferer from cerebral palsy, arrived home in a time of just under 9.5 hours, and 16% never finished! Quite a variation in what might be considered to be a basic locomotor function. A central theme of the present chapter will include consideration of the sources of variation in both skill and ability underlying individual differences in motor performance. Attention will also be given to consistencies in motor behaviour, since the consistencies can be as illuminating as the differences. Such consistencies can illustrate the constraints operating on human motor behaviour at a number of different levels, from simple biomechanical constraints on the system (e.g. you cannot bend your elbow backwards), through limitations imposed by functional synergies, which we will discuss later (e.g. it is difficult to rub one's tummy while at the same time patting one's head), to limitations on the strategy options available for performing a task efficiently (e.g. there are only a limited number of ways one can sensibly attempt to turn on a water tap). In general, it would appear that the more global the level in the hierarchy, the greater the opportunity for variation in the way in which an action is performed, although lower levels in the system have greater freedom to determine the ultimate form of the movement. More will be said of this later.

The study of individual differences has been somewhat of a Cinderella in the motor skills literature, with variations between individuals' performance being considered essentially an inconvenience and classified simply as error

3

variance by experimentalists. Predominantly, only group data have been considered. The reason for the reluctance of researchers to confront the issue is not hard to understand when one is faced with the complications and complexity of attempting to explain the diversity of individual motor performance. This is not to excuse any oversight on the part of researchers. However, such an approach does reflect the fact that we are only beginning to come to any understanding of the complexity inherent in the perceptual-motor system. A concern with understanding the mechanisms and processes that underlie motor skills performance and learning has, for many researchers, relegated the study of individual differences to a subsidiary position. The questions they have been asking relate to the development of general theories of motor control or models of movement, and are different in form from questions concerned with predicting individual performance. It is clear, however, that ultimately failure to consider individual variation reduces explanatory power. For example, one of the most widely recognized findings in the motor skills area is the linear relationship relating the difficulty of a movement (as measured in bits) to the time taken to complete the movement, and is commonly referred to as Fitts' Law[2]. Fitts reasoned that the speed with which movements are made is limited by the information-processing capacity of the motor system. Thus, the information-transmission rate of a specified limb system can be calculated for a given person and task. Fitts' view that the linear relationship results from information-transmission characteristics is not now generally accepted and other models have been developed which lead to Fitts' Law. However, the basic finding of a linear relationship receives support from numerous studies involving a diversity of tasks (see Keele[3] for a review). Moreover, it is often reported that the linear relationship accounts for a large proportion of the variance in *mean* movement times. Some inadequacies have, however, been noted with Fitts' approach[4], and if one considers individual rather than group movement times then the relationship can be seen to deviate markedly from linearity in a number of instances.

While experimental psychologists have typically avoided the issue of individual differences, another group of researchers, termed by Cronbach[5], differential psychologists, have been specifically concerned with the problem. The differential psychologist's interest in such things as genetic variation and early experience as influences on individual performance can be traced to the time of Spearman[6]. Rarely since that time, however, has there been any cross-fertilization of ideas between adherents of the two distinct theoretical positions. As has already been said, failure to consider individual variation ultimately reduces explanatory power, and although adopting a somewhat different approach, some traditional experimentalists are beginning to be concerned with individual differences in such factors as the rate of repetitive activity, which can affect a number of aspects of motor performance[7].

## THE PSYCHOMETRIC APPROACH

The major concern of the differential psychologist is the prediction of individual performance, and more specifically in the area of motor skills, the prediction of motor task performance. The basis of this prediction is usually knowledge about the individual's performance on other tasks. The impetus for this work has predominantly been the need of industry and such organizations as the armed forces to select personnel to operate machinery and complex systems of various types, from lathes to jet aircraft. Selection naturally involves identifying individual differences, and to deal with the problem of predicting performance on the real task on the basis of performance on a test, it is assumed that there are underlying *abilities* which are required for both. The abilities may be seen as completely innate, in which case they are sometimes referred to as capacities, or more usually, it is argued that there is a learned component superimposed on the genetic component, and that this may vary in degree.

Early discussion of abilities revolved around the idea that all motor skills were based on a single motor ability specific to the individual and termed, general motor ability (GMA). Thus, individuals high in GMA were argued to perform well on nearly every motor task, while those low in GMA were supposed to perform badly. The majority of experimental evidence does not support the notion of GMA, and correlations of performance on different tasks are typically low[8]. At an informal level, examples such as the 1984 Olympic decathlete Daley Thompson may be advanced to demonstrate that some individuals do indeed possess a high degree of general motor ability. However, in stressing a capacity argument, the full-time practice behind such performance tends to be neglected. Moreover, one might reasonably doubt whether good track and field performance would transfer to, for example, playing snooker. Seashore's[9] reaction to finding low intercorrelations was to suggest that skills are acquired by a somewhat haphazard trial-and-error process, in such a way that the first fairly successful method of performing the task becomes established in the learner's repertoire. This clearly would lead to large individual differences in the production of movement. As an alternative to GMA ideas, Henry[10] proposed that a very large number of independent abilities underlie motor performance, and that each of the abilities is responsible for only a limited number of movements. There is some evidence for this specificity hypothesis, however, while correlations between motor tasks are low, they are often not near zero as Henry's hypothesis would suggest.

Falling between the GMA and specificity approaches have been Fleishman's ideas concerning motor abilities. Fleishman[11, 12] has been the central figure in the psychometric approach to predicting motor task performance, and for him the development of abilities is a prerequisite for successful performance in a variety of different skills. Thus, abilities are considered to be generally not task specific. Since abilities, like skills, are subject to learning, some distinction needs to be made between them. Fleishman[11] considers that an ability is a 'more general trait of the individual which has been inferred from certain response consistencies (e.g. correlations)', and that abilities are 'fairly enduring traits'. Many abilities he sees as being the product of learning, developing at different rates 'mainly during childhood and adolescence'. We will return to discuss the issue of early learning later in the chapter. Abilities are seen as being person-oriented; thus at a given stage in life they represent 'organismic factors which the individual brings with him when he begins to learn a new task'[13]. On the other hand, skill is for Fleishman a task-oriented term referring to 'the level of proficiency on a specific task or a limited group of tasks'[11]. Characterizing skill in this way we can talk about proficiency attained in various different skills, such as flying an aeroplane, operating a lathe, or playing golf. Although each skill is seen as being specific, it has been argued that they can have characteristics like spatiotemporal patterning in common.

During learning particular abilities change in their relative importance. Considering correlations between measures of performance on trials at different stages of learning a task, it has been found that correlations tend to be lower the greater the separation between trials. This feature of intertrial correlation matrices is known as the superdiagonal form. In simple tasks the correlations tend to zero within an interval of relatively few trials. However, Jones[14, 15] has pointed out that in complex skills the superdiagonal form is less typical and has proposed two complementary processes in skill acquisition. One process occurs in very simple tasks, with a progressive simplification so that individual differences disappear leaving only random error variance, and the other process is in complex tasks, with a progressive combination of simple elements into wholes which may remain to some degree characteristic of the individual and possibly reflect his unique work method.

In 1966 Fleishman discussed abilities and the problems of task taxonomy in terms of 11 psychomotor factors and eight physical proficiency factors. By 1975 the number of factors had risen to 37, but the problems of defining a task largely remain. In any event, the abilities identified only account for a certain proportion of the whole task, while the rest must be accounted for by unknown abilities or other factors intrinsic to the task. For example, Fleishman and Hempel[16] reported that the variance in performance attributed to the 'task specific' factor increased from 10% on the first trial to 45% on the 15th trial, while variance due to the spatial relations factor decreased from 35% to 10% on the same respective trials. Throughout the learning period, however, 25–30% of the variance was unaccounted for by any known factor.

## MOVEMENT AND MOVEMENT OUTCOME

Skill has been defined as 'the learned ability to bring about predetermined results with maximum certainty often with the minimum outlay of time or energy or both'[17]. While such a definition captures only part of the essence of skilled behaviour, skill or ability considered in this way is judged by the degree of success in bringing about a predetermined result. In golf, for example, the desired outcome would be to put the ball into the hole with as few strokes as possible. This overall goal can, of course, have a number of subgoals which may not be precisely defined, for example, driving the ball from the tee so as to place it in a favourable position on the fairway from which the next shot to the hole can be played. The error tolerance for what may be considered a 'favourable position' could be relatively large. The point is, however, that movement is often related to goal-directed activity.

It is important to make the distinction between the form or kinematics of a movement and the outcome of a movement, because the outcome of a movement is often more important than the way we achieve the outcome.

(Kinematic refers to the description of movement in terms of the resultant product of the motor system, that is, motion, considered without reference to force or mass. Motion involves the dimensions of space and time; therefore velocity would be one example of a kinematic variable.) Thus, there is considerable scope for movement variation, both between and within individuals. This naturally can lead to considerable individual differences in movement production. The philosopher Ricoeur[18] describes the situation thus: 'We need to correct radically the opinion that, the "object" of action, the terminus of "realization" is movement . . . Actually, when I act . . . I am concerned less with my body than with the product of the action: the hanged picture, the strike of the hammer on the head of the nail.' Runeson and Frykholm[19] have perhaps put this more succinctly when arguing that, 'Evolutionary pressure has been on achievement, not on the kinematic detail of how we achieve.' It is easy to appreciate the argument that it is the outcome which is more important, rather than producing prescribed movement patterns. If a footballer were given the option of scoring a goal in a somewhat clumsy manner, say off his knee, or missing the goal with a well-struck powerful shot passing over the bar, in most cases there would be little doubt about his choice. However, although outcome is most important, people often value the form of the movement as well. The footballer's ideal choice would presumably be to score the goal in a graceful fashion. Listening to commentators on various sports it is clear that there is an aesthetic quality to the action, in addition to its outcome. Thus, in golf the player may be described as having a 'classic swing', or in cricket the player may produce what is described as a 'beautiful cover drive'. Such description is usually coupled with a successful outcome; however, not all successful outcomes produce such description. In cricket, a snick over the top of the slips for four may not be viewed in the same way as an orthodox square cut for four. A problem arises in such games, when the form of the action is stressed almost to the exclusion of the outcome. An illustration of this has been provided by Hammond[20] in relation to the sport of fencing, in which the traditional approach to coaching had been to stress a particular postural and movement style sometimes at the expense of winning! A few years ago when an English side was, as now, having trouble scoring runs at cricket, a humorous letter appeared in *The Times* suggesting that English batsmen would fare better if they occasionally reversed their bats. Against fast bowling the ball would then either be played into the ground or over the top of the slips for four. Regardless of the outcome, such behaviour would not, however, be considered 'good form' or 'gentlemanly conduct', and in all probability the rules of the game would be changed to outlaw such a ploy. The point is that in games the satisfaction derived from playing (or watching) depends on displaying *skill* within the limitations of the rules of the game, while meeting a challenge that is neither ridiculously easy nor impossibly difficult. Indeed, this is the essence of games. At a gross level the rules of the game limit the action available for achieving a particular outcome, although somewhat paradoxically within the constraints they maximize the range of individual differences displayed. The rules can be extensive. To take but one example, the Book of Rules for golf runs to 87 pages and over 20000 words. In order to prevent the game from becoming too easy and perhaps less satisfying, the game's governing bodies have rules and specifications which prohibit further improvement in the performance of golf equipment. Although a golf ball could be produced which travelled a good deal further, this would tend to reduce the range of skill levels displayed and would reduce the expression of individual differences. To make the game more challenging might then involve a change in the ground rules, for example constructing more bunkers or lengthening fairways. Often the effect of rules is to maximize, within certain limits, the range of skill levels displayed, and hence make individual differences more noticeable. In sporting activities, humans appear interested in performance differences which derive from people, and much less interested in variations due to equipment, although there are exceptions (e.g. motor racing). Governing bodies in all sports are in a continual process of adjusting the rules in an attempt to increase both spectators' and players' enjoyment. This maximization of the opportunity for performance variation between individuals (and teams) may simply be part of a process of social comparison[21, 22], although this is outside of the scope of the present chapter.

The form of a movement and the outcome of a movement may not be as separate as has perhaps been implied. The good form of a movement may contribute to a successful outcome (e.g. playing with a 'straight bat' in cricket), but it will not guarantee it, neither does an ungainly style, which may not be in a 'classic' mould, make failure inevitable. A simple example can be seen in running. In humans the alternate-step gait is used both for running and walking, and with this style of locomotion, whatever the position of one leg, the other leg is always one half cycle out of phase (rather like the pedals of a bicycle). The 'equation of constraint'[23] governing the relationship applies whatever the speed of running, and moreover, holds across individuals. More will be said about equations of constraint later. Similarly, the action of the arms becomes phase-locked to the step cycle of the legs. Thus, there is an invariance and consistency in the relative timing of the components of locomotor movements which applies across individuals. Clearly, however, there are individual differences in running, both in performance and style. The variation between individuals occurs for such aspects as mass of the limbs and body, force which the leg muscles can generate, stride length, etc. Variation can also occur in features which may be incidental to performance, such as whether one runs with one's elbows sticking out or not. These features can give individuals their characteristic styles. As mentioned earlier, however ungainly such an action, if it is incidental to task performance, it may not mitigate strongly against a successful outcome. While these elements can vary between individuals, relative timing of the step cycle varies little[24], except in cases of motor dysfunction, where performance deteriorates markedly.

A more complex example of a less innately programmed action can be taken from the game of golf. Cochran[25] has provided an interesting analysis of the golf swing, and he argues that, 'All highly skilled players must (and do) achieve very similar clubhead conditions at impact, and since these conditions lie near the limits of available power, they must result from swings which are similar in overall pattern.' Thus, the temporal patterning of the swings of different top-class golfers must be essentially similar. The timing of the components of the movement relative to each other may be similar, but certain aspects such as the path the backswing takes relative to the downswing, the angle of the down-swing, and the way in which the hands and wrists act as a pivot for the clubhead, appear open to variation, within limits, without adversely affecting the result. Cochran[25] thus argues that one can meaningfully talk of 'my swing' or 'your swing' or 'Jack Nicklaus' swing', as indeed golfers do. Of course, less experienced golfers may exceed the limits of variation and also may vary considerably in the temporal patterning of their swings, leading overall to poor performance. In contrast, the impression one obtains from watching expert golfers is one of rhythm and smoothness in their swings. Other mannerisms, in a mechanical sense incidental to the task, may characterize individuals or even sports. For example, in golf, individual characteristics may be associated with initiating the backswing, such as Jack Nicklaus' slight turn of the head, or Gary Player's inward press of the right knee. Equivalent mannerisms characterize many sportsmen. Particular initiating characteristics may be quite widely adopted in certain sports, for example, the 'to and fro' rocking motion of the high or long jumper, before initiating the approach run. Such triggering mechanisms, although apparently not necessary in a mechanical sense, nevertheless help the individual to accomplish the mechanically essential movements in a smooth and correct fashion. Such mannerisms are readily noticeable, and we have all been amused by young children who have adopted all the characteristics of a particular sport, or sports personality, while lacking the technique and experience to successfully achieve the desired outcome.

While it has been suggested that there can be latitude for variation in the kinematics or form of movement, and that this to some extent can be independent of outcome, there is another category of activities in which the goal cannot be specified in isolation from the aesthetic quality of the action. For example, in gymnastics, figure-skating, ice-dancing, trampolining and diving, the intrinsic end cannot be identified independently of the means. The form of movement is central to a successful outcome in such activities. It is the case, however, that in most activities the outcome remains of primary importance, with the means of achieving the outcome a secondary factor. A few sports, such as ski-jumping, fall somewhere in the middle of the continuum, between activities involving predominantly aesthetic or predominantly objective measures of performance, with marks being awarded for both style and distance.

## MOVEMENT VARIATION

In the previous section it was argued that the outcome of a movement is, in general, more important than its form. In the present section we will consider the control of movement in more detail, and discuss factors affecting both intra- and interindividual movement variability. In attempting to discuss response organization and movement, a number of aspects of motor behaviour need to be taken into account. First, that the motor system has the ability to achieve functionally the same end result via different movements, involving different muscles and joints (*equifinality* or *motor constancy*). Second, that movements are never exactly repeated (*uniqueness of action*). Performance scores and EMG records indicate that there is variation even when repeating the same response. Learning a response thus involves repeated attempts to achieve the desired result, but without exactly repeating the same movement, and without getting the same feedback. This has led Whiting[26] to observe that acquiring a skill in these terms 'does not mean to repeat and consolidate, but to invent, to progress'. Third, that despite the apparent uniqueness of each movement, the most obvious feature of skilled performance is the consistency and stability of both temporal and spatial structure (*stability and consistency of action*). Fourth, that not only is skilled action consistent and stable, but it is also capable of amendment as a consequence of changes in information available to the performer (*modifiability of action*).

There is not space in the present chapter to consider the various models which have been proposed to deal with these issues (see Sheridan[27] for a review); however, to illustrate the problem let us consider the simple example of holding a cup of tea at a particular position and then moving it towards one's lips. To achieve this one must be able to hold the cup at a particular location in space (the start position) and with a particular orientation (to avoid spilling the tea). It is then necessary to move the cup toward the target, in this case the mouth, in order to make contact.

The position of a static object can be described completely in terms of six dimensions of movement, the three Cartesian coordinates of its location in space, and the three angular coordinates of its orientation at that location. It is necessary to control these six dimensions to place an object, in this case the cup, in a particular position. To avoid spilling the tea it is clear that some degree of precision is required, particularly when one begins to move the cup. Within the arm there are three pivoted points about the wrist, elbow and shoulder joints; if to simplify, we ignore the flexibility of the hand and the ability to move the complete shoulder girdle. Including rotations about the wrist and shoulder the three joints provide us with a total of seven degrees of freedom of movement. This is one degree of freedom more than is necessary to completely control the position of our cup. Since each of the joint angles is continuously variable, there are an infinite number of ways in which we might accomplish the same final cup position. The different joints can be moved varying amounts to achieve the same end position of the hand. In two different movements bringing the hand to the same final position, the individual muscles of the arm could finish at different lengths with the joints at different angles.

While we may not use all of the movement options open to us, we do use more than one. Indeed, the fact that we can achieve the same end result in a number of different ways provides us with flexibility in dealing with the environment. So far we have considered movement related to regulating the seven degrees of freedom based on joint angles. However, it is clear that the patterns of innervation to the limb muscles must be different in different types of movement. Thus, even an ostensibly simple movement taking the hand between two positions in space requires specification of the innervation patterns for many muscles and must be selected from a wide range of possibilities. Over 40 years ago Bernstein[28] (translated in 1967) discussed this issue, terming it the degrees of freedom problem. Bartlett[1] had similarly alluded to the problem.

There are many examples in the literature which illustrate the problem[23]. Controlling even simple movement via the joints may seem quite difficult; however, if what is being regulated are individual muscles then the problem is compounded. Each muscle varies only on the dimension of contractile state, and hence has one degree of freedom. If, to simplify, we ignore the muscles acting as joint stabilizers, then there are 26 muscles involved in arm movement (ten moving the shoulder, six the elbow, four moving the radio-ulna joint and six moving the wrist), producing 26 degrees of freedom that need regulating. Moreover, if, as some theorists postulate, plans are written in terms of individual motor units (or alpha-gamma links) then a conservative estimate is that there are 2600 degrees of freedom to be regulated at a time[23]. The problem does not stop there, however, since even such a simple act as raising one's arm produces reactive forces that require postural preadjustments to maintain balance. Thus, Belen'kii, Gurfinkel' and Pal'tsev[29] conclude from their electromyographic studies that, 'when instructed to move his arm the subject in the standing position at first performs movements with his legs and trunk and only then with his arm.' Such postural preadjustments serve not only to maintain balance, but also to minimize the possibility of damage to the body. Thus, where a job involves unexpected loads, there is often a high incidence of injuries[30]. Postural preadjustments, and indeed movements in general, are based on knowledge and expectations that the performer has about his own system and about the environment in which he is operating. It is important to remember that movements do not occur in a vacuum; the context in which the movement occurs, the task demands, the desired outcome, the expectations of the performer, all affect the final detailed specification of the response. We will return to the issue of knowledge about action later on.

Against this background of potential complexity, how then do we plan, construct, and execute movements? Do we perhaps store in the brain the patterns of innervation for each of the vast array of possible movements? While this is possible, such a system would be highly inefficient in terms of storage and would create further difficulties related to accessing and retrieving the patterns from memory. The complete storage of all movement patterns is most unlikely, and some would argue impossible[31]. It would, therefore, seem desirable to postulate mechanisms which do not require this level of storage. More complete storage of movement patterns may occur in limited instances, for example, in repetitive or highly practised situations. In general, however, it may be more efficient to use a generative process, whereby responses are constructed according to sets of rules or principles appropriate to particular classes of action. By storing a limited set of rules and tailoring the construction process to specific movement conditions (e.g. speed of movement, force against which we are moving, accuracy required, etc.) we can generate many different movements. The concept of a generative process is one component of the schema theory of movement control. The array of possible movements may, however, have constraints placed on the relations between movement at different joints, and hence limit the choice of movements generated. The concept of *synergy* was proposed in the last century by Ferrier[32] and later elaborated by Bernstein[28]. It relates to the idea that motor co-ordination involves a reduction in the number of degrees of freedom of the sensory-motor system by functional groupings of muscles constrained to act as a single unit. Thus, functional synergies are collections of muscles which share a common pool of afferent and/or efferent information and are employed as a unit in a motor task (see Kelso[33] for a review). Ferrier[32] conceived of a synergy as a class of movements having similar kinematics. Others have followed this conception, and recently Kelso, Putnam and Goodman[34] have argued that the chief signature of a *functional synergy* is that, 'the internal timing relations among muscles and kinematic components are preserved invariantly over changes in the magnitude of activity in individual components.' Investigating two-handed movement, where the hands move simultaneously to different targets, they report a strong tendency for the limbs to be co-ordinated as a unitary structure, even when the movements are of different difficulty. For example, an obstacle placed in the path of one limb, but not the other, modulates the space–time behaviour of both limbs. This and other evidence led them to conclude that, 'in multi-joint limb movements, the many degrees of freedom are organized to function temporarily as a single coherent unit that is uniquely specific to the task demands placed on it.' To illustrate this interdependence of limb movements Turvey[35], in a similar vein, points out the difficulty of writing the letter W while making circular movements with a foot.

Related ideas occur throughout the literature, expressed using different terminology. For some, the basic units of movement are termed *co-ordinative structures*[36], although the definition is virtually identical to that given for functional synergies. For example, Michaels and Carello[37] define co-ordinative structures as, 'a group of muscles, often spanning several joints, constrained to act as a functional unit'. Similarly, Turvey and colleagues[23] have discussed such ideas in terms of *equations of constraint*, in an attempt to distinguish movements which occur from movements which are physically possible yet do not occur. Underlying such discussions is the view that much of the co-ordination and control of movement takes place at a relatively low level in the system, thereby reducing the amount of movement control that needs to be computed centrally. Runeson and Frykholm[19] have elegantly stated the basic rationale for this view:

'We must not think of our anatomy as arbitrarily concatenated. Rather, our geometrical proportions, the distribution of mass, the intricate connections of muscles and tendons across the joints, and the elasticity and damping of the tissues have been delicately tuned through evolution to provide adequate constraints. In the dynamic system thus established the options for motion have been reduced substantially toward those conducive to adaptive action.'

Earlier, Bernstein[28] had discussed the way the inertial properties of the limbs can be exploited as natural pendular movements to reduce control and energy expenditure, the basic tenet being that in skilled action muscular force is used only where necessary, to enhance 'natural' movements or to generate required deviations from natural trajectories. An example can be taken from studies of human locomotion. Walking involves a controlled fall forwards, and during the forward swing phase of the leg the muscles are for the most part silent[38]. In the last century Richer[39] had made a similar observation when investigating the quadriceps muscle during the act of kicking. By photographing the leg during motion, he noticed that it was flung by this muscle, which then ceased activity

12

long before the leg completed the movement. Once started the inertial properties of the limb can be used to complete the movement. In quadrupeds an example can be seen of how biomechanical properties such as the mass of the limb/animal affect the form of movement. In running, stride frequency has been found to decrease regularly as the mass of the animal increases, from mice to rats to dogs to horses[40]. In humans, returning to our golfing example, Cochran[25] observes that the expert golfer gives the impression of, 'aiding, adding to, getting the best out of some natural periodic motion of his own particular, club–arm–body system; with additional forces he applies being properly synchronized with the natural movement.' One can readily distinguish the expert golfer from the inexpert golfer, not just in terms of outcome, but also according to the form of the movement, in which the inexpert player often appears to be fighting against natural movements.

It should be clear that anatomical make-up is a potential source of individual differences in movement. Since gender is one source of anthropometric variation this is an obvious source of interindividual movement variation and has been investigated[19]. In general, there are bound to be individual differences in the musculature and in neural mechanisms. For example, Keele and Hawkins[7] report interindividual differences in rates of repetitive activity (tapping) with individuals displaying characteristic general maximum rates. Within individuals the characteristic maximum rates of repetitive activity correlate across muscle groups and limbs (finger, thumb, wrist, arm, foot). Based on Wing's[41,42] timing model, it is possible that maximum tapping rate may be determined by the interaction of variability in the response of the motor system and the cycle time of a postulated central clock. Another source of individual differences in movement has been argued to be related to the co-ordinative structures that the individual habitually employs, and the extent of their activation. Readiness for action may then be seen as, 'a *state* of organization set up throughout the motor system'[19]. Following in the tradition of Koffka[43] and Heider[44], Runeson and Frykholm[19] extend such reasoning to discuss the idea that a person's emotions may be revealed by his or her movements. Hamilton[45] defines personality in terms of, 'preferred methods of responding' and motivation as involving, 'actions towards preferred goals'. Combining such ideas opens up interesting possibilities for integrating traditionally disparate areas of psychology.

Individual differences exist not only for what may be considered essentially ballistic movements, but also for controlled movements requiring a greater degree of accuracy. Where the requirement for movement accuracy exceeds the inherent accuracy of visual translation or the inherent variability in the motor system, then a process of current control is required. This concurrent guidance is typically based on visual feedback (see Sheridan[27] for a review), and individuals differ in their capacity to effectively utilize such feedback. In addition there are differences in the way individuals use knowledge of results (KR) concerning the outcome of a movement to modify subsequent action. There are thus individual differences in practice and experience which at one level affect movement production and at another level affect the available strategy options. We will consider each in turn in the following sections.

## SCHEMA THEORY

While consideration has been given to how movements may be produced and executed and to the factors contributing to intra- and interindividual movement variation, little attempt has been made to consider how performance is modified by experience. It has been suggested that planning and controlling movements must involve a generative process. That is, each movement in a given class is created from the rules governing movements of that class, in the light of the current situation – the position of the limbs, balance and so on. The rules are produced from an abstract representation of the movement class called a schema. There has been much recent discussion of schema theory at levels ranging from the generation of movement[46], to perception and the control of action[47]. Briefly, a schema may be considered to be, '. . . a characteristic of some population of objects (movements), and consists of a set of rules serving as instructions for producing a population prototype'[48]. At different levels schemata may be considered to be the rules for generating movements, for governing actions, and for modifying perception and the attribution of meaning.

At the movement level, Schmidt[46] considers that when an individual makes a movement that attempts to satisfy some goal, he or she stores four things:

(1)  the initial conditions (information about the preresponse state of the muscular system and the environment in which movement is to occur),

(2)  the response specification for the motor programme (specification of elements such as speed of movement, forces involved etc.),

(3)  the sensory consequences of the response produced (an exact copy of interoceptive and exteroceptive information), and

(4)  the outcome of the movement (the success of the response in relation to the intended outcome).

Schmidt argues that the four sources of information are stored together after movement and when a number of similar movements have been made, the individual begins to abstract information about the relationship among these four sources of information. The strength of the relationship among the four stored elements is postulated to increase with each successive movement of the same general type and to increase with increased accuracy of feedback information from the response. This relationship is the schema for the movement type under consideration. Briefly, when an individual is required to make a response of a type for which a schema has already been developed, the schema for the general type of movement is selected, and then the response specification is set for that particular movement.

Evidence in general support of Schmidt's schema theory comes from a number of sources. Glencross[49] found in handwheel cranking, a task similar to turning an old-fashioned grindstone, that the movements were very similar in terms of the onsets of force application even when resistance was added and the radius was changed. Glencross labelled this phenomenon gradation of effort and it appears as if there was a schema for cranking and that changing the quality of the cranking (e.g. less force, more speed, etc.) provided a situation in

14

which the subject apparently used the same schema, but with a different set of response specifications. In another study Glencross[50] noted that while both fast and slow subjects had significantly common patterns of movement, at least in terms of the relative timing of force application, there were considerable individual differences apparent with subjects adopting a variety of synergistic postural adjustments. Thus, while there are common, often task-constrained, elements in the schemata adopted by different individuals, overall they remain specific to the individual, and are dependent on such things as practice, experience, etc. The final form of the movement produced depends in part on the activated co-ordinative structures, as discussed in the last section. Glencross[51, 52] produced further evidence that one schema can apparently be used to effect an appropriate response even though there may be a number of changes in the task conditions. He did not discuss his results in terms of schemata, but independently proposed a two-stage model of motor control to account for them. At one level a motor programme operates in an open-loop fashion, while at another level an executive control system integrates all the feedback arising from the task and controls the motor programme.

A major prediction derived from Schmidt's schema theory is that increasing variability-of-practice on a given task will result in increased (positive) transfer to a novel task of the same movement class. Holding[53] had similarly observed, when discussing transfer of training, that one tendency was toward better transfer from tasks which give wider experience. The basis on which one decides whether movements are in the same class or not is unspecified by Schmidt, and is clearly unsatisfactory. However, using common-sense notions to classify movements, support has been obtained for the variability-of-practice hypothesis, particularly from studies with children, since it is assumed that their schemata are not so well-developed[54, 55].

Catching and hitting a ball can be considered actions that are different each time they are produced. They require remarkably precise predictive visual information, and there is little margin for error. To catch a ball it is necessary to get the hand to the place where the ball will be, to orient the hand correctly, and to start closing the fingers before the ball reaches the hand. For the catcher to use time-to-contact information to predict the arrival of the ball at the hand, the information must be available a sufficient time before contact, so that hand orientation and grasp can be precisely timed. Lee[56] suggests that what the performer is effectively trying to do is precisely fill the time-to-contact interval with reaching out, orienting the hand, and grasping action. He argues that this can be achieved in two ways, either the performer varies the duration of his movement or he keeps duration constant and manipulates the time at which the movement is initiated. Evidence suggests that performers attempt to maintain a constant movement duration and that this tendency increases with practice, at least for predictive type responses[57-60]. In this case, starting the catching movement earlier would only result in greater error. A similar emphasis on constant timing seems to be present when hitting a ball. In studies of the swing of baseball batters[61], and the forehand drive of experienced table-tennis players[62], constant stroke duration seems to be present. In the case of table-tennis players the shots were consistent to within about $\pm 4$ ms. For baseball

15

batters there is variation in the speed of movement of the front foot depending on the speed of delivery, but this in fact has the effect of keeping stroke duration constant[63].

In many sports involving hitting, kicking and catching, it would seem necessary to develop two components: the ability to produce the movement in a sequenced temporal order over a stabilized movement duration, and the ability to integrate the initiation of the sequence with environmental contingencies. The two components may be thought of as relating to *technique* and *experience*. In a varying environment, practised and stabilized technique will not produce good performance without the experience obtained when learning to tailor performance to varying environmental demands (e.g. angle, speed and spin of the ball etc.). It is possible that basic technique for a particular shot could be thought of as the schema or prototype movement, in the sense of Schmidt's use of the term, into which are fed the desired consequences and the initial conditions, determining such things as the release of the shot. While the relative timing of the components of the response is maintained, initiation of the response is varied to meet environmental demands. Experience with a variety of demands could strengthen the schema, although in this case it may not be the movement itself which is altered, but its time of initiation. In Glencross' terms, the motor programme may be maintained while the executive controls its time of initiation.

It would seem necessary that the schema provide information about the spatiatemporal organization of both the micro- and macrostructure of movement. What is meant by microstructure is the temporal organization of the components of movements, which it appears the performer may attempt to stabilize across any variations in performance which occur in a relatively stable environment, i.e. one which does not involve anticipating environmental change. For example, typing or writing slower or faster[64], or making handwriting assume different sizes[65]. Macrostructure refers to the structuring of movement in relation to varied environmental demands. Where such demands vary the performer appears to attempt to maintain the temporal microstructure of movement (e.g. timing of the grasp element in catching), while tailoring the temporal macrostructure to the specific environmental demands (in the catching example, *when* to initiate the response). Thus, the schema would seem to need to operate at different levels, determining both the micro- and macrostructure. Practice in a relatively constant environment may develop technique (e.g. practising a golf swing off a mat on level ground, or practising cricket strokes in front of a mirror) which determines the microstructure, while experience in varied environmental conditions (e.g. golf shots off uneven ground, or cricket strokes made to different speeds of bowling) may develop the macrostructure. Clearly, the amount and type of practice an individual experiences is an important factor influencing motor performance and the expression of individual differences in movement. As was indicated at the beginning of this section, schemata may be considered to operate at different levels, and to be the rules for generating movements, for governing actions, and for modifying perception and the attribution of meaning. We have discussed the schema concept at the movement level in the present section. In the next section we will consider issues relating to knowledge about action, which may be conceived of as representing higher levels in the system.

## KNOWLEDGE AND ACTION

The idea that responses are generated or constructed from abstract representations of general classes of action at higher levels, with the specification of specific details at lower levels affecting the desired outcome is, in various forms, currently popular[35, 66]. This notion of hierarchical motor organization, and discussion of levels of organization, is not new. Since the time of Bryan and Harter[67] and Woodworth[68] this idea has figured prominently in the discussion of voluntary movement and action. Over 40 years ago Bernstein[28] emphasized that actions must be organized in a hierarchical fashion from conscious to peripheral level. More recently, others[69] have, along with Bernstein, argued that there cannot be a direct or even remote correspondence between the representation of action and the detailed form of the movement. Higher levels, variously described as the central, controlling or executive system, are thus argued to have fewer degrees of freedom in determining specific movement details, than the lower levels (effector, mechanical or controlled system). Conversely, higher levels clearly have more freedom in determining the overall action. The context in which the movement occurs, the task demands, the desired outcome, the expectations of the performer, all affect the final detailed specification of the response. This can be conceived of as a pyramidal structure, with global decisions at the apex, and the fine details of how this is actually accomplished in terms of the movement structure, toward the base. Thus, the kinematic shape of movements unfolds as a result of the interplay of many factors, and is unlikely to be the same, even for successive movements with the same outcome. Once the decision to act has been taken, the number of ways movement can be structured in order to achieve the goal is immense, as we have already discussed. The hierarchical view does not mean, however, that higher levels necessarily control lower levels. In attempting to understand 'executive ordering' and 'plans for action', Lashley[70] discussed the integration of levels and the transfer of control between them. The concept of transfer of control is important because, as Broadbent[71] points out, it avoids a rigid view of levels and hierarchies. For, rather than higher levels necessarily incorporating and controlling lower levels it becomes necessary to understand the influence of one level on another, and to recognize that control can shift between levels, or even appear to reside at several levels of complexity simultaneously, with processes occurring in parallel at different levels.

Miller, Galanter and Pribram[72] in their classic cognitive-behavioural representation of action conceptualize the organism as having a 'Plan', stating that, 'A Plan is any hierarchical process in the organism that can control the order in which a sequence of operations is to be performed.' Thus a Plan, a determinate sequence of operations, can be visualized as the programme of the organismic computer. Integrated with the Plan is the cognitive component of the behavioural system known as the 'Image', and is 'all the accumulated, organized knowledge that the organism has about itself and its world'. Clearly, this 'knowledge' may be tacit in the sense that we may not know the rules for a particular action, e.g. riding a bicycle[73], yet nevertheless be able to ride. Control of the process of riding could be considered to be at a different level from the action of riding. The notion of control residing at different levels in the system has been termed by some a heterarchical view[74]. The development of an action plan is unlikely to reflect a rigid and ordered sequence, but rather a flexible building up of any particular act. To quote Newell[75], 'Action plans are continually being updated as a consequence of the interaction of the performer with the environment. There is a dynamic link between perception and action, in which knowing facilitates doing, and doing fosters knowing.'

Before considering the traditional approach adopted in the literature to developmental trends in skilled action, let us briefly consider some of the dramatic effects higher level strategy changes can have on performance. The literature on the development of strategies is not comprehensive, and is particularly scarce when dealing with the processes employed by children in acquiring motor skills (see Wade[76] for a review). There are finite limits to the performance of the human motor system, but it is clear that by a change of strategy or tactics, tasks potentially constrained by these limits can nevertheless be accomplished. What one may witness in the progression of skilled performance is a change in strategy or tactics designed to circumvent or ameliorate the constraints placed upon performance by the human motor system. For example, in playing a fast sequence of notes a bagpipe player can slide his finger past a hole on the chanter to close and reopen it more quickly than his muscles can make a reversing movement of the finger. Similarly, in playing a long and fast series of ascending or descending notes on the piano, it is clearly easier to run one's finger along the keyboard (*glissando*) than attempt to produce the notes by individual finger movements. Such 'tricks' are used to accomplish tasks which are near the limits of motor performance and which would otherwise be difficult or impossible. In a similar way, a person with a motor disability may compensate, by strategic changes in the way that a task is performed. It is instructive to observe the way in which an individual who has suffered the loss of an upper limb can continue to cope in a remarkably successful way with the environment. Strategic changes of a global nature can also be seen to occur with the advancement of skill. For example, in playing squash, the beginner after having mastered the ability to hit the ball with a reasonable degree of success, often proceeds to a situation in which he appears to chase the ball around the court, covering a lot of ground to no good effect. Later in learning a change of strategy takes place, in which the player begins to predict in advance the position of the ball, and while appearing to slow down, is actually more effective in task performance. This process of anticipation is clearly important in many complex and co-ordinated actions. A final example can be seen in relation to the recently popular craze of 'Space Invader' video games. In the initial stages of learning the player masters the controls and becomes proficient at shooting the 'Invaders' and dodging their missiles. In later stages of proficiency comes the realization that shooting at the Invaders at random is less efficient than shooting the end lines (the reason for this is that when the end line of Invaders reaches the end of the television screen they move down the screen bringing them nearer to their invasion of Earth!). This change of strategy on the part of the player, while not requiring a higher degree of motor control, radically improves performance. Obviously, it is possible to short-circuit this learning process by instruction[26], in which case one may adopt an advanced strategy more rapidly. When after early childhood one has by experience acquired a degree of knowledge about oneself and the environment, there is another way to short-circuit a trial-and-error learning process. This is by the use of mental practice. Using this technique positive transfer has been shown from mental practice to physical perform-ance[77, 78]. Although a controversial area, it is not unreasonable to suppose that by practising mentally one might establish appropriate performance strategies, at least early in learning. Indeed, theories of skill acquisition have an early 'cognitive phase'[79] or 'verbal-motor stage'[80]. Another source of individual differences emerges here, since individuals can differ in their ability to image or mentally practise.

The investigation of developmental trends in skilled action has traditionally been dominated by the issue of capacity. Capacity or structural factors (e.g. that physical parameters and brain activity co-vary with age) are seen as direct reflections of maturational influences and are discussed in biological terms. The explanation for differences in motor performance over age, and the times of appearance of various phylogenetic skills, are frequently discussed in terms of capacity based on maturation, rather than in terms of experience and knowledge. While it seems self-evident that maturation contributes significantly to the onset of phylogenetic skills, Newell and Barclay[81] have recently con-tended that exclusive capacity arguments are less than clear-cut. Indeed, there is evidence that experiential factors can affect the development of even funda-mental actions. For example, Zelazo, Zelazo and Kolb[82] reported that exercising the stepping reflex early in life can accelerate the onset of self-controlled walking in infants. Similarly, Bower[83] demonstrated the role of experience in facilitating the onset of reaching and grasping skills. At a more general level, recent con-ceptions suggest that what practice and experience gained from it do, is to yield an increasing number of situations and patterns which people recognize and which prompt various response routines[84]. For example, Chase and Simon[85] briefly presented 24 chess pieces arranged according to a real midgame position. A chess master could reproduce about 16 of the positions, a class A player about eight, and a novice only four. The superior performance of the chess master was, however, specific to chess, since the performance of the master was no better than the novice when the chess pieces were randomly arranged. This view of practice relates to Fleishman's[13] work suggesting that with practice, skill in a task becomes more specific to itself, and less predictable by other perceptual-motor factors. While this may be true at one level, practice and experience can at another level contribute to the general knowledge base of the organism. Such argument parallels the distinction made by Miller et al.[72] between the Plan and the Image, between Piaget's[86] operative and figurative knowledge, between Newell and Barclay's[81] conception of strategies and knowledge, and between what others have referred to as procedural and declarative knowledge. Knowledge gained by experience may even be related to personality if one defines the latter in terms of 'preferred methods of responding'[45].

In a further study, Chi[87] showed that 10-year-old children who were chess experts could remember chess positions better than skilled but less knowledge-able adult chess players. However, this was only the case for meaningful chess positions. When the positions were random typical developmental trends were found, with adult performance superior. Thus, explanations of performance differences based on chronological age and capacity factors may provide only a partial account. There are a number of sources of evidence that practice and experience can overcome performance deficits traditionally attributed to capacity limitations. For example, Mowbray and Rhoades[88] showed that with prolonged practice, reaction time in a four-choice situation could equal that in a two-choice task. More recently, Laszlo and Bairstow[89] have shown that kinaesthetically undeveloped children can be trained to a higher level of kinaesthetic performance, and that this transfers to improvement in their drawing skills.

We will turn now to consider briefly the wider issue linking motor performance and development with general cognitive growth. A number of theories concerning intellectual growth propose that early motor development is the foundation upon which cognitive development is built. Theories of cognitive growth based on voluntary motor activity take a variety of forms. Bruner[90] proposed that human beings construct models of their world through action ('enactive representation'), through imagery ('iconic representation'), and through language ('symbolic representation'), *in that order*. The implication is that if the child has not been able to represent past events through appropriate motor responses then iconic and symbolic representation do not develop. Kephart[91] even more explicitly draws the connection between motor learning and perceptual and cognitive development. He argues that, 'Through these first motor explorations, the child begins to find out about himself and the world around him, and his motor experimentation and his motor learning become the foundation upon which such knowledge is built.' Over 30 years earlier Piaget had argued along similar lines. Such approaches can be summarized by Piaget's statement that, 'Knowledge is derived from action . . .'[92]. For teachers, implications have been interpreted in such statements as, 'Children do not learn by sitting passively in their seats . . .'[93], and that, 'The preschool child . . . should be given tasks that allow him to act on objects'[94]. Clearly, however, children born with severe neuromuscular impairment are prevented from going through a similar phase of development, and yet, there are very severely handicapped persons who are cognitively normal[95,96]. Such individuals pose a potential problem for the outlined theories of cognitive development.

There is, in general, little evidence concerning the interaction of severity of sensory-motor impairment with cognitive development[97]. If, however, the IQs of cerebral-palsied individuals are taken as an approximation, then it is clear that this group score much lower than normal. One study reviewed by Cruickshank, Hallahan and Bice[98] indicated that 35% of spastic quadriplegics had IQ scores over 70, only about 1% scored over 100, and about 0.4% scored over 120. Less totally involved groups (e.g. paraplegics) had, in general, higher IQs. Such data do not, however, support the contention that motor activity is needed for cognitive growth since low IQs in handicapped individuals may relate directly to the brain damage underlying the motor dysfunction. Moreover, problems relate to accurately assessing IQs in such individuals.

In one of very few studies attempting to measure directly the effects of motor impairment on cognitive function, Melcer and Park (1967) (quoted in Goldenberg[97]) investigated the development of action concepts in cerebral-palsied children. Along with other measures, they modified the Peabody Picture Vocabulary Test so that each card contained both an object representation of the vocabulary item and an action representation of the item, e.g. a ball versus someone playing with a ball. They summarized their findings along the lines that cerebral-palsied children are deficient in perceptual-motor ability, and that they do not develop concepts of actions in the same ratio to object concepts as children who are not motorically handicapped. Melcer and Park conclude that their results support theories suggesting that sensory-motor experience in infancy is one of the main factors in conceptual development, although as the authors recognize many problems attend such a conclusion. The findings of their study should come as no surprise, although one may question their conclusions. As Neisser[47] points out, 'In one respect, discussions of object concepts are bound to be misleading no matter what theoretical view eventually prevails.' Such concepts implicitly suggest that the function of perception is to inform us about things as 'mere objects', geographically and physically defined. While this is true, it is not the complete picture. As Neisser[47] continues to argue,

'In the normal environment most perceptible objects and events are *meaningful*. They afford various possibilities for action, carry implications about what has happened or what will happen, belong coherently to a larger context, possess an identity that transcends their simple physical properties. These meanings can be, and are, perceived.'

Gibson[99] attempted to deal with the perception of meaning through the concept of 'affordance'. He argued that all the potential uses of objects (the activities they afford) are directly perceivable. Invariant properties of the optic array specify that, for normals, the floor affords walking, the pen affords writing and so on. These aspects of optical structure are different from those that specify position, shape or motion, but are argued to be no less objective. Such a formulation suggests that, while there is a general knowledge base dependent upon features of the environment, what an object appears to afford (or to mean) depends on who is perceiving it. From the vast array of potential uses and meanings that every optic array specifies, Neisser argues that the meaning perceived depends on, '... the individual's schematic control of information pickup'. In Neisser's terms, interpretation of meaning depends on the activated schemata. For example, whether one processes an individual moving an arm about at a surface level, or whether one attributes specific meaning to the movement – a wave of greeting – depends on the activated schemata. Do I expect to meet someone, etc.?

Experience and interaction with the environment affect the development of schemata. Clearly, if one's interaction with the environment is at a more static level then it is not surprising that cerebral-palsied children are deficient in the development of action schemata. The actions simply do not have the same meaning or significance as for the motorically active individuals. At a more specific level, Whiting[26] has argued that one's experience with particular skills leads to the build-up of a conceptual model of the system one is controlling. In Fowler and Turvey's[100] terms this is described as 'attunement'. Such a model is the outcome of successive discoveries about the structure of the skill (i.e. it is dynamic), and it enables the performer to, '... appreciate the interaction of the main parameters in the system and to predict the consequences of any control action he may take'[101]. Such statements capture the essence of motor control: that the primary function of movements is to provide the organism with control of the environment. Such control involves predictive ability which is developed via interaction with, and experience of, the environment. What many motorically handicapped individuals lack is any control of their environment. It is no wonder that this, coupled with severely restricted environmental experience, contributes to problems with cognitive development.

Returning to developmental theories outlined earlier. It may be argued that it is not movement *per se* that primarily contributes to development, but the opportunity this provides to link actions with consequences, to connect cause and effect, to develop schemata. Lack of environmental control not lack of movement may more severely restrict cognitive development. It may then be that those severely physically handicapped individuals indicated as being 'cognitively normal'[95, 96], are a minority who have achieved some consistent control of the environment. The fundamental concept underlying theories of learning is *feedback*. That information is fed back to the organism concerning the consequences of action, and on the basis of this information later performance is modified. If action is lacking or restricted, and if feedback is lacking or distorted by noise in the perceptual-motor system, then it is no surprise that learning will be severely impaired.

At a general level, differences in the experience of individuals will lead to differences in action and movement production. While there are clearly individual differences in initial potential, when watching an outstanding performance, there is a tendency to undervalue the years of practice and experience that result in the culmination of skilled performance.

# References

1. Bartlett, F. C. (1932). *Remembering*. (Cambridge: Cambridge University Press)
2. Fitts, P. M. (1954). The information capacity of the human motor system in controlling the amplitude of movement. *J. Exp. Psychol.*, **47**, 381–91.
3. Keele, S. W. (1981). Behavioral analysis of movement. In Brooks, V. B. (ed.) *Handbook of Physiology, Section 1, The Nervous System, Volume II, Motor Control, Part 2*. pp. 1391–414. (Bethesda, MD: American Physiological Society)
4. Sheridan, M. R. (1979). A reappraisal of Fitts' Law. *J. Motor Behav.*, **11**, 179–88
5. Cronbach, L. J. (1957). The two disciplines of scientific psychology. *Am. Psychol.*, **12**, 671
6. Spearman, C. E. (1927). *The Abilities of Man*. (London: Macmillan)
7. Keele, S. W. and Hawkins, H. L. (1982). Explorations of individual differences relevant to high level skill. *J. Motor Behav.*, **14**, 3–23
8. Marteniuk, R. G. (1974). Individual differences in motor performance and learning. In Wilmore, J. H. (ed.) *Exercise and Sports Sciences Review*. Vol. 2. (New York: Academic Press)
9. Seashore, R. H. (1951). Work and motor performance. In Stevens, S. S. (ed.) *Handbook of Experimental Psychology*. pp. 1341–62. (New York: Wiley)
10. Henry, F. M. (1968). Specificity vs. generality in learning motor skill. In Brown, R. C. and Kenyon, G. S. (eds.) *Classical Studies on Physical Activity*. (Englewood Cliffs, NJ: Prentice-Hall)
11. Fleishman, E. A. (1964). *The Structure and Measurement of Physical Fitness*. (Englewood Cliffs, NJ: Prentice-Hall)

12. Fleishman, E. A. (1975). Taxonomic problems in human performance research. In Singleton, W. T. and Spurgeon, P. (eds.) *Measurement of Human Resources*. (London: Taylor and Francis)

13. Fleishman, E. A. (1966). Human abilities and the acquisition of skill. In Bilodeau, E. A. (ed.) *Acquisition of Skill*. pp. 146-67. (New York: Academic Press)

14. Jones, M. B. (1969). Differential processes in acquisition. In Bilodeau, E. A. (ed.) *Principles of Skill Acquisition*. pp. 141-70. (New York: Academic Press)

15. Jones, M. B. (1970). A two-process theory of individual differences in motor learning. *Psychol. Rev.*, **77**, 353-60

16. Fleishman, E. A. and Hempel, W. E. Jr. (1955). The relation between abilities and improvement with practice in a visual discrimination reaction task. *J. Exp. Psychol.*, **49**, 301-12

17. Knapp, B. N. (1964). *Skill in Sport*. (London: Routledge and Kegan Paul)

18. Ricoeur, P. (1966). *Freedom and Nature: The Voluntary and the Involuntary*. (Illinois: North-Western University Press)

19. Runeson, S. and Frykholm, G. (1983). Kinematic specification of dynamics as an informational basis for person-and-action perception: expectation, gender, recognition, and deceptive intention. *J. Exp. Psychol.: Gen.*, **112**, 585-615

20. Hammond, W. (1975). A systems-analysis of fencing. In Whiting, H. T. A. (ed.) *Readings in Sports Psychology*. pp. 138-51. (London: Lepus Books)

21. Tajfel, H. (ed.) (1978). *Differentiation between Social Groups: Studies in the Social Psychology of Intergroup Relations*. (London: Academic Press)

22. Turner, J. (1975). Social comparison and social identity: some prospects for intergroup behavior. *Eur. J. Soc. Psychol.*, **5**, 1-3

23. Turvey, M. T., Fitch, H. L. and Tuller, B. (1982). The Bernstein perspective. I. The problems of degrees of freedom and context-conditioned variability. In Kelso, J. A. S. (ed.) *Human Motor Behavior: An Introduction*. pp. 239-52. (Hillsdale, NJ: Lawrence Erlbaum)

24. Grillner, S. (1975). Locomotion in vertebrates: central mechanisms and reflex interaction. *Physiol. Rev.*, **55**, 247-304

25. Cochran, A. J. (1979). The golfer. In Singleton, W. T. (ed.) *Compliance and Excellence. The Study of Real Skills*. Vol. 2. pp. 199-221. (Lancaster: MTP Press)

26. Whiting, H. T. A. (1980). Dimensions of control in motor learning. In Stelmach, G. E. and Requin, J. (eds.) *Tutorials in Motor Behavior*. pp. 537-50. (Amsterdam: North-Holland Publications)

27. Sheridan, M. R. (1984). Planning and controlling simple movements. In Smyth, M. M. and Wing, A. (eds.) *The Psychology of Human Movement*. pp. 47-82. (New York: Academic Press)

28. Bernstein, N. A. (1967). *The Coordination and Regulation of Movement*. (London: Pergamon Press)

29. Belen'kii, V. Ye., Gurfinkel', V. S., and Pal'tsev, Ye. I. (1967). Elements of control of voluntary movements. *Biophysics*, **12**, 154-61

30. Andersson, G. (1979). Low back pain in industry: epidemiological aspects. *Scand. J. Rehabil. Med.*, **11**, 163-8

31. Kugler, P. N. and Turvey, M. T. (1979). Two metaphors for neural afference and efference. *Behav. Brain Sci.*, **2**, 305-12

32. Ferrier, D. (1886). *The Functions of the Brain*. (London: Smith, Elder)

33. Kelso, J. A. S. (1981). Contrasting perspectives in order and regulation of movement. In Long, J. and Baddeley, A. (eds.) *Attention and Performance IX*. pp. 437-57. (Hillsdale, NJ: Erlbaum)

34. Kelso, J. A. S., Putnam, C. A. and Goodman, D. (1983). On the space-time structure of human interlimb co-ordination. *Q. J. Exp. Psychol.*, **35A**, 347-75

35. Turvey, M. T. (1977). Preliminaries to a theory of action with reference to vision. In Shaw, R. and Bransford, J. (eds.) *Perceiving, Acting and Knowing: Towards an Ecological Psychology*. pp. 211-65. (Hillsdale, NJ: Erlbaum)

36. Easton, T. A. (1972). On the normal use of reflexes. *Am. Sci.*, **60**, 591-9.

37. Michaels, C. F. and Carello, C. (1981). *Direct Perception*. (Englewood Cliffs, NJ: Prentice-Hall)

38. Mochon, S. and McMahon, T. A. (1980). Ballistic walking. *J. Biomech.*, **13**, 49-57

39. Richer, P. (1895). Note sur la contraction du muscle quadriceps dans l'acte de donner un coup de pied. *C. R. Soc. Biol. (Paris)*, **47**, 204–5
40. Heglund, N. D., Taylor, R. C. and McMahon, T. A. (1974). Scaling stride frequency and gait to animal size: mice to horses. *Science*, **186**, 1112–13
41. Wing, A. M. (1977). Perturbations of auditory feedback delay and the timing of movement. *J. Exp. Psychol.: Hum. Perception and Performance*, **3**, 175–86
42. Wing, A. M. (1980). The long and short of timing in response sequences. In Stelmach, G. E. and Requin, J. (eds.) *Tutorials in Motor Behavior*. pp. 469–86. (Amsterdam: North-Holland Publications)
43. Koffka, K. (1935). *Principles of Gestalt Psychology*. (London: Routledge and Kegan Paul)
44. Heider, F. (1958). *The Psychology of Interpersonal Relations*. (New York: Wiley)
45. Hamilton, V. (1983). *The Cognitive Structures and Processes of Human Motivation and Personality*. (Chichester: Wiley)
46. Schmidt, R. A. (1975). A schema theory of discrete motor skill learning. *Psychol. Rev.*, **82**, 225–60
47. Neisser, U. (1976). *Cognition and Reality*. (San Francisco: Freeman)
48. Evans, S. H. (1967). A brief statement of schema theory. *Psychonomic Sci.*, **8**, 87–8
49. Glencross, D. J. (1973). The effects of changes in direction, load, and amplitude of movement on gradation of effort. *J. Motor Behav.*, **5**, 207–16
50. Glencross, D. J. (1973). Temporal organisation in a repetitive speed skill. *Ergonomics*, **16**, 765–76
51. Glencross, D. J. (1975). The effects of changes in task conditions on the temporal organisation of a repetitive speed skill. *Ergonomics*, **18**, 17–28
52. Glencross, D. J. (1977). Control of skilled movements. *Psychol. Bull.*, **84**, 14–29
53. Holding, D. H. (1965). *Principles of Training*. (London: Pergamon Press)
54. Carson, L. M. and Wiegand, R. L. (1979). Motor schema formation and retention in young children: a test of Schmidt's schema theory. *J. Motor Behav.*, **11**, 247–51
55. Moxley, S. E. (1979). Schema: the variability of practice hypothesis. *J. Motor Behav.*, **11**, 65–70
56. Lee, D. N. (1980). Visuo-motor coordination in space-time. In Stelmach, G. E. and Requin, J. (eds.) *Tutorials in Motor Behavior*. pp. 281–95. (Amsterdam: North-Holland Publications)
57. Alderson, G. J. K., Sully, D. J. and Sully, H. G. (1974). An operational analysis of a one-handed catching task using high speed photography. *J. Motor Behav.*, **6**, 217–26
58. Schmidt, R. A. and McCabe, J. F. (1976). Motor program utilization over extended practice. *J. Hum. Movement Stud.*, **2**, 239–47
59. Sharp, R. H. and Whiting, H. T. A. (1974). Exposure to occluded duration effects in a ball-catching skill. *J. Motor Behav.*, **6**, 139–47
60. Sharp, R. H. and Whiting, H. T. A. (1975). Information-processing and eye movement in a ball-catching skill. *J. Hum. Movement Stud.*, **1**, 124–31
61. Hubbard, A. W. and Seng, C. N. (1954). Visual movements of batters. *Res. Q.*, **25**, 42–57
62. Tyldesley, D. A. and Whiting, H. T. A. (1975). Operational timing. *J. Hum. Movement Stud.*, **1**, 172–7
63. Fitch, H. L. and Turvey, M. T. (1978). On the control of activity: some remarks from an ecological point of view. In Landers, D. M. and Christina, R. W. (eds.) *Psychology of Motor Behavior and Sport*. pp. 3–35. (Champaign, Ill.: Human Kinetics)
64. Terzuolo, C. A. and Viviani, P. (1979). The central representation of learned motor patterns. In Talbott, R. E. and Humphrey, D. R. (eds.) *Posture and Movement*. pp. 113–21. (New York: Raven Press)
65. Viviani, P. and Terzuolo, C. A. (1980). Space–time invariance in learned motor skills. In Stelmach, G. E. and Requin, J. (eds.) *Tutorials in Motor Behavior*. pp. 525–33. (Amsterdam: North-Holland Publications)
66. Greene, P. H. (1972). Problems of organization of motor systems. In Rosen, R. and Snell, F. M. (eds.) *Progress in Theoretical Biology*. Vol. 2. (New York: Academic Press)
67. Bryan, W. L. and Harter, N. (1897). Studies in the physiology and psychology of the telegraphic language. *Psychol. Rev.*, **4**, 27–53
68. Woodworth, R. S. (1899). The accuracy of voluntary movement. *Psychol. Rev.*, **3** (Suppl. 2), 1–114

69. Turvey, M. T., Shaw, R. E. and Mace, W. (1978). Issues in the theory of action: degrees of freedom, coordinative structures and coalitions. In Requin, J. (ed.) *Attention and Performance VII*. (Hillsdale, NJ: Erlbaum)
70. Lashley, K. S. (1951). The problem of serial order in behavior. In Jeffress, L. A. (ed.) *Cerebral Mechanisms in Behavior*. pp. 112–36. (New York: Wiley)
71. Broadbent, D. E. (1977). Levels, hierarchies and locus of control. *Q. J. Exp. Psychol.*, **29**, 181–201
72. Miller, G. A., Galanter, E. and Pribram, K. H. (1960). *Plans and the Structure of Behavior*. (New York: Holt)
73. Polanyi, M. (1958). *Personal Knowledge: Towards a Post-Critical Philosophy*. (London: Routledge and Kegan Paul)
74. McCullock, W. S. (1945). A heterarchy of values determined by the topology of nervous nets. *Bull. Math. Biophys.*, **7**, 89–93
75. Newell, K. M. (1978). Some issues on action plans. In Stelmach, G. E. (ed.) *Information Processing in Motor Control and Learning*. pp. 41–54. (New York: Academic Press)
76. Wade, M. G. (1976). Developing motor learning. In Keogh, J. and Hutton, R. S. (eds.) *Exercise and Sport Science Reviews IV*. (Santa Barbara: Journal Publishing Affiliates)
77. Kohl, R. M. and Roenker, D. L. (1983). Mechanism involvement during skill imagery. *J. Motor Behav.*, **15**, 179–90
78. Richardson, A. (1967). Mental practice: a review and discussion (Part I). *Res. Q.*, **38**, 95–107
79. Fitts, P. M. and Posner, M. I. (1967). *Human Performance*. (California: Brooks/Cole)
80. Adams, J. A. (1971). A closed-loop theory of motor learning. *J. Motor Behav.*, **3**, 111–49
81. Newell, K. M. and Barclay, C. R. (1982). Developing knowledge about action. In Kelso, J. A. S. and Clark, J. E. (eds.) *The Development of Movement Control and Co-ordination*. pp. 175–212. (Chichester; Wiley)
82. Zelazo, P., Zelazo, N. and Kolb, S. (1972). 'Walking' in the newborn. *Science*, **177**, 1058–9
83. Bower, T. G. R. (1974). *Development in Infancy*. (San Francisco: Freeman)
84. Chase, W. G. and Chi, M. T. H. (1981). Cognitive skill: implications for spatial skill in large scale environments. In Harvey, J. (ed.) *Cognition, Social Behavior, and the Environment*. pp. 111–36. (Hillsdale, NJ: Erlbaum)
85. Chase, W. G. and Simon, H. A. (1973). The mind's eye in chess. In Chase, W. G. (ed.) *Visual Information Processing*. pp. 215–81. (New York: Academic Press)
86. Piaget, J. (1970). *Structuralism*. (New York: Harper Row)
87. Chi, M. T. H. (1978). Knowledge structures and cues. In Siegler, R. S. (ed.) *Children's Thinking: What Develops?* (Hillsdale, NJ: Erlbaum)
88. Mowbray, G. H. and Rhoades, M. U. (1959). On the reduction of choice reaction times with practice. *Q. J. Exp. Psychol.*, **11**, 16–23
89. Laszlo, J. I. and Bairstow, P. J. (1983). Kinaesthesis: its measurement, training and relationship to motor control. *Q. J. Exp. Psychol.*, **35A**, 411–21
90. Bruner, J. (1964). The course of cognitive growth. *Am. Psychol.*, **19**, 1–15
91. Kephart, N. (1971). *The Slow Learner in the Classroom*. (Columbus: Merrill Publishing)
92. Piaget, J. (1971). *Science of Education and the Psychology of the Child*. (New York: Viking Press)
93. Pulaski, M. A. B. (1971). *Understanding Piaget*. (New York: Harper and Row)
94. Ault, R. L. (1977). *Children's Cognitive Development: Piaget's Theory and the Process Approach*. (Oxford: Oxford University Press)
95. Jordan, N. (1972). Is there an Achilles' heel in Piaget's theorizing. *Hum. Dev.*, **15**, 379–82
96. Kopp, C. B. and Shaperman, J. (1973). Cognitive development in the absence of object manipulation during infancy. *Dev. Psychol.*, **9**, 430
97. Goldenberg, E. P. (1979). *Special Technology for Special Children*. (Baltimore: University Park Press)
98. Cruickshank, W. M., Hallahan, D. P. and Bice, H. V. (1976). The evaluation of intelligence. In Cruickshank, W. M. (ed.) *Cerebral Palsy: A Developmental Disability*. (Syracuse: Syracuse University Press)
99. Gibson, J. J. (1966). *The Senses Considered as Perceptual Systems*. (Boston: Houghton Mifflin)

100. Fowler, C. A. and Turvey, M. T. (1978). Skill acquisition: an event approach with special reference to searching for the optimum of a function of several variables. In Stelmach, G. E. (ed.) *Information Processing in Motor Control and Learning*. pp. 1–40. (New York: Academic Press)
101. Whitfield, D. C. (1967). Human skill as a determinant of allocation of function. In Singleton, W. J., Easterby, R. S. and Whitfield, D. C. (eds.) *The Human Operator in Complex Systems*. (London: Taylor and Francis)

# 2

# Personality theory and movement

## *John Brebner*

---

## INTRODUCTION

Considering the volume of work published separately in the two areas of personality and movement it is surprising that relatively few studies are concerned with individual differences in movement. In part this must be due to the fact that most personality theories are concerned with attitudes and verbal expressions of mental states rather than motor behaviour. But it is also the case that studies of movement tend to be concerned with specific movements and their central control mechanisms rather than the organism as a functioning whole. Even those studies which look at motor behaviour as an expression of the internal state of the individual tend to regard gestures and movements as a sort of library of communication possibilities revealing emotional states like anxiety, aggression or sexual interest, rather than as enduring characteristics of personality. This may be because, despite an early belief that expressive style reflected personality[1], more recently it has been argued that it can be dangerous to assume expressive style means consistency in other behavioural areas[2].

Where differences in general movement between different types of individual have been researched[3], it is the age, or the sex, of the individual which has been seen as typifying their movements, not their personalities. The few studies which relate expressive movement and personality are dealt with below but there appears to be something of a gap in the literature on movement and the question is whether movement is relevant for theories of personality or not. Because controlled movement depends on musculature it is not surprising that Sheldon's[4] analysis of temperament produced major components which differed, among other items, on being typically relaxed (viscerotonia), assertive (somatotonia) or restrained in posture and movement (cerebrotonia). Beyond that, however, even Sheldon, who measured the physique of his subjects so meticulously, described temperament in terms of general traits. In doing so he was following a tradition which goes clear back to the Greek 'Character' writers the last of whom, Theophrastus, wrote short sketches of undesirable character types[5]. These character sketches described not individuals but types of people recognizable through examples of their general behaviour, e.g. talkativeness,

27

boorishness, faultfinding, and some of Sheldon's descriptions of his traits such as 'lust for power', or 'indifference to pain', although based on correlational studies, take a somewhat similar form.

However, it is when we concern ourselves with objective measures of movement, such as the speed and force with which movements are made, the frequency of occurrence of voluntary movements, their amplitude, or the effects of inhibiting movement, that some current personality theories depart from this venerable tradition and predict more specific behavioural differences between individuals with different personality structures. The theories which are relevant are those concerned more with the responsiveness of the individual to environmental changes than their attitudes. By far the most important of these is Hans Eysenck's, in which the person is characterized on three main dimensions of personality, Extraversion (E), Neuroticism (N) and Psychoticism (P), and one minor dimension which is measured by the Lie Scale of the Eysenck Personality Questionnaire (EPQ). During the last 40 years Eysenck has developed two of the most influential theories of personality within experimental psychology. The main theoretical concern of both of these has been the search for a universal cause underlying the behavioural attributes of introversion–extraversion. Other aspects of Eysenck's theorizing, such as his views on N or P, are closely interwoven with his theories of E and, while the reason for concentrating upon E in this chapter is that it is more directly relevant to movement than the other personality dimensions, it should be made clear that this is only part of Eysenck's theoretical position.

His earlier theory[6] related E to the Hullian[7] notion of reactive inhibition which was conceived of as an inhibitory state or drive not to respond which built up as a function of responding and the amount of work that involved. With repeated similar responses, reactive inhibition would build up as a function of the number of responses until the inhibitory state overcame the drive to respond, at which point responding would cease. Unlike conditioned inhibition in Hullian learning theory, reactive inhibition dissipated spontaneously if no work was being performed, so that after a period of time the drive to respond would re-assert itself and responding would begin again. Eysenck suggested that extraverts (Es) generated reactive inhibition more quickly than introverts (Is) did, and dissipated it more slowly, so that over a wide range of tasks Es' responses could be seen to be suppressed by reactive inhibition, giving way to alternative behaviours not affected by the reactive inhibition, or being replaced by an involuntary rest pause until the inhibition dissipated. This theory was eminently testable and hundreds of experiments were performed within this explanatory framework.

The main thrust of research altered, however, in 1967 when Eysenck[8] offered a second theory of extraversion. In this theory differences in the strength of the effect of the ascending reticular activating system, exercising a general tonic, priming effect on the cortex, were proposed to underlie I–E differences in behaviour. Es were proposed to be characteristically below an 'optimum' level of arousal, so that they sought stimulation to increase their arousal. Is were generally above an 'optimum' level and sought to reduce the level of stimulation acting upon them, whether emanating from their own behaviour or from external sources. This explanation in terms of arousal level has also produced an enormous volume of research, and, as in the case of the reactive inhibition theory, the balance of evidence has supported Eysenck's view.

## A NEW MODEL OF EXTRAVERSION

In 1971 Eysenck[9] brought together several studies of motor behaviour which are of interest here. However, before reviewing these, the attempt to unify these two explanations into a single theory by Brebner and Cooper[10] needs to be outlined. The amalgamation of Eysenck's two explanations was achieved by suggesting that the central mechanisms could be in one of two states, excitation or inhibition, thus deliberately following Pavlov's[11] original view, and that either could be separately induced by the demands for stimulus (S)-analysis or for response (R)-organization acting on the organism. Excitation manifested itself behaviourally in the tendency to continue and augment current response activities; inhibition showed in behaviour as the tendency to cease or attentuate responding. R-organization, like S-analysis, refers to a central process which precedes the emission of a response. By allowing that the feedback from actually responding should be treated as stimulation, and that Es were prone to generate inhibition from S-analysis, whereas their I-counterparts in contrast produced excitation, it was possible to incorporate the reactive inhibition explanation into Brebner and Cooper's new model. In the model Es and Is also differed with respect to R-organization with Es producing excitation from this process while, for Is, inhibition resulted from R-organization.

Various experiments have tested the new model[12-15] and because it brings together two well-tried theories it is not surprising that findings have favoured it. Some of the experiments predicted differences in the speed and frequency of responding of Is and Es based on whether task-demands were biased towards S-analysis or R-organization and the effect of this for Is and Es respectively. In very general terms the model predicts that, because they generate excitation from R-organization but inhibition from S-analysis, Es should make faster and more frequent responses of a motor nature than Is do. Is, on the other hand, should persist more in perceptual activities and the analysis of sensory information which, however, necessarily involve some motor responses, e.g. of an orienting sort, and in the creation of response-mediated feedback stimulation.

Two other complicating factors need to be taken into account in this attempt to relate the personality of an individual in the terms of the new model to their characteristic movement tendencies. First, at any moment, the responsiveness of an individual results from the overall balance of inhibition–excitation deriving from all the demands they experience for S-analysis and R-organization. Hence, it is entirely possible to have Is and Es equally responsive for different reasons if, for example, the former derive as much excitation from S-analysis as they do inhibition from R-organization, and the opposite is true for the latter group of Es. Under such conditions, however, differences in performance between the groups may still be expected if what is measured by the experimenter depends more upon excitation in one of the two central processes than the other. Secondly, precisely because of their respective inherent biases towards S-analysis and R-organization, Is and Es may adopt entirely different strategies in performing the same task. It is, for example, possible that Is might more readily use cautious, 'data-driven, bottom-up' strategies in complex perceptual tasks such as reading reversed and inverted print, whereas Es might tend to choose to work in a more rapid, 'global-features, top-down' manner, trading accuracy for speed under these conditions. Es would be predicted to perform more poorly than Is if the task set was one of the proofreading sort, but better than Is if the task set was to obtain the meaning of a sentence quickly.

It is theoretically important to consider factors like these above, and if they do complicate attempts to make broad generalizations about the ways Is and Es differ in their performance, this should be offset by increased predictive and explanatory power. Although alternative sugestions have been made, including the possibility that differences at the level of the sensory and motor neuron might underlie differences in S-analysis and R-organization in the Brebner–Cooper model[16] – strategies like those outlined above, which result from an inherent central bias toward S-analysis or R-organization seem more likely to underlie I–E differences in speed and frequency of movement in any particular task. In drawing attention to the critical need to distinguish between S-analysis and R-organization the model requires that situations and tasks be fully analysed for the effects they create.

## S-ANALYSIS AND R-ORGANIZATION

The importance of motor processes in maintaining responsiveness in Es is accepted by Eysenck and some of his colleagues in their comprehensive review of personality and sporting activities[17] where they write, 'extraverts (and high P scorers) are more likely to take up sports, and to excel in them, because their low arousal level leads them to seek sensory stimulation *through bodily activity* (sensation seeking),' (my italic). But the distinction between the effects of generating stimulation from activity and those of organizing responses, which is central in the new model, is not made. Instead, for these authors, responses are organized for the stimulation they give rise to. However, later in their paper they point to an interesting difference between Is and Es in their strategies on a pursuit rotor task[18]. Trying to match a moving stimulus which followed a triangular track, Is adopted a strategy of frequently comparing the relative positions of their marker and the stimulus, using a corrective movement to hit the target. This resulted in many short periods ('hits') when the subject was on target. Es behaved differently. Their strategy involved paying less attention to immediate differences between target and marker than to the future track of the target which they had learned and, therefore, could achieve longer times on target by matching the velocity of the target along the sides of the triangular track. These longer periods on target were necessarily fewer in number. What is more interesting here is that, as Eysenck[17] points out, E's performance appears to have been controlled by a central motor programme, depending on stored information about the target's future movements to set up a similar movement and hold to it, while Is operated by using current sensory information (the visual mismatch between target and marker). Although the strategy of velocity matching depends partly upon target shape[19], with a triangular target the two personality groups thus adopted differing strategies involving organizing a continuous movement (Es) or relying on frequently performed S-analysis of the relative positions of target and marker (Is). This result reflects Is' bias to S-analysis and Es' to R-organization and shows that, following the model, where excitation can be derived either from frequent S-analyses and the feedback stimulation from many discrete responses, or by organizing more complex, integrated, continuous responses, it is Is who opt for the former approach and Es who choose the latter. When velocity matching is not possible Es have been shown to be less accurate in pursuit rotor tasks than Is, but also to evidence a greater reminiscence effect[20].

Under different experimental conditions Es have been shown to emit more frequent responses[12, 13]. The first of these experiments[12] showed Es responded more often than Is on trials when a signal to respond was withheld following a warning signal. In other words, Es tended to make commissive errors. If one interprets this as a prepared motor programme, begun by the warning signal, running to a conclusion, this would explain Es' errors of commission while Is' failure to make such errors is in line with their proposed greater dependence upon S-analysis. The other result[13] showed Es responded more frequently, and with more response runs in which response latencies kept decreasing or reached a maximum speed. But the time to the first response was also shorter for Es in this task which allowed the free inspection of projected 35 mm slides, indicating again Es' bias in favour of R-organization processes at the expense of S-analysis. Given such a bias it would be predicted that Es would perform less well than Is at tasks demanding continuous S-analysis, e.g. at vigilance tasks. Moreover, on the new model, this difference between the personality groups would be expected to become apparent in the course of time on task as inhibition from S-analysis built up for Es. Eysenck's suggestion that Es are in a state of chronic underarousal would lead to the expectation that differences would be apparent between Es and Is from the outset of the task.

More generally, the new model would assume that, left to themselves, Es would generate excitation through R-organization which would manifest itself, under everyday conditions, in a higher degree of motor activity. This generalization accords with non-psychologists' modal conception of Es as individuals who are alert, talkative, active, outgoing and who react strongly and quickly when people or events affect them. But, when placed in controlled conditions, Es can be shown to lose this characteristic responsiveness. The first experiments carried out to test the model[10] investigated the effect on reaction times of a task low on R-organization demands but requiring regular attention to the occurrence of an infrequent visual signal to respond which appeared every 18 s. Under these conditions it was Es whose reaction times became slower with time on task. This result shows there is more to E than appears in the everyday conception of it as well as supporting the model which predicted it.

Other findings along the same lines, showing Es' performance decreases relative to that of introverts only after time on task, can be cited. Some of these, e.g. in which their subjects' hands were partially immobilized and they were

31

asked to tap at a rate of five taps per second for 1 minute[21], could be explained in terms of the build-up of response-mediated S-inhibition during this demanding task, but other findings, e.g. that Es' performance at a vigilance task which did not require much in the way of response movements declined only after prolonged exposure to the task[22], seem better understood in terms of S-analysis producing inhibition for Es but excitation for Is. Still other findings provide further support for the model provided assumptions made about the relative demands for S-analysis and R-organization are correct. As an example of these, the experimental result[23] that, under white noise of about 80 dB, Es' performance at Ammons' version of the Tsai–Partington test[24] declined with time on task, may be due to inhibition from S-analysis. This particular task involves visually searching for successive numerals which are randomly distributed on a page, then connecting them up by drawing a line from one to the next. It seems likely that such a task loads more heavily on S-analysis than R-organization because responses are only made after a successful search which may inspect many numerals particularly at the start of the test. This, however, is an assumption and this experiment[23] also exemplifies the problem of interpreting previous research tasks in terms of the new model.

The studies of movement brought together by Eysenck[9] include one in which subjects moved a control knob sideways from a central starting point in response to a simple or complex pattern of visual stimuli[25]. Two identical sets of stimuli were located on the left and right halves of a display screen. Five stimuli, arranged vertically, were used. From the bottom they were – three coloured lights, white, green, red – then the words 'yes' and 'no'. The instructions were to move the knob out to, then back from a position under that of the white light if it occurred on its own, or if it was accompanied by the green light or the word 'yes'. But, if the red light or the word 'no' appeared, the knob had to be moved to and from the position on the opposite side from the stimuli. There were two conditions in the experiment, 'simple' in which only the white light ever appeared, and 'complex' in which all the lights were used. In the 'complex' condition every fifth stimulus was the white light by itself. Three test periods in the order A. simple, B. complex, C. simple, were given during which responses to the white light on its own were recorded.

The measures taken included (1) the maximum extent of the movement, (2) the time between passing the same points on the outward and homeward movements, and (3) the former measure divided by the latter to give the amount of movement per unit of time. Among the subjects tested were a group of 11 Es and a similar sized group of Is. Both these groups had high N scores. The results for these two subject groups adapted from ref. 25 are shown in Table 2.1.

*Table 2.1    Average amount of movement per unit of time (from Venables, 1955)*

|  | Condition | |
|  | Simple | Complex |
| --- | --- | --- |
| Es | 5.73 | 5.29 |
| Is | 4.71 | 5.35 |

In terms of the model, since the response remained the same in both conditions, so did the demand for R-organization, but because the complexity of stimulus information varied, the loading on S-analysis is greater in the complex condition. Under these conditions Es would be predicted to be less responsive in the complex condition than in the simple one because of greater S-inhibition, but Is, generating S-excitation in the complex condition, should be more responsive in that condition than in the simple one. Table 2.1 shows the average amount of movement per unit of time for Es and Is in the simple and complex conditions. From the table it can be seen that the pattern of results is as predicted. In that study the conclusion was that it was premature to provide a theoretical basis for the data obtained, but perhaps some 30 years later the Brebner–Cooper model can do so retrospectively.

These results depend in part on the fact that the time between passing the same points on the outward and homeward journeys is greater for Es in the complex condition than it is in the simple while the reverse is true for Is (see Table 2.2).

*Table 2.2   Average times between outward and homeward moves (from Venables, 1955)*

|     | Condition |         |
| --- | :---: | :---: |
|     | *Simple* | *Complex* |
| Es  | 3.79 | 3.92 |
| Is  | 4.50 | 3.83 |

Using the same sort of apparatus a separate study[26] also found Es responded with more extensive movements than Is did, and in other studies not primarily directed at the extent of movement[27], Es were observed to use more wide-ranging movements than Is. This result is interesting because the extent of the movement was directly related to the degree of distraction–distortion of auditory verbal material being attended to, and it may be that tendency to choose over a wide range and test the conditions 'vigorously as compared with the timid and limited' responses of Is, results from their R-excitation. The fact that E correlated positively and significantly with the number of shifts in the level of distortion–distraction chosen seems to support this view since it is clearly not merely the level of complexity of stimulation which is being sought by Es, otherwise they would choose the optimally stimulating and hold to it. Change and variety of stimulation is a likely factor in this result, but so is the tendency to make more frequent as well as larger responses.

A more recent experiment[28] gives results similar to those previously obtained[25]. This experiment involved varying the complexity of a discrimination task and of the response required in order to change the demands for S-analysis and R-organization and vary them independently. The task was to discriminate whether a triangle or square was embedded in a random pattern of dots displayed on a computer-controlled video. Greater complexity was achieved by increasing the density of the masking dots which made the discrimination more difficult. The response made was either the simple pressing of one of two response keys or the more complex one of pressing four keys using the index, middle, ring and little finger in that order. Two sets of keys were used: one for the left hand, one for the right. In this way the first response was always a choice response between index fingers. The measures recorded were reaction time, i.e. time to first response, movement time in the complex response conditions only, i.e. time between first and fourth responses, and the number of incorrect discriminations. The timed results are shown in Table 2.3.

Table 2.3    Mean reaction times (ms). (Data from Khew, 1984)

|  | Response | |
| --- | --- | --- |
|  | Simple | Complex |
| Simple discrimination | | |
| Es | 487 | 472 |
| Is | 530 | 518 |
| | | |
| Complex discrimination | | |
| Es | 2220 | 2589 |
| Is | 1883 | 2893 |

As far as accuracy of discrimination is concerned there were no differences between Es and Is and for the simpler discrimination average accuracy ranged from 99.2% correct to 100%. For the more complex discrimination mean accuracy varied between 77.8% and 81.5%. This raises the question of whether the degree of S-analysis (or R-organization for that matter) which any particular task involves can be quantified before performing the task. Apart from the case where the same operation is repeated a number of times, the answer is that one can only make ordinal judgements that a task is more or less demanding. To discover how much more demanding requires that a pilot study be performed and, if necessary, the task adjusted so that the phenomenon under study is allowed to reveal itself. Obtaining the right strength of the phenomenon one is studying is necessary in any theory-testing exercise, but it is sometimes ignored leading to incorrect conclusions; more often relativities are assumed. Because it is important in the model to set the demands for both S-analysis and R-organization at the right levels most of the experiments designed to test it have been preceded by pilot studies[10, 12–15].

What Table 2.3 shows is that the simple discrimination task, carried out with near perfect accuracy, did not overload the capacity of Es relative to Is, rather Es' tendency to R-excitation makes them respond faster. When faced with the more demanding discrimination, however, Es' reaction times are slower than Is' when only a simple response is required in line with S-inhibition affecting them, but when the more complex response is added, Is' performance becomes slower than Es' supporting the view that they are deriving inhibition from

R-organization but Es are deriving excitation. Looked at as a pattern, it is difficult to see how any other model of E could explain the shifts in performance that follow the manipulations of stimulus and response components of this study.

A further finding which involved maintaining a response rather than making a movement[29] can also be regarded as supporting the model. This is the finding that, asked to maintain a force of two thirds of their previously determined hand-strength for as long as possible on a dynamometer, Es held the response for an average of 9.04 s longer than Is. Since only two sets of three trials separated by 13 min were given, it seems unlikely that R-mediated S-inhibition would exert any strong influence in this experiment. However, the result is what would be expected if Is tended to generate R-inhibition but Es R-excitation as they attempted to continue their holding of the dynamometer setting.

A complementary finding[30] demonstrated that E male undergraduate subjects were superior to Is when required to pedal on a bicycle ergometer at 30 km/h. A total of eight trials was given each separated by 1 min except that, because the task was so difficult a 5 min rest was allowed between the fifth and sixth trial. In this very highly responsive task Es began by performing very much better than Is in line with what the model would predict. But also consistent was the finding that Es' performance was more affected than Is' across trials although in all trials they performed significantly longer than Is. This result is expected on the basis that R-mediated S-inhibition is greater for Es, who are in any case responding for longer because of their R-excitatory tendency, and the inhibition does not dissipate entirely during the short rest pauses. The difference in performance times between the first and second halves of the experiment was a massive 193 s for Es in comparison with only 54.5 s for Is[30]. The improvement following the longer rest pause is also of interest with Es improving by 20 s to the Is 5.7 s. Clearly under these conditions Es remained more responsive than Is. The data were considered to show Es had greater physical strength, possibly related to their body build, but this was not measured or controlled. The point that Es withstand pain better than Is was also made. However, continuing to inflict pain on oneself to reach a higher level of arousal seems inherently unlikely since pain would usually be assumed to create more than optimum arousal even for Es. Rather, it seems necessary to assume higher thresholds for pain, related not to the search for increased arousal, but to the attenuating effect S-inhibition has on stimuli for Es, perhaps particularly so when reinforced by R-mediated S-inhibition. Unfortunately, this clear picture is marred by one report[31] that in a study of 20 Es and a similar number of Is, which involved four measures of persistence including leg persistence and dynamometer persistence, it was Is who were significantly more persistent. This result may be due to mixing two forms of persistence, physical and ideational, since the other persistence measures were problem solving and continuous addition, and it may be that Is performed very much better at these two latter tasks. Certainly, an earlier study of ethnically similar students[32] found that Es correlated positively with persistence when they replicated[29].

Hendry[33] adopted the approach of assigning British Psychology students to different groups according to their involvement in physical, sporting activities, and comparing these groups on E and N. In descending order of degree of physical activity the three groups were labelled Active-competitive, Active-recreational and Non-participating. Table 2.4 gives the mean E scores for men and women in those three groups. From the table it is evident that there is a positive relationship between E scores and physical activity. In terms of N, the competitive group appeared to score lower than the other two groups, but in a multiple regression analysis N failed to reach a significant level whereas E was significant ($p < 0.05$).

Table 2.4   Average E scores of students grouped by the degree of their physical activity. (From Hendry, 1975)

|        | Active-competitive | Active-recreational | Non-participant |
|--------|--------------------|---------------------|-----------------|
| Women  | 13.07              | 11.72               | 10.15           |
| Men    | 13.77              | 12.43               | 10.00           |

These results are in agreement with an earlier study[34] which used the 16PF test and showed a positive relationship between general athletic ability (i.e. sports participation, explosive strength, stamina and co-ordination) and tough-minded extraversion. This result was supported by the finding that children who were more intelligent, extraverted and tough-minded tended to be better at tests of motor co-ordination, speed and agility[35]. However, in an extension of the original study, the tough-minded component failed to appear again although the link between E and general athletic ability was confirmed. Other studies support this conclusion showing that in a selected group of highly skilled table-tennis players there were three times as many Es as there were Is[36]. Among players of average ability there were equal numbers of Es and Is, but among those who stated that they were extremely poor at ball games Is outnumbered Es by more than two to one. An investigation[37] into the personality of 100 English children who were swimmers and 100 who were not found that swimmers scored significantly higher on E as measured by the Junior Eysenck Personality Questionnaire, again implicating E in sporting participation. Complicating matters, however, is the finding in Hawaii that 176 female novice swimmers were more introverted than a group of 264 female students enrolled in basic movement, golf and tennis courses[38].

While it is interesting that E should correlate positively with physical, sporting activity, it is difficult to analyse most sports into their relative demands for S-analysis or R-organization. Moreover, factors like physique, skill and learning opportunities are difficult to control. Nevertheless, it seems reasonable to conclude that Es show a stronger tendency to choose physical, sporting activities, and this could be related to their R-excitatory tendency.

## EXPRESSIVE GESTURE

Returning to the question of expressive gesture and personality, consideration of which has been delayed until findings on the greater frequency and extent of movement for Es could be reviewed, it can now be suggested that, in free response situations, Es will express themselves with more expansive and more frequent movements. To some extent we already know this from experiments where Es' preferred rate of pressing a set of five response keys was faster than that of Is[39]; or as previously outlined in ref. 13. What is being expressed in such studies is argued to be Es' tendency to R-excitation, Is' to R-inhibition, in so far as the tasks set allow these to show in behaviour. However, other studies implicate factors other than E when what is being expressed is emotionality, though they may interact with E. One[40] is cited[9] as showing that Es high on anxiety show less graphic expansiveness (measured by the amount of a page covered by subjects asked to doodle designs to express the mood of pieces of jazz music to which they had just listened) than Es low on anxiety. Is showed the reverse effect. The explanation suggested is a symbolic one involving anxious Is, 'covertly seeking to move toward others and therefore being more expansive graphically', while anxious Es are 'covertly seeking to move away from others and therefore being more constricted graphically'. However, an alternative interpretation which may be offered is that being anxious is associated with higher levels of stimulation, some of which arise internally, therefore anxious Es will develop S-inhibition, but anxious Is S-excitation, and this will reflect in their graphic responsiveness. This view has the advantage of avoiding the need for responses to symbolize movement toward and away from other people.

Although using Guilford's[41] scales rather than Eysenck's, gestural amplitude has been found to be a consistent feature of motor responses, and also measures like step length and free leg movement were positively correlated with E[42]. In this study using children as subjects no differences were observed between the sexes. In a later study in which the results supported the view that communicative gesture is a unitary and stable dimension of behaviour[43], the further point is made that it differs from graphic communication and is related to emotional stability. It may be argued, then, that emotional states, whether chronic or temporary, serve to over-ride or at least interfere with motor behaviour characteristic of other personality dimensions.

While E has usually been a variable of secondary interest in studies of personality and expressive movement, some interesting results have, nevertheless, been obtained. For example[44], that an individual's own E 'leaks through' their video-taped role-playing of a Mathematics' teacher supposed to be E or I[44]. The correlations among raters for a variety of different presentations of information, e.g. sound only, video only, head obscured, sound and video, were high, around 0.8, showing that naive raters agreed closely in their assessments. One of the consistent findings is that Es tend to speak more often, shown for young female occupational therapy students[45], and for groups of men and women conversing with either male or female confederates of the experimenter[46]. This is scarcely unexpected, but from a theoretical point of view it is important to understand this in terms of a more general explanation of behavioural differences between Es and Is. Speaking more often in social situations is an important aspect of Es' characteristically greater sociability, or social extraversion, and it can be regarded as deriving from their R-excitatory tendency. This tendency, which favours not only speaking more but also other responses, underlies social extraversion and impulsiveness in Es as far as our model is concerned.

37

Social interactions can be inhibited by anxiety, and it is a possibility that Es are less anxious socially because of their successful learning experiences. However, another feature of social extraversion deriving from R-excitation is Es' speed of responding, and it may be argued that Is' R-inhibitory tendency not to respond, or to take longer to organize responses, can serve as a handicap in social interactions. Since there is some evidence that verbal fluency in children is positively related to their E scores, and that anxiety scores on the Children's Manifest Anxiety Scale were not relevant to the boys' performance though it did affect the girls[47], fluency may have been a function of R-excitation in those subjects.

Another feature of social behaviour which has been related to E is the frequency of looking at another individual. Es tend to look more often when interacting with another person, though not for longer periods[46]. Against this latter finding, which could show Es simply making more frequent responses, must be set the result[48] from testing Es', 'neutrals'' and Is' behaviour while discussing one of the TAT pictures for a 3 min period (the same length of time over which data were recorded in ref. 46). It was found that both average and total eye contact time were a function of E. However, it appears that female Is were better than female Es at discriminating which of seven points on the upper halves of their faces another person was looking at[49]. While the carry-over of such findings from the laboratory to everyday social situations is far from guaranteed, the possibility is raised that, even though they initiate fewer visual contacts by looking at other people, Is tend to process more non-verbal information than Es. On this argument, Is' S-excitatory proneness may be affecting their own verbal performance.

Clearly, there are some fine-grain effects which remain to be researched more fully, but the picture which is emerging seems to have a certain coherence, and it supports the view that Es and Is can be characterized by their expressive gesture even though emotional states may interfere with or overlay this.


## CONCLUSION

While not every attempt to relate personality and movement has been dealt with in this selective review, for example refs. 50, 51, the conclusion[52] concerning movement requirements of different personality types, that, 'This approach would not appear to have been developed to any great extent', may no longer be justified even though this short chapter is only one step in that direction. Empirical support for the new model has been demonstrated in many forms of behaviour[10,12-15] but they all involve S-analysis and R-organization. It could be suggested that pointing to the importance of distinguishing between these processes should be unnecessary in psychological explanations since as long ago as 1868 Donders attempted to separate and measure the time taken by the processes concerned with discriminating between stimuli and selecting one of a set of possible responses[53]. More recent work in reaction times has tended to confirm the existence of stages in processing information to arrive at an appropriate response[54, 55], but the truth is that while some areas of psychology, e.g. learning theory and the study of cognitive processes, have been receptive to discoveries in other fields, personality theorizing has been less open to such developments. The main bridges which allow traffic between personality theory and other areas of experimental psychology are those built by Pavlov and Eysenck, or influenced by them. The new model attempts to continue in this tradition in the belief that this has proved the most fruitful and lasting approach to the study of differences in the behaviour of people with differing personality structures.

## References

1. Allport, G. W. and Vernon, P. E. (1933). *Studies in Expressive Movement.* (New York: Haffner)
2. Mischel, W. (1968). *Personality and Assessment.* (New York: Wiley)
3. Runeson, S. and Frykholm, G. (1983). Kinematic specification of dynamics as an informational basis for person-and-action perception: expectation, gender recognition, and deceptive intention. *J. Exp. Psychol: Gen.,* **112,** 585–615
4. Sheldon, W. H. (1949). *Varieties of Delinquent Youth: an Introduction to Constitutional Psychiatry.* (New York: Harper)
5. Theophrastus (1970). *The Character Sketches.* Translated by Anderson, W. (Kent State University Press)
6. Eysenck, H. J. (1957). *The Dynamics of Anxiety and Hysteria.* (London: Routledge & Kegan Paul)
7. Hull, C. L. (1943). *Principles of Behaviour.* (New York: Appleton-Century-Crofts)
8. Eysenck, H. J. (1967). *The Biological Basis of Personality.* (Springfield, Ill.: Thomas)
9. Eysenck, H. J. (1971). *Readings in Extraversion–Introversion. 3. Bearings on Basic Psychological Processes.* (London: Staples)
10. Brebner, J. and Cooper, C. (1974). The effect of a low rate of regular signals upon the reaction times of introverts and extraverts. *J. Res. Pers.,* **8,** 263–76
11. Pavlov, I. P. (1927). *Conditioned Reflexes.* Translated by Anrep, G. V. (London: Oxford University Press)
12. Brebner, J. and Flavel, R. (1978). The effect of catch-trials on speed and accuracy among introverts and extraverts in a simple RT task. *Br. J. Psychol.,* **69,** 9–15
13. Brebner, J. and Cooper, C. (1978). Stimulus- or response-induced excitation. A comparison of the behaviour of introverts and extraverts. *J. Res. Pers.,* **12,** 306–11
14. Katsikitis, M. and Brebner, J. (1981). Individual differences in the effects of personal space invasion: a test of the Brebner–Cooper model of extraversion. *Pers. Individual Differences,* **2,** 5–10
15. Tiggemann, M., Winefield, A. H. and Brebner, J. (1982). The role of extraversion in the development of learned helplessness. *Pers. Individual Differences,* **3,** 27–34
16. Stelmack, R. M. and Plouffe, L. (1983). Introversion–extraversion: the Bell-Magendie law revisited. *Pers. Individual Differences,* **4,** 421–7
17. Eysenck, H. J., Nias, D. K. B. and Cox, D. N. (1982). Sport and personality. *Adv. Behav. Res. Ther.,* **4,** 1–56
18. Eysenck, H. J. and Frith, C. D. (1977). *Reminiscence, Motivation and Personality.* (London: Plenum Press)
19. Frith, C. D. (1971). Strategies in rotary pursuit tracking. *Br. J. Psychol.,* **62,** 187–97
20. Shamberg, N., Baker, S. and Burns, J. (1969). Reminiscence and pursuit rotor performance in introverts and extraverts. *Br. J. Soc. Clin. Psychol.,* **8,** 375–82
21. Wilson, G. D., Tunstall, O. A. and Eysenck, H. J. (1971). Individual differences in tapping performance as a function of time on task. *Perceptual and Motor Skills,* **33,** 375–8
22. Keister, M. E. and McLaughlin, I. (1972). Vigilance performance related to extraversion-introversion and caffeine. *J. Res. Pers.,* **6,** 5–11

23. Di Scipio, W. J. (1971). Psychomotor performance as a function of white noise and personality variables. *Percept. and Motor Skills*, **33**, 82
24. Ammons, C. H. (1960). Temporary and permanent inhibitory effects associated with acquisition of a simple perceptual-motor skill. *J. Gen. Psychol.*, **62**, 223–45
25. Venables, P. H. (1955). Changes in motor response with increase and decrease in task difficulty in normal industrial and psychiatric patient subjects. *Br. J. Psychol.*, **46**, 101–10
26. Rachman, S. (1961), Psychomotor behaviour and personality with special reference to conflict. *Unpublished PhD thesis.* (University of London)
27. Morgenstern, F. S., Hodgson, R. J. and Law, J. (1974). Work efficiency and personality: a comparison of introverted and extraverted subjects exposed to conditions of distraction and distortion of stimulus in a learning task. *Ergonomics*, **17**, 211–20
28. Khew, K. (1984). Personal communication
29. Costello, C. G. and Eysenck, H. J. (1961). Persistence, personality and motivation. *Perceptual and Motor Skills*, **12**, 169–70
30. Shiomi, K. (1980). Performance differences between extraverts and introverts on exercises using an ergometer. *Perceptual and Motor Skills*, **50**, 356–8
31. Chinnian, R. and Murphy, V. N. (1969), Personality and persistence. *Trans. All-India Inst. Ment. Health*, **9**, 51–8
32. Singh, S. D., Gupta, V. P. and Manocha, S. N. (1966). Physical persistence, personality and drugs. *Ind. J. Appl. Psychol.*, **3**, 92–5
33. Hendry, L. B. (1975). Personality and movement: a university study. *J. Hum. Movement Stud.*, **1**, 19–23
34. Kane, J. (1968). Personality and athletic ability. *Swimming Tech.*, **5**, 79–81
35. Kirkendall, D. R. (1970). The multivariate relationships between selected facets of motor performance and personality profiles in preadolescent children. *Proceedings of Indiana University Sesquicentennial Symposium in Physical Education.* (Bloomington: Indiana University Press)
36. Whiting, H. T. A. and Hutt, J. W. R. (1972). The effects of personality and ability on speed of decisions regarding the directional aspects of ball flight. *J. Motor Behav.*, **4**, 89–97
37. Williams, J. G. (1970). Personality factors and the acquisition of swimming skills. *Pap. Psychol.*, **4**, 10–11
38. Meredith, G. M. and Harris, M. M. (1969). Personality traits of college women in beginning swimming. *Perceptual and Motor Skills*, **29**, 216–18
39. Howarth, E. (1963). Differences between extraverts and introverts on a button-pressing task. *Psychol. Rep.*, **14**, 949–50
40. Wallach, M. A. and Gahm, R. C. (1960). Personality functions of graphic constriction and expansiveness. *J. Pers.*, **28**, 73–88
41. Guilford, J. P. (1959). *Personality.* (New York: McGraw-Hill)
42. Bruchon, M. (1969–1970). Gestural amplitude and personality. *Bull. Psychol.*, **23**, 426–7
43. Bruchon, M. (1972–1973). An expressive modality of personality: communicative gesture. *Bull. Psychol.*, **26**, 4–21
44. Lippa, R. (1976). Expressive control and the leakage of dispositional introversion-extraversion during role-played teaching. *J. Pers.*, **44**, 541–59
45. Campbell, A. and Rushton, P. (1978). Bodily communication and personality. *Br. J. Soc. Clin. Psychol.*, **17**, 31–6
46. Rutter, D. R., Morley, I. E. and Graham, J. C. (1972). Visual interaction in a group of introverts and extraverts. *Eur. J. Soc. Psychol.*, **2**, 371–84
47. Tapasak, R. C., Roodin, P. A. and Vaught, G. M. (1978). Effects of extraversion, anxiety, and sex on children's verbal fluency and coding task performance. *J. Psychol.*, **100**, 49–55
48. Mobbs, N. A. (1968). Eye-contact in relation to social introversion–extraversion. *Br. J. Soc. Clin. Psychol.*, **7**, 305–6
49. Ellgring, J. H. (1970). Judgement of glances directed at different points in the face. *Z. Exp. Angewandte Psychol.*, **17**, 600–7
50. North, M. (1972). *Personality Assessment Through Movement.* (London: Macdonald and Evans)
51. Whiting, H. T. A. (1973). Personality and movement behaviour. In Brooke, J. D. and Whiting, H. T. A. (eds.) *Human Movement – A Field of Study.* pp. 189–95. (London: Henry Kimpton)

52. Warburton, F. W. and Kane, J. E. (1966). Personality related to sport and physical ability. In *Readings in Physical Education*. pp. 61–89. (London: Physical Education Association)
53. Donders, F. C. (1968). Translated by Koster, W. G. Reprinted (1969). On the speed of mental processes. *Acta Psychol.*, **30,** 412–31
54. Sternberg, S. (1969). The discovery of processing stages: extensions to Donders' method. In Koster, W. G. (ed.). *Attention and Performance*. Vol. 2. (Amsterdam: North-Holland)
55. Welford, A. T. (ed.) (1980). *Reaction Times*. (London: Academic Press)

# 3
# Perceiving people through their movements

## Sverker Runeson

What can be known about a person from observing his or her movements? If there is to be any knowing at all of this kind there must exist *relations of specificity* between properties of movements and persons; movements must contain *information* about that which moves.

Can there be such informative relations? To find out we need to know what determines the shape of our movements. To common understanding, the issue is trivial. As acting persons we see ourselves as sovereign controllers of our movements. Although we usually do not care too much to tailor the manner of our movements, we feel able to do so whenever we wish.

In this view there could not be much information in our movements, except of course about how we *wish* to move, including what we might want to express by our movements. Hence, one does not usually recognize the possibility of strong and comprehensive connections between movements and the properties of the person. It therefore seems up to each one of us to give *expression* to our properties or states while relying on cultural conventions for the meaning of the expressive movements. We might say that the relations of specificity implied in this are *soft* since conventions are variable and one is free to omit expressions completely or even to provide false, deceptive, expressions. Although on a very different time-scale, the same argument applies to the expressive movements installed by biological evolution (cf. Darwin's *The Expression of the Emotions in Man and Animals*). Hence, the selection of movements that have come to express the various organismic conditions is arbitrary and deceptive expressions occur also in this context (e.g. birds feigning a broken wing to detract the attention of a predator from their offspring).

Work on social perception has sometimes claimed that facial movements or movements of hands and feet can reveal emotions or intentions and studies have shown that observers can make some use of such cues in judging other people. However, these phenomena are viewed as leaks in an essentially tight system, exceptions to the overall rule of complete movement control[1-3]. Social functioning, in this context, takes on a character of arbitrariness, as an expression-playing game.

There are reasons to call this popular view into question. First, it is biologically unsound. In the life of animals, perceiving *true* characteristics of other animals, for instance, their strength, agility, alertness, emotions, intentions, individual identity, or group membership, are very often of critical importance. Expressions might be satisfactory for communication among co-operative individuals but social functioning entails just as much relating to indifferent or antagonistic creatures. Optional and fakeable expressions would seem to comprise too soft a basis for such important functions. Thus the prevalence of a strong need for accurately perceiving other animals suggests that animals will have developed in such a way that available information is well-used.

The second and most important reason for a new approach derives from considerations of information available in movements. In approaching this issue, one is well advised to realize that arguments or proofs for the *non*-existence of information can never be strongly founded when one is dealing with systems of natural complexity. One can only say that the scientific search (as conducted) for the target information (as construed) has so far been unsuccessful. The history of perception research is marked by an issue of this kind. At least since Berkeley's *New Theory of Vision*, philosophers and psychologists have claimed to have proven that the patterns available at our senses are fundamentally ambiguous. In perception textbooks it appears in the form of issues such as the celebrated size/distance and shape/slant invariances. A variety of mental functions such as learning, association, thinking, or inferencing, have been called upon to do supplementary work on the incomplete or meaningless products of perception.

Initiated by the work of James J. Gibson[4-6], recent more realistic analyses have shown the inadequacy of established opinion. For instance, it has been demonstrated that the changing pattern of light that reaches the eye of a moving person, the so-called *optic array*, contains reliable information about sizes and distances of objects and the general three-dimensional layout of the environment. Thus the old puzzle of the informational support for 'depth perception' has been resolved in a positive way. At the same time it was shown that the optic array also specifies one's own location and locomotion (by foot or vehicle) and that it provides excellent information for maintaining balance and controlling approach movements[7,8]. Armed with such discoveries, perception research can now proceed to study whether and how the perceptual systems make use of the rich and naturally available information. For instance, experiments have shown that optical information about one's own motion is in fact used by the visual system, and the way it is used makes vision stand out as the dominant proprioceptive and kinesthetic sense[9-11]. Crucial parts of this new platform for understanding perception are, for instance, the insight that we only need to consider natural conditions; cluttered natural conditions usually provide better information than 'simple' hypothetical or laboratory environments. The available information may be in extremely complex form. Complexity, however, is not an intrinsic property of the real world but is relative to the power of the conceptual tools used to describe and analyse reality. Seemingly very complex information might therefore be used in a simple and direct way by a perceptual system that is functionally adequate for the task (e.g. a 'smart mechanism'[12-14]).

The above examples of *firm* information for perception concern the non-animate environment and the perceiver's relation to the environment. Is a similar change of scene also possible in the field of person perception? I think it is, and in what follows I will briefly present recent theoretical and empirical work that supports this presumption. Consider the studies by Robert Shaw and co-workers[15,16] of perception of people's age and recognition of individual identity despite age changes. Although growth and ageing alters all features of the human profile they were able to show that all the changes can be captured by a single mathematical transformation applied to the profile. Because of this lawfulness in the process of growth (cf. d'Arcy Thompson's *On Growth and Form*) there exists a principled basis for distinguishing the higher-order identity-carrying structural properties of profiles from the effects of age transformation. Furthermore, a variety of empirical studies have shown that this possibility is made good use of by our visual system. The work by Shaw *et al.* sets a model for how one may reach an understanding of our ability to perceive a stable and recognizable environment despite the extreme variability of the patterns available at our senses. In line with the theme of the book, however, the treatment of the issue will be in terms of the information made available by the lawfulness of human movement.

## THE CONTROL OF MOVEMENT: AN EMERGING VIEW

Let us return to the question of how the shape of our movements is determined. Is it really the case that we have full control over all the details of the spatio-temporal trajectories of each part of our body? Certainly not! Try writing the letter 'W' while making circular movements with the foot[17]. Or try flapping your hand back and forth without moving the wrist[18]. You will find both exercises almost impossible. Why? The case of performing unrelated movements with hand and foot demonstrates an absence of independent concurrent central control over the limbs. The second case additionally points out the role of mechanics in our movements. Each impulse (the action of a force, e.g. from a muscle, over an interval of time) necessarily goes with a reactive impulse in the opposite direction. Thus, while the active impulses flap the hand the *reactive* impulses are transferred to the upper end of the lower arm. Because the effective mass at the wrist is not very large, sizeable opposite movements of the wrist will occur. To extinguish these movements would require the muscles operating the elbow and shoulder joints to produce precise amounts of opposed impulses distributed in a special and smooth way over the time course of the event. No doubt the muscles would have the necessary strength for it but, once again, we do not seem to possess that kind of control over our motor system.

One might be tempted to regard the above type of phenomena as peculiarities or exceptions. There is no warrant for doing so, however. In fact, it has been shown that the sort of central motor control entailed by the popular view is not even possible in principle: the magnitude of the task of centrally controlling a system expands in explosive fashion when its mechanical complexity, the number of *degrees of freedom*, increases beyond a few. Centralized control of a system such as the human body with its well over 100 degrees of freedom (i.e. the elbow joint has two dimensions of movement, the shoulder has three, etc.) certainly exceeds the capacity of any conceivable controlling device. This is the so-called *degrees-of-freedom problem*, put forth by physiologist Nicolai Bernstein[19], who also laid the foundation for a new approach to the understanding of motor action (for an introduction, see ref. 20). As will be shown below, this emerging view is especially useful for the study of the relations between person properties and movement.

When a movement is actually performed it does have a detailed shape. We must therefore ask: if the detailed shape of our movements is not determined by central neural control, then how is it determined? It might seem that it is not determined at all, that the uncontrolled details get settled at random. However, such a view would arise from a neglect of the *mechanical* properties of the body and the laws of mechanics that apply to it. It is as simple as this: a purely mechanical system, without any controlling functions, nevertheless behaves in perfectly lawful ways. In particular, a mechanical system similar to our body, consisting of several relatively rigid sections connected in hinge-like fashion, constitutes a system of pendulums and mass-spring oscillators. If the proportions and other parameters of such a system are well-tuned, as they no doubt are in the case of our bodies, its *free mechanical movements* will exhibit a number of valuable characteristics. Not only does the considerable mass of the various body members lead to a smoothing of the movements, the combination of the mass of the segments and the elasticity and damping provided by the muscles and other tissues sets up *damped mass-spring oscillators* throughout the body. Far from being quirks in the system, such oscillators in themselves behave in a manner that takes us an important bit of the way towards realizing the purpose of the motor system: goal-directed, intentional action. For instance, the oscillators tend to reach the target (resting position) independently of where they start and do so even if they are perturbed *en route*. When damping is low we get oscillation; at critical damping we get a single movement with a smooth start and a smooth stop at the target position. Spring stiffness determines the speed of the movement. Thus, by setting just three parameters, resting length, stiffness, and damping, a mass-spring unit can be made to execute all sorts of movements to a target: fast or slow, repetitive or singular. And for disturbances the movements may get subjected to, first-order compensation is inherently provided[21, 22].

These properties of mass-spring systems and other types of oscillators, such as the limit-cycle oscillator, have made them attractive and plausible for inclusion in models of our motor system. Since, as said above, our body members *are* such systems, mechanically speaking, there are only two possibilities: either the oscillatory and other mechanical characteristics are exploited positively in the shaping of movements or they are suppressed by very precisely controlled muscular effort[23]. The traditional view of motor control must not only come up with an account of how central control can occur, it must also specifically deny that the free movement components have any role and explain how they are counteracted by neural control so as not to appear in the resulting movements – clearly a less parsimonious approach. The emerging view can take the more promising route of saying that the role of central control in human movement is to *harness* the free movements by, for instance, setting the parameters (tuning) of the mass-spring units and linking them together into functional units, so-called *co-ordinative structures*, appropriate for the current task[24].

A further discussion of these matters will be deferred until the concluding section of this chapter. Let us just note that what we get is a very much decentralized system of control and one in which the mechanical properties of the body have an important role. It follows that we can neither control nor monitor the details of our movements. Central control of movement appears to have a role similar to that of an executive at an industry plant: he is in control of the goals of the operations and monitors progress relative to that. But he neither has the competence, capacity, nor channels to give meaningful orders at lower levels. If he nevertheless ventures to try he may just cause malfunction. His instructions may be useful in starting up a new production line but operations will remain slow and cranky until the shop people begin to ignore him and find their own ways of doing their jobs. (No need to explain how this metaphor applies to skilled action – we have all experienced its various aspects!)

## FROM MOVEMENT TO INFORMATION: THE KSD PRINCIPLE

If mechanical properties of the body (mass and its distribution among the limbs, geometrical proportions, etc.) have an important role in shaping movement, could this relation hold in reverse? Mechanical science distinguishes kinematics from dynamics, where *kinematics* is motion described as such while *dynamics* is motion treated in terms of what causes or constrains it, the causal aspect of movement. In these terms we can state our problem as whether kinematics, the movements, specify dynamics, the causes of the movements. In an earlier work[18], we refer to this possibility as *Kinematic Specification of Dynamics*, or the *KSD-principle* for short. If it can be shown to hold, then a wealth of useful information about the person turns out to be available.

The dynamic factors involved in generating a person's movements include, as we have seen, first of all the geometrical and mechanical proportions of the person's body. Since people differ in anatomical make-up there would be a basis for recognizing people by their movements, either their *individual identity* or their *category membership*: men/women, physically fit/unfit, etc. Furthermore, the person's *intentions* and *expectations* also have a dynamic role in shaping the movements. Such 'hidden' inner properties or states could therefore be specified to the extent that they influence the generation of movements. By the same token, *emotions* or *personality* characteristics could probably influence the states of action-readiness that prevail in the body, and hence be potentially perceivable (see concluding section below).

The procedure for analysing the tenability of the KSD-principle is a very technical one, involving a sizeable hypothetical system of differential equations accounting for how the dynamic factors of the human body generate kinematic patterns. Instead of plugging in values for all the dynamic parameters, as one would do to predict movements, we want to treat the movement parameters as given by observation and solve for the dynamic factors. A strictly formal treatment might not have been accomplished; however, an examination of the prospects for its solvability has given reasons to expect that the KSD-principle holds true in a manner relevant for the functioning of perceptual systems[18]. Three circumstances are particularly favourable. First, when observed values for displacement and its derivatives (velocity and acceleration) are available the remaining equations are no longer in differential form. Second, by observing movements over time as many sets of observations as required may be obtained while the dynamic factors remain constant. Thus, we can increase the number of equations without increasing the number of unknowns. Third, if the mass-spring model of movement control is adopted (or more advanced versions of it[25]) the equations will be relatively free from terms that are explicit functions of time (force functions). This follows from what we discussed above on the absence of finely time-graded muscular action and the consequent prevalence of free mass-spring-like movement components.

For an intuitive grasp of the issue, we may consider whether a particular movement could be generated from another set of dynamic parameters (constellation of causal factors). There are many dynamic factors involved in generating human movements. Hence, if the value of one were to change, could not some of the others be changed at the same time in such a way as to restore the shape of the original movement?

This represents the human movement version of the general issue of specificity v. non-specificity in the information available for perception. If *substitutability* holds among causal factors in generating the patterns that reach our senses then the patterns cannot specify which of two or several constellations of causal factors gave rise to a particular pattern. On closer analysis such arguments turn out to be based on invalid implicit assumptions of additivity and unidimensionality. In the case of human motion the argument might be reasonable provided one focuses on a single, simple parameter of motion, say the speed of a particular movement. Lifting an empty box is usually faster than lifting a heavy one but intentionally one could slow down the lifting of the empty box. Thus, the effect of a change in one factor (box weight) would be cancelled by a change in another dynamic factor (the lifter's intention). The argument loses its seeming validity, however, as soon as one takes into account the well over 100 degrees of freedom of the human body and that most action involves movement at most joints. While lifting the light box slowly one will not experience the same inertial and reactive forces as with the heavy box and the preparatory and compensatory movements that necessarily occur throughout the lifter's body will be different. What we can learn from this example, is that the human kinematic pattern, because of its multidimensionality, has an enormously large theoretical variability which at least equals, perhaps vastly transcends, the variability of the dynamic factors. If we consider human movement patterns in detail, the number of kinematically different ways in which a particular goal-directed action can be performed is so large that the chance of two different persons, or the same person in different states of intention or emotion, performing it in the same way is negligibly small. Consequently, the actually occurring kinematic pattern *is* indeed specific for the conditions that generated it. Notice how the complexity of the human body, its large number of degrees of freedom, which presented such a burden for the control system, becomes a boon for perception. The specification power of human kinematics, its capacity for conveying information, turns out to be exceedingly large.

Although the KSD-principle has not been proved in the strict sense, it has gained sufficient support to warrant a revised approach to person perception. Biological evolution, of course, only requires that available information is sufficient to develop perceptual systems that are geared to it. Rare or hypothetical instances of non-specificity and malfunction have been of no consequence. Indeed, the possibility itself that firm information about people might be available is sufficient to prompt at least the following:

(1) Experimenters can no longer assume that firm information is non-existent and proceed to study expressions etc. without specifically controlling for kinematic information.

(2) Old work in the general area of social psychology and person perception must be re-examined to determine whether subjects have picked up or been influenced by kinematic information about true conditions, in particular through kinematics, conflicting with the information deliberately administered by the experimenters or acting accomplices.

(3) Experiments exploring what information can be picked up from human kinematics should be undertaken.

## FROM INFORMATION TO PERCEPTION

The demonstration of *available* information, as per the KSD-principle, is not sufficient to establish the actual role of human movement in person perception. We must also test whether and how it is *used* in perception and how it might relate to our use of other kinds of information. There are several possible reasons why available information might not be used:

(1) The information might reside in indiscriminably small parametrical variations in the kinematic pattern.

(2) We might not have the perceptual sensitivity for the particular kind of information, either because we have not educated our perceptual skills for it or because we as humans are inadequately equipped for it.

(3) We do not attend to it at the moment, either because it has not caught our attention, we are not interested in it, or other information emitted by the person is more salient (e.g. expressive movements).

In order to do experimental studies in this area one stands in need of a methodology which allows isolated presentation of the kinematics of people in action. A very useful method for this is the so-called *point-light technique*, introduced in the field by Gunnar Johansson[26]. In the more recent version of it people are dressed in black and fitted with patches or bands of retroreflectant tape at the main joints of the body and around the forehead. Their activities are videotaped while illuminated with a floodlight placed as close to the camera lens as possible. In this way, the patches get rendered in supercontrast and are the only things visible if the intensity control is turned down on the monitor. Consequently, normal room illumination can be left on during recording sessions.

The original studies with this technique[26] revealed a remarkable sensitivity of our visual system to the human kinematics as displayed through a dozen or so bright patches on a screen. Stationary, they just look like dissociated patches but when they begin to move, within a fraction of a second one sees a human being engaged in walking, dancing, doing push-up exercises, etc. The impression is so vivid that viewing the scene at the normal intensity setting usually does not strike one as adding much information!

Collision Events

The question then becomes, can anything be seen besides that it is human and the sort of activity being performed? The question was triggered by the results of investigations of visual perception of non-animate events such as collisions. Using the above-mentioned dynamics v. kinematics distinction it had been shown that in linear collisions between objects, the kinematics, comprised in this case by the velocities of the two objects directly prior and following the collision, uniquely specifies two dynamic properties of the objects: the ratio of their masses (i.e. how heavy one is relative to the other) and the effective damping characteristics of the materials of which they are made[27]. Investigations then showed that observers of simulated collision events could in fact make use of this information[28]. Thus, it has been established, both theoretically and empirically, that supposedly invisible internal dynamic properties of objects can be perceived visually when the objects are involved in events. In other words, event perception involves perceiving dynamics. Could this hold for animate events too?

Perceiving the Weight Lifted by Another Person

In our initial studies addressing this question[29] the event chosen consisted of action by a person on an object, the lifting and handling of a box. The weight of the box was varied and observers viewing patch-light recordings of lifter and box were asked to judge the weight of the box. Thus, although the variable to be judged was an 'invisible' property of the object, the information was provided essentially by the kinematic pattern of the lifter. When lifted, the mass of the box becomes one of the dynamic factors that generate the kinematic pattern, and hence should be specified according to the KSD-principle. The judgements obtained were surprisingly accurate (Figure 3.1). In a follow-up study with lifters shown live in normal illumination, weight judgements made by observers came close to matching the accuracy of the judgements made by the lifters themselves (Figure 3.2)!

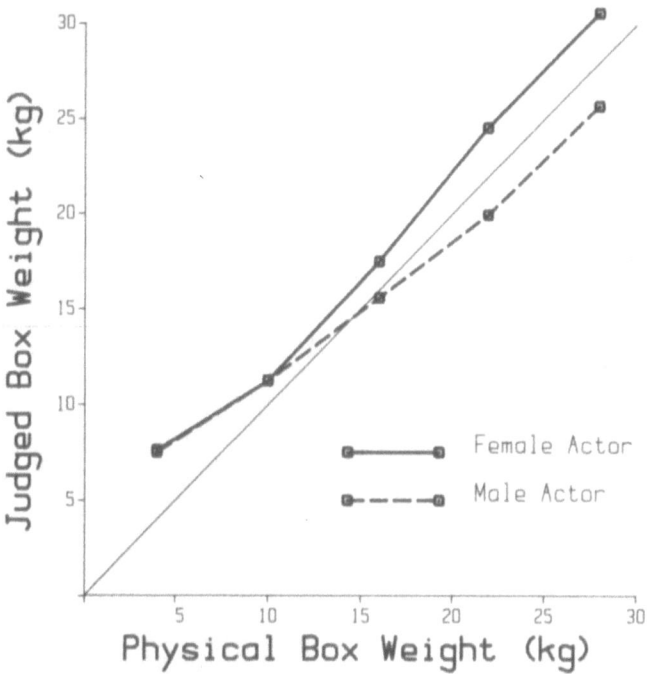

*Figure 3.1   Results of box weight judgements made by observers of patch-light video displays of two persons ('actors') lifting and carrying a 50 × 40 × 25 cm plywood box. Each plot point is the average of 48 judgements: 12 observers judging four different recordings of the same weight/actor combination. The difference in slope between the two curves is best accounted for by differences in weight and stature between the two actors: a box of a given weight has larger effects on movements and posture on the shorter and lighter person, and thus will be easier to discriminate. Pooled standard deviations were 4.1 kg for the male actor and 3.4 kg for the female. (For full results, see ref. 29.)*

Perceiving the Movement of an Invisible Thrown Object

Another study with a similar technique[18] displayed side views of people throwing a sandbag at targets placed at varying distances on the floor, usually beyond the edge of the screen. Neither the targets nor the sandbag were fitted with reflex tapes, hence the main joints of the thrower were the only things visible. Nevertheless, the observers were able to judge the length of the throws with good precision (Figure 3.3). In a conventional perspective of what perception is about, this result is perplexing: how can one judge the movement of an invisible object towards an invisible target outside the edge of the screen! Indeed, the bag was much larger than needed for the amount of sand it held and was grabbed around its neck and thrown by swinging it back and forth at least once before releasing it. Thus, the mass of the thrown object was only loosely attached to the

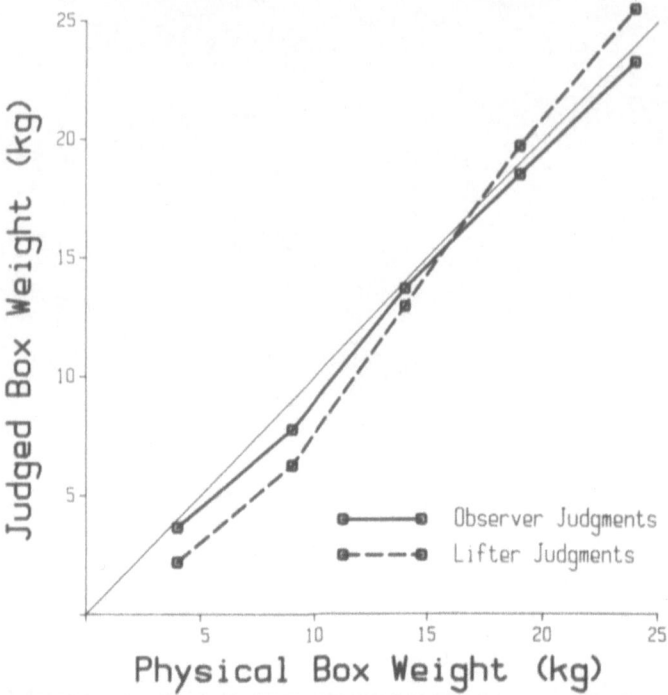

*Figure 3.2 Results of experiment comparing visual and haptic[5] box weight judgements made by seven pairs of subjects. Haptic judgements were made by the lifter after each lifting of the box; visual judgements were made by the pair-mate after observing the same event live in normal room illumination. Standard deviations were somewhat higher in the observers' judgements, 3.1 kg as compared to 2.0 kg for the lifters' judgements. (For full results, see ref. 29.)*

thrower and concentrated about 20 cm below the hand. The light-patch nearest to the mass was at the thrower's wrist. Arguing from the KSD-principle, on the other hand, the sandbag and its intended trajectory are two additional dynamic factors involved in generating the total integrated kinematics of the event. The kinematics should, therefore, specify them as well and with a suitable perceptual system we could perceive them.

Perceiving Person Properties

The results of the 'invisible throw' experiment are especially worthy of attention because of a possible extension. If human kinematics can specify *external* invisible sources of influence on movements so effectively, and we are perceptually so adept at using such information, then it may be possible to have kinematic specification and perception of *internal* invisible sources. If anything, we should be even more sophisticated at perceiving this, given its higher biological relevance.

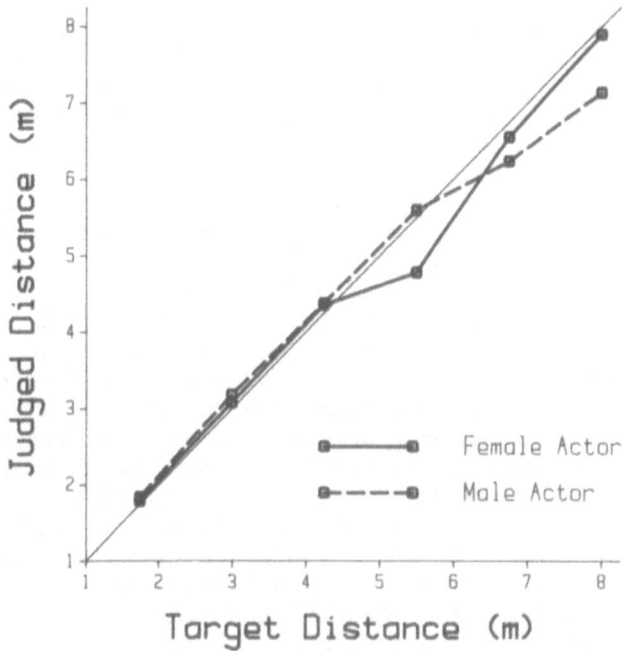

*Figure 3.3   Results of 'invisible throw' experiment. Observers judged the distance a sandbag was thrown after watching patch-light video recordings of the movements of the thrower. There was no light patch on the sandbag. The male actor was an adult well-trained ski-instructor of height 183 cm and weight 72 kg. The female actor was a 14-year-old girl, 158 cm tall, weight 49 kg. To anchor the observers' judgement scale a few standard throws with each of the actors were presented and their actual length (4.25 m) was reported to the observers. Pooled intra-observer standard deviations ranged from 0.50 to 1.68 m. (For full results, see ref. 18.)*

A first set of internal or personal properties worth testing in this context is the anatomical characteristics of people. One may assume that each individual has a unique composition of anatomical measures: skeletal geometry, mass distribution, etc. It follows that each one of us also exhibits unique kinematic patterns in everything we do. In principle, it should therefore be possible to recognize individual persons by observing their actions. Furthermore, there are statistical differences in anatomical make-up between categories of people, for instance, between men and women[30]. Even such distinctions are therefore likely to be specified in the kinematics and are potentially available to perception.

The first evidence to suggest that human movement could support perception of identity and gender was brought forth by Cutting and co-workers[31, 32]. Their actors (i.e. people recorded with the patch-light technique) were shown walking once across the screen after which observers had to judge whether it was a man or woman or which of six friends, including the observer, it was. The six scenes were judged several times and the average correctness of the judgements was calculated. In both cases, there were significantly more correct judgements than pure guessing would have given. Still, the figures remained a fair amount lower than what normally is implied by recognition of one's friends or accurately identifying gender: 38% correct naming of six friends and 63% correct gender identification.

Applying the KSD-principle to these studies offers an explanation why the results may underestimate the information that observers can get from human kinematics. The displays were very brief, only a few steps, and the activity simple and undemanding on the action capabilities of the actors. In the limiting case, when people are not moving at all, there is, of course, no kinematics that can convey information. When movement begins there is kinematics but the speed or vigorousness makes a difference in how discriminable the important aspects of it are. Following the KSD-principle, one is led to expect that it is the free (ballistic) components and the preparatory and compensatory components that are of special significance. The free components are relatively less prevalent in slow movements, since the kinematic shape of the movements can then be controlled to a higher degree. As to preparatory and compensatory components, they vary with at least two things; bodily proportions, which is what we are investigating, and the accelerations involved in the movements. Roughly, we may say that these two factors combine in a multiplicative fashion and therefore higher accelerations, that is more vigorous action, should tend to enlarge the crucial aspects of the kinematics, which in turn would make them easier to discern. A series of studies were therefore undertaken in which recognition of gender and individual identity was tested with recordings displaying people involved in extended (30–60 s) and varied activities. Care was taken to include actions that required impulsive exertion (jumping, throwing) and precision (balancing on a beam). The number of actors was increased whereas repeated displays of the same recorded scenes were omitted to prevent recognition based on irrelevant details of the scenes.

Recognizing Individual Persons

The results of the identification studies[33, 34] generally demonstrated improved recognition. Thus among eight to ten actors, recognition varied between 35% and 49% correct, a significant improvement over earlier results given that the chance level is lower when the number of actors to identify is larger. Similar figures were also obtained with children (classmates) at the age of 11 as actors and observers. When the children were tested at the age of 14 with the recordings made 3 years earlier their performance was somewhat better than at age 11, despite the particularly rapid anatomical changes that had occurred between tests. Moreover, two pupils had joined the class after the first occasion, and thus had not seen their classmates at the age when initial recordings were made, nor had they been tested before. Nevertheless, they scored about equal with the other children, indicating that individual identity in anatomical make-up and movement is preserved during the period.

## Recognizing Gender

For our first gender recognition study[18], 20 persons were recorded: ten males and ten females, half of whom were adults, half 11-year-olds. All these recordings were shown in random order and the figure obtained for gender recognition was 75%, a considerable improvement over the previous gender study. There was no difference between recognizing gender of children and adults – gender differences obviously also appear in movements before puberty.

## Expression and Deception

At this point we directed our attention to the possible role of expressions, in particular deceptive expressions. It had often been suggested that, especially in studies concerning gender and box lifting, the observers might be fooled by miming of the opposite sex or the weight of the box. Applying the KSD-principle we found reasons to be sceptical of such expectations. Neither the box weight nor the anatomical make-up changes when deception is attempted. What we may call the *appearance-intention* factor is the only thing that changes, from neutral to deceptive, and considering it as a dynamic factor suggests that it should be specified as such rather than corrupt specification of the true gender or weight factors. Thus, in turning to intentions we are moving on to study the specification through movement of *mental* states, considered as dynamic factors in the generation of human movement.

The view from the KSD-principle points out an important methodological precaution that must be observed in testing the effects of deception. If real gender and intended gender, or real and intended box weight, are different dynamic factors which may be distinctly perceivable, then the usual instruction to judge 'gender' or 'weight' will be ambiguous since there are two things visible in the displays that fit the description. Whichever way the observers understand it, the experimenter will not know whether the results refer to the real or the intended aspect. A straightforward way to handle the problem is, of course, to ask observers to judge *both* the real and the appearance-intention factor.

## Faking Lifted Weight

To prepare for the box weight deception experiment, three students practised with boxes loaded with various weights and alternatingly tried to fake the same weights with empty boxes. Recordings of their action with the truly loaded boxes were then made and mixed with recordings of faking attempts. For each scene, observers were asked to judge the real weight of the box and, if different, the intended weight. The results conformed well with expectations. The faking attempts had only a minimal effect on the real-weight judgements whereas it led observers to judge intended weight quite precisely. In other words, observers of the kinematic displays had little problem disentangling real from intended weight (Figure 3.4).

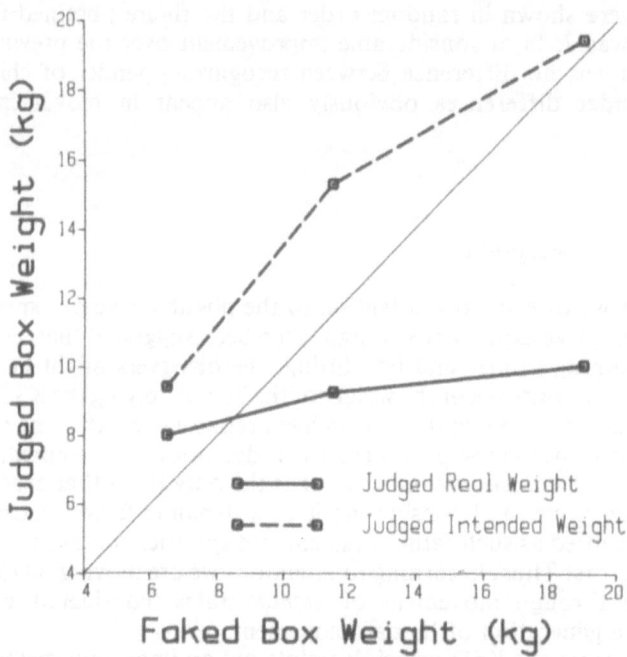

*Figure 3.4   Results of box weight deception experiment. Three actors (psychology students) were recorded with the patch-light technique trying to lift and carry the empty box so as to give the impression it weighed 6.5, 11.5 and 19 kg, respectively. These recordings were mixed with recordings in which the box was actually loaded to these weights (results not shown here). For each display, observers gave two judgements: actual weight of box and the weight-impression intended by the actor. (For full results, see ref. 18.)*

Gender Expression and Deception

For the gender expression and faking experiment ten actors were recorded performing the same action programme under three different conditions. First, the *natural* condition in which they were told that observers would be trying to identify their activities from the point-light displays. In this way we tried to prevent gender related self-awareness in the actors. Second, the *emphatic* condition was recorded. The actors were told that the study was in fact concerned with gender recognition from movement and were asked to give a slight emphasis to their gender-typical movements so as to be more convincing to the observers. Third, they were required to elude the observers by adopting a movement style characteristic of the opposite sex and we recorded the *deceptive* condition. After each new instruction the actors practised for a few minutes before recordings were taken.

The experimental procedure followed the same outline as in the weight-faking experiment. The 30 recordings were presented to observers in a mixed order and they were asked to judge both the real gender of the actor in each scene and the gender appearance-intention (natural, male, female). Thus the observers knew that attempts at fooling them could occur. The results for real gender recognition under the 'natural' condition were better than had been obtained before, 85.5% correct. In the 'deceptive' condition the figure dropped, but only to 75.5% correct. This result might have been taken to indicate a marginal deception effect. However, the figure obtained in the 'emphatic' condition turned out to be even lower, 67.5% correct. This surprising figure stems especially from the female actors for whom recognition in the 'emphatic' condition was down to 56% while it remained at 79% for the male actors. The best way to understand the results is probably that the two expressive (i.e. non-natural) conditions made the actors self-conscious about gender and that this added factor causes some confusion on the part of the observers. One may observe that in the previous gender recognition study the actors were informed about the purpose of the study before they were recorded. The figure obtained then was 75%, thus falling in line with the non-natural conditions of the present experiment. Knowing that one's movements will be examined for their content of gender-typical characteristics could quite possibly make people self-aware and add a special character to the movements, possibly a tenseness or inhibition. To the observers, that might suggest that 'something is going on here'. In particular with the dual task of judging both real and acted gender, these conditions may divert the observers' attention somewhat away from real gender which might be sufficient to cause a drop in the recognition figures. There were also indications that interference between the two tasks occurred at the judgement stage. Thus observers might have implicitly applied 'rules' saying, for instance, that 'it must be a man because a woman wouldn't act female in such a crude way'.

The results of the gender appearance-intention judgements are rather complicated to present. Suffice it to say that intentions were reported in 60% of the cases where it was actually present (i.e. where the actors were operating under an intention instruction) and that when it was correctly reported it was accurate in identifying gender-portrayal in 76% of the cases. It would seem that recognition of appearance-intentions is less easy than recognition of real gender. However, some of the imperfections of the results are probably due to lack of compliance of the actors with the instructions or due to their lack of expressive skill. In communicating by expressions, skilled actors or mimics would no doubt be more successful. Whether they would also be very successful in deceiving people about real gender or box weight is open to doubt, however. We can conclude that, to a considerable extent, observers are able to separately discern real and expressed gender, that is, one could often see that 'this is a man acting male', 'this is a woman acting male', etc., and that these cases can be distinguished from cases of men or women going about their business without expressing gender. Once again we have found evidence that undercuts the prevailing presumption that person perception is based on optional expressions rather than on firm information about actual conditions.

In a follow-up study the same recordings were administered to new observers with the single task of judging just 'gender' for each person appearing in the displays. No mention was made of the possibility of deceptive or expressive action on the part of the actors. In this way we wanted to make a comparison between our dual task design and a conventional deception experiment. Clear-cut differences between the two experiments appeared. Although the 'natural' condition gave the same result as before (84.6% correct), the 'emphatic' condition was now up at 84.1% correct judgements. The 'deceptive' condition, on the other hand, led to 66.3% correct judgements. Hence, no reversal of the judgements appeared as a result of the deceptive action but a substantial increase in the proportion of errors was recorded. These results would therefore have fitted the traditional view of gender perception fairly well if it was not for what we already knew from the previous results. No doubt the apparent support for a traditional view obtained in the follow-up experiment is a methodological artifact, arising from the ambiguity of the term 'gender' as used in the instructions.

## Consequences for Social Psychology Research

The above findings cast severe doubt on the relevance of experiments in which accomplices are used to enact the experimental conditions. If, as it seems, the kinematics of the accomplice reveal true conditions, the subjects are placed in an ambiguous situation and one can not know to what extent the results reflect the subjects' reaction to the true or the enacted conditions or perhaps to the ambiguity as such. Similar objections would apply to experiments in which subjects are studied 'interacting' with people they know only by written descriptions.

## Perceiving Expectation

A small experiment has been devoted to perception of another mental state, *expectation*. Two actors were recorded approaching a box on the floor, lifting it and carrying it forwards to a table, very much as in the first weight-lifting experiment. In this case, however, the actors knew well which weight to expect since there was no lid on the box and they had made a test lift immediately before. When the recordings were shown to observers in the experiment the display was interrupted precisely at the moment the box began to rise from the floor. Thus, the box was never seen to move, nor was the actor seen while moving it. Only the preparatory movements were seen. Three box weights had been used: 3, 13 and 23 kg. The observers were asked to rate them as light, medium, or heavy based on observations of the interrupted displays. The results showed clearly that discrimination of the boxes was possible. For the lighter and shorter actor 80% of the judgements were correct while for the other actor the judgements were 46% correct (each of the results were significant at $p < 0.001$).

The way one can understand these results is to take into account the bio-mechanical necessity of adjusting posture and movement *in proportion* to the weight of the box. To be most efficient much of the adjusting is done in advance of the beginning of the lift, based on the lifter's expectation concerning the weight. When the weight is well-known, pre-adjustments will occur full blown; when the weight is not so well-known adjustments will be more restricted. Thus the movements can be expected to specify not only the lifter's expectation but also the degree of certitude of expectation.

The occurrence of pre-adjustments of posture is a universal feature of our action system[35,36]. Through reactive effects virtually all movements threaten to disturb our balance and posture, and the system is therefore designed so that each action *includes* the necessary postural compensations. Thus, the system does not have to wait for sensory feedback concerning the reactive effects before it can compensate. Active and reactive effects are related through laws of mechanics and the action system is organized to take advantage of this. In this way, all movement is whole-body movement.


## A DYNAMICS-ORIENTED PERSPECTIVE ON MOVEMENT AND PERCEPTION

The series of experimental studies reviewed above yields a first round of evidence to suggest that kinematic information about another person can be used in visual perception. Furthermore, observers exhibit an ability to perceive true conditions and expressions as distinct from each other, irrespective of whether the expressions are intended to emphasize or to deceive about true conditions. The development of the KSD-principle provides a theoretical basis for these results and a vehicle for considering possible contributions to other fields, in particular to the study of individual differences in movement.

It follows from the KSD-principle and its backing in mechanics, bio-mechanics, and action theory that virtually all *physical* characteristics of a person influence movements. When it comes to *mental* characteristics, the same no doubt holds for specifically action-related characteristics such as intentions and expectations and for expressive intentions. However, the prospects for extending the principle to less obviously action-related characteristics seem very good. We may say that any state or characteristic of a person that has physio-logical aspects or consequences that could influence the action system are within reach. The question then is, which characteristics could actually fulfil this requirement? The trend away from detailed central control conceptions of the motor system, and their replacement with the mass-spring and co-ordinative structures' type of model, opens the way for a wide scope of influences in which the unfolding kinematic shapes of the movements are understood as a dynamic product of a multitude of factors. These include, notably, states of organization that prevail across the system. Co-ordinative structures are thought of as functional connections which are set up at lower (spinal) levels, each linking the action of several muscle groups or joints to function as a unit for as long as the co-ordinative structure remains in effect. Internally, co-ordinative structures consist of enforced relations or ratios of activity between the muscle components, similar to the way the two ailerons of an aeroplane are always linked to move in opposite phase to each other, thus forming a unitary control for roll manoeuvres as seen from the pilot's end[24]. However, unlike the permanent organization of the aeroplane roll control, human co-ordinative structures are replaced or modified as one engages in or prepares for different actions.

What is important here is that co-ordinative structures are set up more or less *in advance* of action, and thus may prevail in the system for extended periods even when the person is not moving at all. When movement is initiated the kinematics will be constrained by the prevailing co-ordinative structures whether the action taken is the one for which the prevailing co-ordinative structures are appropriate or not. The latter case may seem strange but is realized when the person has to do corrective movements following, for instance, a disturbance of balance, a surprise, or a sudden change of intention.

By a small extension of the above we may come to expect that the configuration of co-ordinative structures that prevails in a particular person will exhibit some kind of constancy over longer periods and some correlation with the variation in condition of the person. We can think in terms of the person's repertoire of co-ordinative structures or in terms of tendencies to activate certain types of co-ordinative structures rather than others, and we can think in terms of a set of default co-ordinative structures characteristic of the person. It appears to offer a rich conceptual basis for establishing links between dynamic (causal) aspects of the action system and psychological domains such as emotion and personality. Possibly, one may attempt even to explicate emotion or personality in terms of co-ordinative structures and other concepts that current action theory provides.

## CHOOSING DESCRIPTORS FOR MOVEMENT

Generally, it follows from the KSD-principle that the issue of *whether* individuals differ in movement in a way that bears a meaningful relation to their characteristics can be settled immediately since a positive answer is implied by the KSD-principle itself. Movements *are* specific to all those aspects of the person that influence the movements. However, one must pay for this by accepting that the properties (variables) of the movements (kinematics) that are specific in this way are *not simple*. Rather, they are in the form of *complex invariants definable over the total kinematic pattern*. Since the precise composition of these invariants is as yet unknown, they cannot simply be selected from action theory and used in attempts to correlate movement and personality.

Tough as this may seem, the KSD-principle also allows us to pinpoint the negative consequences of using simple movement measures (frequencies or amplitudes of selected movements, stride length, speed, etc.) in such studies. All such measures are co-determined by many dynamic factors. Thus the effects of the few dynamic factors we may be interested in are merged with all the others (as explained above, substitutability does hold for simple measures). If the other dynamic factors are brought under control, reasonably high correlations between movement measures and known person properties may be obtained, but if they are allowed their natural variation, correlations will tend to vanish. The point is that the level of correlation obtained under controlled conditions may reveal nothing about the actual strength of the relationship – it merely indicates the degree of abnormal constraints on the situation that the studies employ. In summary, using inappropriate movement descriptors inevitably yields weak and noisy results. They can be made spuriously stronger by standardizing the situation but then the validity of the results is correspondingly weakened (for similar arguments, see refs. 36, 37).

The KSD-principle points to an alternative method: measuring relevant complex invariants instead. It is in their nature that they need not be influenced by other factors, hence correlation should, in principle, be perfect with the person-properties to which they are specific. The problem is, of course, that we do not know what these measures are. Is it then meaningful to try this approach? Yes it is, and this kind of predicament is not unusual in science. Scientists frequently spend extensive effort on contriving new conceptualizations, novel descriptors, and methods for observation and measurement so as to be better able to handle the phenomena under study. There is no warrant for letting the shortcomings of traditionally available descriptive systems and techniques permanently restrict the contents of one's field of study.

The study of 'depth' perception provides an analogous case. For a long time, relations between stimuli and perceptions emerged as weak and unstable. This in turn led to a proliferation of theorizing about how the perceiving of even basic things like form, size, and distance of objects were determined by the observer through, for instance, experience, learning, culture, volition, or needs (e.g. 'transactionalism', 'new look in perception'). It is through sophisticated analyses of what information is in fact available, including the introduction of the complex invariant conception, that these subjectivistic excesses are discarded. It turns out that the old results of weak relations between the environment and perception were artifacts of the experimental conditions. Perception had been tested under conditions that did not contain the relevant informational invariants and/or the tasks given to the subjects were not of the kind that the perceptual systems are fit to handle.

It took the application of more advanced geometrical-optical conceptions (e.g. flowfields and cylindrical co-ordinate systems[7,8]) to bring forth relevant informational invariants for perceiving the spatial layout of the environment. For studies of the psychological sides of human movement the field of action theory or motor control and co-ordination will be a natural support in developing relevant movement descriptors. The study of human movement, whether for its role in person perception or for its dependence on person properties, has much to gain by following the development in this field.

Generally, the chances of making progress in a scientific endeavour are contingent upon the adoption of appropriate descriptors. The descriptors provided by Newtonian mechanics have proven very successful in several branches of science and technology. Despite this, they possess no privileged properties that make them capture reality in a more fundamental or objective way than other conceivable systems of descriptors[27, 38]. The challenge for the human movement field, therefore, is to develop a more useful system of descriptors, a system that distinguishes those occurrences that need to be treated distinctly and at the same time avoids distinguishing those that are best treated as equivalent. As a first step we should consider whether the descriptors should focus on the kinematic or the dynamic aspects (or perhaps cut across this distinction[39]). Such an option is already available within the Newtonian framework. Thus, mechanical events such as linear collisions can be described either kinematically (four velocities) or dynamically (masses, damping factor, initial conditions). The KSD-principle says that these two descriptions contain the same information since one can be 'translated' into the other[18, 27].

Because of the large number of degrees of freedom, a conventional kinematic description of human movement will be extremely cumbersome, yet, as a rule, none of the measures it consists of will be very useful as such. How can we figure a dynamic alternative for describing human movement? It should describe the dynamic factors involved in generating the movements, and thus should have two parts:

(1)  the intentional part, what the person is doing (e.g. walking, jumping, hammering a nail, reaching for a cup, expressing true or false emotion); and

(2)  the personal and situational part (properties and states of person and situation).

As mentioned above, the KSD-principle entails a fundamental equivalence in coverage between kinematic and dynamic descriptions; the complete event can be captured either way. Ideally, there is no loss of information in choosing one rather than the other. In practice, however, the situation is different since conversions between them are possible only if the description converted from it is complete, and for a complex system completeness cannot be achieved. However, if we choose a descriptive system that contains descriptors aimed directly at the entities we are interested in, usually on the dynamical side, then we should not need a complete description of the event since there is no need to do conversions. The description is useful as it is, piece by piece.

The choice of descriptors entails more than deciding on kinematics or dynamics. Within each of these domains we can choose or design different sets of descriptors. Thus, in treating expectations, intentions, and other person properties as dynamic factors, we have already gone beyond what is provided by Newtonian dynamics. On the kinematic side we probably need to do the same (for examples, see refs. 13, 38, 40, 41).

The above discussion has brought attention to some issues involved in developing adequate descriptors for human movement. Unfortunately, it is hardly surprising that conciliation of issues is not achieved. Groping for new and more useful descriptors is a crucial and delicate part of scientific endeavour and is likely to remain an area of interest.

## USING PERCEPTION AS A MEASURING DEVICE

Our theoretical development together with the empirical results lead to a methodological suggestion. Although we are not very well able to explicitly define the informative invariants in human movement we know that they exist and as perceivers we seem to be able to *use* them implicitly in perceiving other people. Thus, our visual system could be treated as a practical instrument for measuring such invariants. The sensitivity and reliability of this instrument may not be as good as we would wish. However, it could often surpass ordinary measurements in being eminently appropriate for the task, that is, by yielding measurements of good *validity*.

A problem with using perceptual observation to measure movement is that observers cannot report on the movements as such (if, by that, we mean conventional kinematic descriptions). They can only report on them in terms of their dynamic aspects, the causal factors, which may include person characteristics. This may be less of a problem than it at first seems, given the principled equivalence of kinematic and dynamic descriptions. The logic is this: if an observer can correctly report on properties of seen persons we can be certain that the information for it is available and that it can be perceptually used. Hence, if presentation was of kinematics only, as with some version of the point-light technique, we should be able to conclude that the person properties identified are specifically involved in shaping the movements.

In using perception as a measuring method one should also be aware that perceptual functioning has very much the character of *skills*. By appropriate experience, new informational invariants available at the senses can be detected and sensitivity to them can be heightened. In particular, we may change from using simplified to more advanced versions of the invariants. Perceptual skills can often be driven far beyond the ordinary level through special interests and training, as in connoisseurship. Skilled observers could therefore be expected to obtain more precise and more delicate information from human movements. In all likelihood, there are many categories of people who have already developed such skills: sport coaches, dance and acting teachers, clinicians, etc. For such groups of people it would be of interest to test, and use, their abilities on displays of human kinematics, using the point-light or similar technique. Although the removal of the non-kinematic information would generally suggest a lowering of perceptual performance it remains an exciting hypothetical possibility that in some cases the effect might be the opposite. This would follow from the firm and unfakeable nature of kinematic information. Assuming that other information available in a full display of a person in action is less reliable, the removal thereof would help the observer attend to the kinematic information, thus possibly obtaining a truer impression of the observed person.

## AN ALTERNATIVE TO THE 'LEAK' METAPHOR

Our discussion has provided reasons for the existence of strong relations between human movement and characteristics of the person. Clearly human kinematics provide more than 'leaks' of truth in an enclosure of expression. We should, therefore, conclude by suggesting an alternative metaphor that better captures what we have arrived at:

> Our movements are like a river. They provide a steady flow of information about our true conditions. Expressive movements are like eddies and bubbles with which we adorn the surface. As perceivers we can attend either to the flow of the river or to what flows with it just as we can attend either to actual properties of a person or to the communicative expressions. To be at the theatre would then be like travelling on a raft carried by the river: although we know very well that the river is really flowing, that the theatre has a true place in space and time, and that the actors are real people with true characteristics, all that matters for a while is the movement stirred *within* the framework of the flowing river or the theatre.

## ACKNOWLEDGEMENT

The research reviewed and the writing of this chapter was supported by a grant to the author from the Swedish Council for Research in the Humanities and Social Sciences (HSFR).

## References

1. Ekman, P. and Friesen, W. V. (1969). Nonverbal leakage and clues to deception. *Psychiatry*, **32**, 88–106
2. Ekman, P. and Friesen, W. V. (1974). Detecting deception from body or face. *J. Pers. Soc. Psychol.*, **29**, 288–98
3. Lippa, R. (1976). Expressive control and the leakage of dispositional introversion-extraversion during role-played teaching. *J. Pers.*, **44**, 541–59
4. Gibson, J. J. (1950). *The Perception of the Visual World.* (Boston, MA: Houghton Mifflin)
5. Gibson, J. J. (1966). *The Senses Considered as Perceptual Systems.* (Boston, MA: Houghton Mifflin)
6. Gibson, J. J. (1979). *The Ecological Approach to Visual Perception.* (Boston, MA: Houghton Mifflin)
7. Lee, D. N. (1974). Visual information during locomotion. In MacLeod, R. B. and Pick, H. L. (eds.) *Perception: Essays in honor of James J. Gibson.* pp. 250–67. (Ithaca, NY: Cornell University Press)
8. Lee, D. N. (1980). The optic flow field: the foundation of vision. *Philosophical Trans. R. Soc. London, Series B*, **290**, 169–79
9. Lee, D. N. and Aronson, E. (1974). Visual proprioceptive control of standing in human infants. *Perception Psychophys.*, **15**, 529–32.
10. Lishman, J. R. and Lee, D. N. (1973). The autonomy of visual kinesthesis. *Perception*, **2**, 287–94
11. Lee, D. N. (1977). On the functions of vision. In Pick, H. L. and Saltzman, E. L. (eds.) *Modes of Perceiving and Processing Information.* pp. 159–70. (Hillsdale, NJ: Erlbaum)
12. Runeson, S. (1977). On the possibility of 'smart' perceptual mechanisms. *Scand. J. Psychol.*, **18**, 172–9
13. Runeson, S. and Bingham, G. P. (1983). Sight and insights: contributions to the study of cognition from an ecological perspective on perception. *Uppsala Psychological Reports* (Serial No. 364)

14. Turvey, M. T., Shaw, R. E., Reed, E. S. and Mace, W. M. (1981). Ecological laws of perceiving and acting: in reply to Fodor and Pylyshyn (1981). *Cognition,* **9**, 237–304
15. Shaw, R. E. and Pittenger, J. B. (1977). Perceiving the face of change in changing faces: implications for a theory of object perception. In Shaw, R. E. and Bransford, J. D. (eds.) *Perceiving, Acting, and Knowing.* pp. 103–32. (Hillsdale, NJ: Erlbaum)
16. Pittenger, J. B. and Shaw, R. E. (1975). Aging faces as viscal-elastic events: implications for a theory of nonrigid shape perception. *J. Exp. Psychol.: Human Perception and Performance,* **1**, 374–82
17. Turvey, M. T. (1977). Preliminaries to a theory of action with reference to vision. In Shaw, R. E. and Bransford, J. D. (eds.) *Perceiving, Acting and Knowing: Towards and Ecological Psychology.* pp. 211–65. (Hillsdale, NJ: Erlbaum)
18. Runeson, S. and Frykholm, G. (1983). Kinematic specification of dynamics as an informational basis for person and action perception: expectation, gender recognition, and deceptive intention. *J. Exp. Psychol.: Gen.,* **112**, 585–615
19. Bernstein, N. (1974). *The Co-ordination and Regulation of Movements.* (Oxford: Pergamon Press)
20. Kelso, J. A. S. (1982). *Human motor behavior: an introduction.* pp. 1–58, 237–87. (Hillsdale, NJ: Erlbaum)
21. Kugler, P. N., Kelso, J. A. S. and Turvey, M. T. (1980). On the concept of coordinative structures as dissipative structures. I Theoretical lines of convergence. In Stelmach, G. E. and Requin, J. (eds.) *Tutorials in Motor Behavior.* pp. 3–47. (Amsterdam: North-Holland)
22. Kelso, J. A. S., Holt, K. G., Kugler, P. N. and Turvey, M. T. (1980). On the concept of co-ordinative structures as dissipative structures. II Empirical lines of convergence. In Stelmach, G. E. and Requin, J. (eds.) *Tutorials in Motor Behavior.* pp. 49–70. (Amsterdam: North-Holland)
23. Turvey, M. T., Fitch, H. L. and Tuller, B. (1982). The Bernstein perspective. I. The problems of degrees of freedom and context conditioned variability. In Kelso, J. A. S. (ed.) *Human Motor Behavior: An Introduction.* pp. 239–52. (Hillsdale, NJ: Erlbaum)
24. Tuller, B., Turvey, M. T. and Fitch, H. L. (1982). The Bernstein perspective. II. The concept of muscle linkage or coordinative structure. In Kelso, J. A. S. (ed.) *Human Motor Behavior: An Introduction.* pp. 253–70. (Hillsdale, NJ: Erlbaum)
25. Saltzman, E. L. and Kelso, J. A. S. (1983). Skilled actions: a task dynamic approach. *Haskins Labs Status Reports Speech Research* (Serial No. 76)
26. Johansson, G. (1973). Visual perception of biological motion and a model for its analysis. *Perception Psychophys.,* **14**, 201–11
27. Runeson, S. (1983). On visual perception of dynamic events (Originally published 1977). *Acta Universitatis Upsaliensis: Studia Psychologica Upsaliensia* (Serial No. 9)
28. Todd, J. T. and Warren, W. H. (1982). Visual perception of relative mass in dynamic events. *Perception,* **11**, 325–35
29. Runeson, S. and Frykholm, G. (1981). Visual perception of lifted weight. *J. Exp. Psychol.: Human Perception and Performance,* **7**, 733–40
30. Krogman, W. M. (1962). *The Human Skeleton in Forensic Medicine.* (Springfield, Ill.: C. C. Thomas)
31. Cutting. J. E. and Kozlowski, L. T. (1977). Recognizing friends by their walk: gait perception without familiarity cues. *Bull. Psychonomic Soc.,* **9**, 353–6
32. Kozlowski, L. T. and Cutting, J. E. (1977). Recognizing the sex of a walker from a dynamic point-light display. *Perception and Psychophysics,* **21**, 575–80
33. Frykholm, G. (1983). Perceived identity. I Recognition of others by their kinematic patterns. *Uppsala Psychological Reports* (Serial No. 351)
34. Frykholm, G. (1983). Perceived identity. II. Learning to recognize others by their kinematic patterns. *Uppsala Psychological Reports* (Serial No. 352)
35. Belen'kii, V. Ye., Gurfinkel', V. S. and Pal'tsev, Ye. I. (1967). Elements of control of voluntary movements. *Biophysics,* **12**, 154–61
36. Reed, E. S. (1982). An outline of a theory of action systems. *J. Motor Behav.,* **14**, 98–134
37. Brehmer, B. (1984). Brunswikian psychology for the 1990's. In Lagerspetz, K. M. J. and Niemi, P. (eds.) *Psychology in the 1990's: In honour of Johan von Wright.* pp. 383–98. (Amsterdam: North Holland)
38. Runeson, S. (1974). Constant velocity – not perceived as such. *Psychol. Res.,* **37**, 3–23

39. Runeson, S. (1983). Kinematic specification of dynamics, and dynamic event perception: their meaning and consequences. Presented at the *2nd International Conference on Event Perception,* June 9–13, Vanderbilt University, Nashville, TN
40. Runeson, S. (1975). Visual prediction of collision with natural and nonnatural motion functions. *Perception Psychophys.,* **18,** 261–6
41. Bingham, G. P. and Runeson, S. (1983). On describing what is perceived: seeing 'velocity' vs. seeing 'push' in moving objects. Presented at the *Autumn Meeting of the International Society for Ecological Psychology,* October 29, Trinity College, Hartford, CT

# 4

# Reminiscence as a factor in the learning of skilled movements

## *Hans J. Eysenck*

---

### SKILLED LEARNING AND REMINISCENCE

Skill in movement has to be acquired, and to acquire such skills is a lengthy and complicated business. A baby has to spend many months in order to learn to toddle, and finally to walk, and sportsmen spend years of arduous training, often many hours a day, in order to perfect their ability to hit or kick a ball accurately, perform the correct movements in jumping or throwing, and in the development of other movement skills. Psychologists can look upon such developments of skilled movements, and the individual differences inevitably shown therein, from either a *macroscopic* or a *microscopic* point of view[1]; in other words, we may look at the actual training that occurs in the development of sporting abilities, under everyday life conditions (macroscopic), or we may study in the laboratory certain theories concerning the development of movement skills (microscopic). A review of work in the macroscopic field, particularly as far as it is concerned with individual differences, is given in the monograph on *Sport and Personality* by Eysenck, Nias and Cox[1]. Here we will be concerned with a particular microscopic phenomenon which is fundamental to an understanding of the problem in question.

William James pointed out, many years ago, that we learn to skate in the summer and to play tennis in the winter. What he meant was that increments in our ability to perform these sports (and others, too, of course) occur when we are not in fact practising. In other words the practice in skating we put in during the winter, or the practice in tennis we put in during the summer, lie shallow until long rest pauses occur (for skating in the summer, for tennis in the winter), and it is during these rest pauses that improvement occurs. Such improvement in performance, following a period of rest rather than immediately following a period of exercise, is called *reminiscence*[2]. Historically this phenomenon was discovered by Kraepelin and his students in the 1890s, although Ballard[3] has been credited with the discovery of this phenomenon. It was actually Oehrn[4], a student of Kraepelin, who first explicitly demonstrated it experimentally, but English-speaking psychologists seem to be unaware of the existence of the many German studies antedating the work of Ballard and others.

While the phenomenon of reminiscence is easily reproducible in the experimental laboratory, it is much more difficult to discover in everyday life. Indeed, William James was quite wrong in his suggestion about ice-skating and tennis; the phenomenon of reminiscence is overlaid by the long-term loss of ability consequent upon lack of practice, and tennis players and skaters as well as learners of other sportive activities, need several weeks to recover from the effects of a lengthy rest. If anything, there is a *loss* of performance during long rest, and even in laboratory tasks quite short rest periods can produce forgetting, i.e. a decrement in performance. Reminiscence clearly is not the only factor operating in everyday life events; other factors too must be taken into account.

While reminiscence is easy to characterize, it is less easy to find a satisfactory definition. Hovland[5] defined it in terms of increments in *learning* which occurred during a rest period; he added the warning that before reminiscence 'can be considered a fundamental *learning* phenomenon, explanations offered in terms of fatigue, motivation, and artifacts of measurement must be eliminated.' Osgood[6], on the other hand, defined reminiscence as 'a temporary improvement in *performance*, without practice', and says that, 'The term ... refers to the objective fact of improved performance' (italics added). It is of course through performance that learning is usually indexed, and to that extent the two definitions may be considered equivalent, but it is also true that modern learning theory makes a radical distinction between learning and performance; learning may or may not issue on performance, depending on various conditions which require careful investigation.

Most empirical work on reminiscence in the laboratory has been done using the pursuit rotor, and an example from an experiment using this instrument will illustrate the main features of reminiscence. Essentially the pursuit rotor consists of a rotating disc, usually similar to a gramophone, but made of bakelite; inset in this disc is a small metal plaque, roughly the size of a dime, which constitutes the target. The subject of these experiments attempts to keep a metal stylus, hinged in order to prevent pressure being exerted on the disc, in touch with the target, a task much more difficult than it appears at first. On-target and off-target periods are recorded electrically, and the score is usually stated in time-on-target during 10 s periods. There are, of course, many different ways in which the apparatus can be constructed, i.e. variations in size of disc, size of target, speed of rotation, shape of stylus, etc., and there are many ways in which the experimental paradigm can be varied.

Consider a report by Denny[7], who administered a pursuit-rotor task to two groups of 18 subjects each; one group worked *continuously* for 16 min, the other group worked continuously for 5 min, received 5 min of rest and then worked continuously for 12 min more. The results of the experiment are shown in Figure 4.1. It will be obvious that the two groups pursue quite divergent courses after the rest pause. The experimental group shows an *increase* from the 10th to the 11th 30 s trial of 8%, i.e. from 14% to 22%, while the control group shows no change of any kind from the 10th to the 11th trial; this is an instance of *reminiscence*.

Clearly there are other differences also between the two curves subsequent to the imposition of a rest pause. First, there is a sharp rise immediately after rest; this we shall call postrest upswing (PRU). This is sometimes attributed to

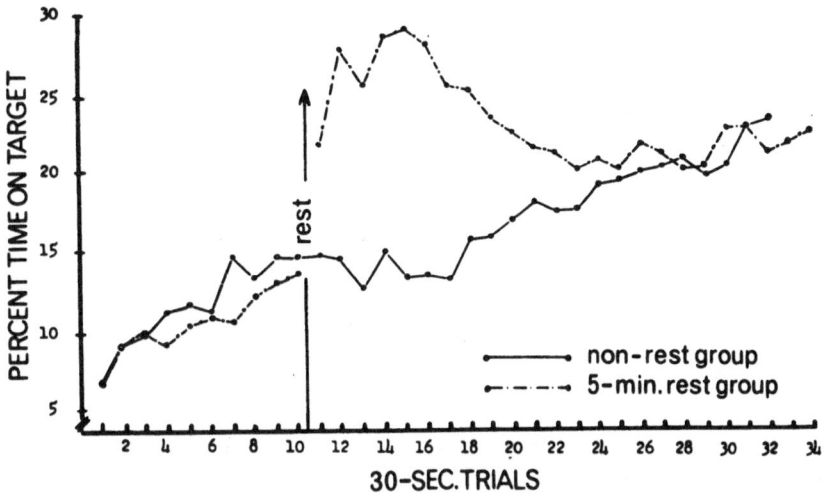

*Figure 4.1 Reminiscence on the pursuit rotor, also showing postrest upswing, postrest downswing, and the eventual meeting of the rest and control groups. Taken with permission from Denny[7]*

reinstatement of the set to perform the task in question, or 'warm-up'; this notion was introduced in this connection by Hoch and Kraepelin[8], and widely popularized by Thorndike[9] in the English-speaking countries. It is also sometimes known as 'warm-up decrement'[10].

PRU is followed in turn by a levelling of performance, followed in turn by a gradual decline; this may, by analogy, be called postrest downswing (PRD). Finally, this decline is arrested and a slow, regular upswing is resumed which seems to run at roughly the slope and level of the control group, which has continued to improve slowly with a roughly linear slope throughout. Clearly, any proper theory of reminiscence must do more than account for the reminiscence effect itself; PRU and PRD are equally clear-cut consequences of the interpolation of a rest pause, and a worthwhile theory of reminiscence must also cover these effects.

The length of the rest pause is clearly an important feature in determining the strength of the reminiscence effect. Consider Figure 4.2, which shows the results of an experiment carried out by Eysenck and Cookson[11], who administered the inverted-alphabet printing task, in which the subject is required to print the letters of the alphabet upside-down. 2560 boys and 2679 girls, aged between 10 and 11 years, were administered the test: Twelve 1 min periods of massed practice were followed by a variable rest (0, 1, 5, 10 and 60 min, respectively), and the rest was in turn followed by another 5 min of massed practice. There is clearly some learning prerest, as shown in the first three trials, but then there is performance decrement, bringing the terminal score almost down to the initial level (a fatigue inhibition effect?). The rest produces a marked reminiscence effect, proportional to the length of the rest period. This time there is no PRU, but only PRD.

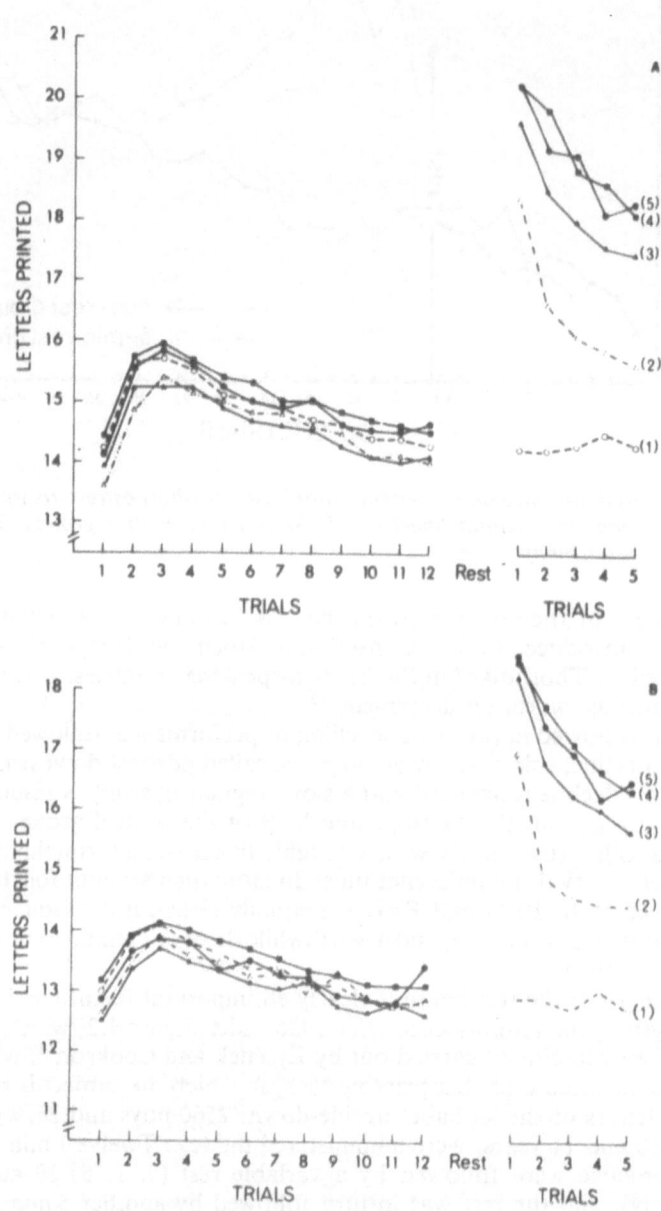

*Figure 4.2   Reminiscence on the inverted alphabet printing task, showing effect after rest pauses of 0, 1, 5, 10 and 60 min, respectively. Data are for boys (a) and girls (b). Taken with permission from Eysenck and Cookson[11]*

## THEORIES OF REMINISCENCE

The concept of 'fatigue' has been mentioned in the last paragraph; this is a very complex concept, which may be related to deterioration in muscular performance, mental performance, etc. Muscular fatigue can be ruled out in practically all the studies of reminiscence that have been carried out in psychological laboratories; the amount of work done puts very little stress on the muscular system, and as far as muscular performance is concerned most if not all subjects could continue well beyond the period in question. Mental fatigue is a different matter, but unfortunately the concept is not a very clear one, and itself in need of elaboration and explanation.

From the beginning there have been two types of theories to account for reminiscence. Kraepelin himself favoured a kind of *inhibition* theory. According to this type of theory, which was later on embraced and much extended by Clark Hull[12], inhibition is set up during the first work period, and this manifests itself in a decline in performance which prevents the effects of learning becoming obvious. This inhibition, which may be considered a kind of mental fatigue, or perhaps a kind of neural fatigue, dissipates during the rest period, allowing the effects of learning to become apparent in performance. This theory has been developed in particular by Ammons[10, 13, 14], and was widely accepted during the 1950s and 1960s.

An alternative hypothesis, that of *consolidation*, was developed by Mueller and Pilzecker[15] and applies quite generally to all memory phenomena. According to this theory we must make a distinction between short-term memory and long-term memory. Short-term memory is mediated essentially by reverberating cortical circuits, maintained over short periods of time; in order to lay down the foundations of long-term memory these must be *consolidated*, i.e. transformed into chemical traces within cortical nerve cells. According to Walker's[16] theory of the work decrement, consolidation and performance are antagonistic, and cannot easily co-exist. Hence during the original work period little consolidation occurs; it is left to the rest period to make possible consolidation, and this manifests itself as the reminiscence phenomenon. The consolidation theory is a viable alternative to the Kraepelin–Hull inhibition theory, and explains many phenomena which cannot be explained by the inhibition theory[2]. Before looking at the problems which arise for both theories, it may be useful to look at certain ascertained facts which require to be explained by any theory.

In Figure 4.1 we compared massed practice, on the one hand, with a massed practice broken up by a rest pause, on the other. Obviously there is a close relation between this work on reminiscence and work on massed and spaced practice, and Kraepelin suggested that among the control groups there should be one which allowed no fatigue-inhibition to arise, i.e. a group given spaced practice. Figure 4.3 shows the results of an experiment[17] which contrasts spaced practice with massed practice broken up by two rest pauses. In this experiment on the pursuit rotor the lower set of curves presents the mean time-on-target scores during successive 10 s intervals of 50 subjects; three sets of 30 massed trials are separated by 10 min rest pause. The upper set of curves consist of 10 s trials separated by 30 s rest pauses; after 300 and again after 600 s this group

71

was also given 10 min rest pauses. Kraepelin would have explained the very marked improvement in performance of the distributed group as due to practice (learning). The failure of the massed group to achieve equally good performance he would have considered due to fatigue (inhibition). This fatigue disappeared during rest, thus producing the reminiscence effect, denoted $I_R$ in Figure 4.3 after Hull's symbolic representation of reactive inhibition. The failure of the lower curve to reach the upper curve even after rest Kraepelin would have explained in terms of his semipermanent fatigue (inhibition); this effect is denoted $sI_R$ in Figure 4.3 after Hull's symbolic representation of conditioned inhibition, which is also supposed to be permanent (unless extinguished by suitable experimental manipulation). The rapid postrest rise (PRU) Kraepelin would have attributed to the regaining of set lost during rest (warm-up); PRD he would have attributed to the rapid accumulation of fatigue, possibly adding semipermanent fatigue to that due to the resumption of practice. The failure of reminiscence to appear in the distributed group would not have surprised him, in view of the lack of fatigue accumulated by that group, with its frequent long rests.

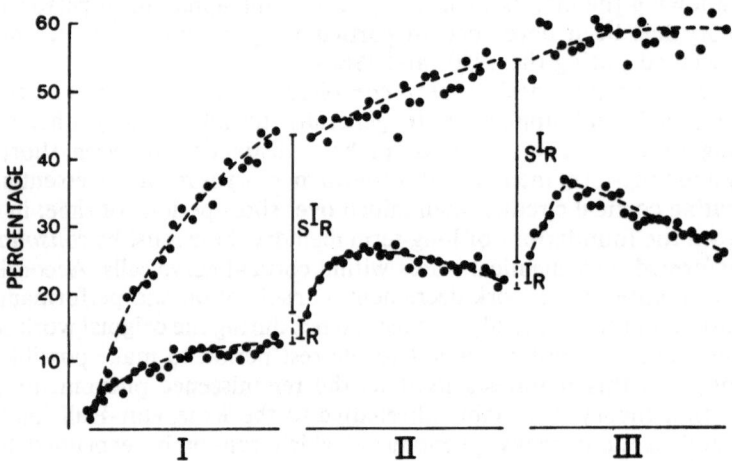

*Figure 4.3  Pursuit-rotor scores obtained during massed (lower curves) and spaced (upper curves) practice. Taken with permission from Eysenck[17]*

## THE AMMONS MODEL

During the inter-war period many experiments were reported on the reminiscence phenomenon, using many different types of apparatus and procedure. These experiments added a good deal to our knowledge of the phenomena in question, but little to our theoretical understanding. The all-embracing learning theory of Hull rekindled interest in reminiscence, particularly as Ammons[10, 13] and Kimble[18-20] attempted to provide a quantitative model for reminiscence in motor learning. Ammons advocated the production of 'miniature models' and 'small-scale theories'; Kimble has made a more determined attempt to align his theories with the more ambitious ones of Hull. Ammons begins his discussion by presenting a figure (Figure 4.4) which is extremely useful and illustrates in detail the phenomena which must be explained in any workable theory of reminiscence. Curve A represents the curve of performance we would obtain under conditions of massed practice if no special rest periods were introduced; this can be obtained by the use of a control group, or by extrapolation. Normally this 'curve' is a straight line, usually less steep than shown in Figure 4.4. If a rest is introduced, performance does not resume at level G (predicted level of performance on first postrest trial if there had been no rest), but at level F. The difference between G and F is often used as a measure of reminiscence, but as we shall see Ammons prefers another measure. From F to H there is a rapid rise in the curve of performance; this is often referred to as 'warm-up', but the more neutral term 'postrest upswing' seems preferable as already explained. After H the curve of performance declines again (postrest downswing) until it reaches point L; this declining section is fitted by the straight line B, which is extrapolated backwards to point C. This point is located at the first postrest trial. After reaching L performance picks up again and proceeds as if rest period, reminiscence, PRD, and PRU had been nothing but a bad dream. The point D is also defined in the figure; this might be visualized as a level of performance reached after the same amount of practice (in seconds) as G, but with perfectly spaced practice. These are the main features and points introduced by Ammons; others are described in detail in the figure caption itself.

We come now to the definition of certain theoretical variables. The first of these is 'warm-up decrement', defined as the 'decrement on any trial due to the necessity for the subject to "warm-up" after rest'. This is measured as the difference between points C and F; Ammons used the symbol $D_{wu}$ for this concept. It should of course be noted that this is essentially the inverse of warm-up, being the decrement in performance due to failure of warm-up to have taken place. 'At any trial $D_{wu}$ will be the vertical difference between line B and the postrest performance curve where line B is higher.' The second decremental variable to be defined is $D_{Wt}$ – 'the amount of temporary work decrement dissipated over rest. This is the difference between points C and G in Figure 4.4. . . . Decrement is present at all points in practice but can only be measured by the introduction of a rest period sufficiently long to insure its relatively complete dissipation. Then by eliminating $D_{wu}$ (by extrapolating line B backward) it is possible to estimate the total temporary work decrement present at the end of the last prerest trial. Reminiscence or gain over rest is due to this dissipation of temporary work decrement. No implication is intended that temporary work decrement is due to fatigue as commonly defined. $D_{Wt}$ can be seen to be similar to Hull's $I_R$' (Ammons[10]). In this definition of $D_{Wt}$ Ammons thus includes the major part of his general theory; reminiscence is due to recovery from some form of inhibition which keeps prerest practice under massed conditions from reaching its proper level (i.e. the level it would have reached under optimally spaced conditions).

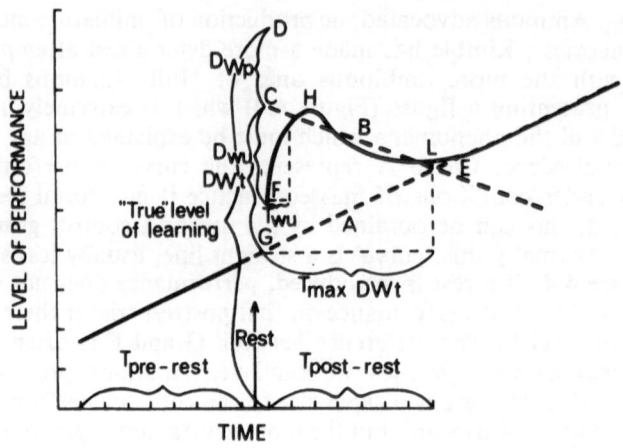

*Figure 4.4   Representation of certain rotary pursuit variables.* A = *extrapolation of prerest performance curve;* B = *straight line fitted to the relatively decremental segment of the postrest performance curve;* C = *level of line B at first postrest trial – estimated performance level if there were no* $D_{wu}$; D = *'true' level of learning – performance level if there were no* $D_{Wp}$, $D_{Wt}$, *or* $D_{wu}$; E = *intersection of B and A – point at which maximum postrest* $D_{Wt}$ *is reached;* F = *actual performance level on first postrest trial;* G = *predicted level of performance on first postrest trial if there had been no rest;* H = *relative high point reached early in postrest performance;* L = *relative low point in postrest performance at the end of the 'decremental' segment;* $T_{prerest}$ = *time spent practising before rest;* $T_{postrest}$ = *time spent practising after rest;* $D_{Wp}$ = *permanent work decrement on first postrest trial* (D–C *where all temporary work decrement has dissipated over rest);* $D_{Wt}$ = *amount of temporary work decrement dissipated over rest;* $T_{max\,DWt}$ = *time to reach a maximum level of work decrement after rest;* $D_{wu}$ = *initial decrement in postrest performance curve due to necessity for subject to 'warm-up' after rest; and* $T_{wu}$ = *time to overcome 'warm-up' decrement after rest. Taken with permission from Ammons*[10]

A third variable is needed to complete Ammons' system; this is $D_{Wp}$ or permanent work decrement. On the first postrest trial this will be the difference between points C and D in Figure 4.4, providing there is no temporary work decrement remaining after rest.... There will be an amount of $D_{Wp}$ at every point in performance, which can be measured only by introducing a rest to eliminate the decremental effects of temporary work decrement completely and comparing initial postrest performance corrected for $D_{wu}$ with that of a control group with short trials and long rests. The difference, by definition, would be due to $D_{Wp}$. $D_{Wp}$ is thus similar to Hull's $sI_R$. This, Ammons tells us, 'completes the isolation and definition of variables'; but as already noted, it does more than that. We are already committed to an inhibition type of theory; Ammons' nomenclature and choice of variables have predetermined the direction in which the theory to be proposed must proceed. Note that Ammons does not present any argument in favour of this inhibition theory; it is taken for granted that this type of theory is the only type of theory applicable to data of this kind. 25 years after the event it is easier to see how Ammons drew a mathematically straight line from an unwarranted assumption to a possibly erroneous conclusion.

Ammons goes on to present a series of what he calls 'assumptions'; these are essentially parametric laws indicating how a given variable will behave over time, or as another variable is changing. These assumptions are partly based on empirical evidence, partly intuitive; they clearly owe much to the grander design of Hull's system. Deductions are made from these assumptions, and these deductions have led to a good deal of empirical work.

Ammons followed up his theoretical work (or perhaps in point of time preceded it!) in large scale experimental studies which have become classics. By and large these tend to bear out his theories in considerable detail. Kimble's theory of reminiscence is in many ways similar to Ammons, which is not surprising as both are ultimately based on Hullian notions. It may be worth while to look at Kimble's classic statement of Hullian inhibition theory, called by Kimble the 'two-factor theory of inhibition'.

## KIMBLE'S TWO-FACTOR THEORY

The theory distinguishes between reaction inhibitive ($I_R$) and conditioned inhibition ($sI_R$); the former is essentially a negative drive state, resembling fatigue in that it results from all effortful behaviour and dissipates during rest, while the latter is essentially a habit of resting, reinforced by the dissipation of $I_R$, which serves the purpose of drive reduction. 'Since pauses, however slight, serve as reinforcements, it follows that the response of resting will become conditioned to whatever stimuli are present in the learning situation.' We thus have two inhibitory factors, a drive and a habit, in which the drive component provides the motivational basis for the development of the habit. Since the general characteristics of drives and habits are known, we can predict that $sI_R$ 'must be a positive growth function of the number of reinforcements', leading to $D_{Wp}$. (This statement, and the term 'permanent work decrement' used by Ammons to characterize this concept, must not be allowed to mislead us. Habits are permanent only if nothing is done to extinguish them; when an appropriate process of extinction, through lack of reinforcement or in some other way, is applied then of course the situation changes completely, and 'permanence' disappears. Ammons made this error in arguing from his 'switching' experiment that the results disproved the existence of $D_{Wp}$; this is true only if the changes introduced through the switching of the conditions of distribution did not lead to extinction of $sI_R$.)

The negative drive, $I_R$, would be expected to accumulate at some increasing function of the amount of effort previously expended, but there is a clear ceiling to this increase. When negative drive ($I_R$) reaches the level of positive drive (D), the total effective drive is zero, and consequently performance would be expected to stop, in conformity with Hull's generalized equation: $sE_R = D \times sH_R$. Thus a short involuntary rest pause (IRP in our terminology[2]) will occur. During this pause $I_R$ will dissipate, and presumably, once $I_R$ is reduced

75

to below the critical level, the organism driven by motivation to perform the task at hand will resume work and continue working until the critical level of $I_R$ is reached again. Then it will rest, reducing $I_R$; start work again, increasing $I_R$ and so on. What will eventually happen is that a state of equilibrium will be reached in which the organism rests long enough to keep $I_R$ at or slightly below some constant specific level. Clearly, since $I_R$ is a negative drive, acting antagonistically to the other drives in the learning stiuation, then the greater the motivation driving the subject to learn the task at hand, the greater the amount of inhibition which must be accumulated to produce the resting response. Kimble uses this general argument to account for the fact, observed by Ammons and himself, that there is a decrease in the amount of reminiscence later in the course of learning. He argues that as the S approaches the motivational goal set him by E (becoming proficient at the task), so his drive is reduced. This reduced $D^+$ counterbalances a weaker inhibition ($D^-$), and this weaker inhibition is then indexed as a low reminiscence score.

These are the classical statements of reminiscence theory as derived from Hull, and similar in many ways to the principles introduced by Kraepelin. The theory has been very influential, and certainly accounts for many of the observed facts. Before looking at an alternative theory, it may be interesting to look at the influence of motivation on reminiscence. This is particularly interesting as in everyday life experience motivation plays an extremely important part in deciding on the degree of success or failure of a given person in acquiring a set of motor habits.

## REMINISCENCE AND MOTIVATION

Kimble[19] had suggested that motivation-produced differences in tolerance for $I_R$ are responsible for differences in reminiscence. The theory was taken up by Eysenck and his colleagues in a series of studies which began by supporting the inhibition hypothesis, and ended up by throwing much doubt upon its adequacy and validity. In these studies Eysenck made use of a special type of motivator to produce high-drive and low-drive groups. Previous workers had used ego- vs. task-oriented instructions; competitive feelings of 'losers' as opposed to 'winners'; verbal encouragement and instructions; social vs. isolated conditions. Eysenck used real-life motivation, as opposed to these laboratory-type artificial motivators; a detailed description of the method is given in *Experiments in Motivation*[21]. Briefly, the low-motivation group consists of industrial apprentices at a large motor company; these adolescent boys are tested under task-oriented conditions, in that they know that the results are of interest only to the experimenter, not to the company, that whether they do well or not will not in any way affect their future standing in the company. The high-motivation group consists of candidates who have applied to the same company to be taken on to their apprentice course, and who are being extensively tested and interviewed; they are highly motivated to do well in the experimental tests (which are included among the selection tests proper, but which are not being used for selection purposes) because the training course has a high reputation, guarantees a highly paid job at the end, and because for many young school dropouts it presents a unique opportunity of gaining access to the highly skilled working class.

Predictions concerning the superior performance of highly motivated groups as opposed to poorly motivated groups thus contrast applicants for a training course with youngsters who a year or so ago were actually accepted for the course; this comparison inevitably reduces the chances of finding such effects of motivation because (a) whatever abilities are involved in the test are possibly also involved in the tests which constitute the selection procedure, so that the low-motivation group would be slightly superior in ability, and (b) the high-motivation group is somewhat younger, and during adolescence there is probably a slight gain on most perceptual and visuomotor tests with age. Neither difference is likely to be large; age differences in performance are known to be quite small after the age of 15 or so, and of course all the candidates would have left school and be 16 years of age or older. Also it is well known that perceptual and motor tasks of different kinds do not correlate at all highly together; neither do they show much correlation with intelligence. Thus selection on IQ tests and pegboard and other motor tests would not make much if any difference to performance on the pursuit rotor. We would thus expect there to be only slight differences, if any, due to the selection process, and those that did exist would go counter to the hypothesis that high motivation would lead to better performance. A large body of evidence has in fact been collected under these experimental conditions, ranging from eye-blink conditioning to paired-associate learning, and from mirror drawing to multiple-choice reaction[21, 22]; the results unambiguously demonstrate large and predictable differences between high- and low-drive groups on these and many other types of test. It seems quite clear that the experimental conditions are such as to produce differences in motivation which justify us in calling the groups thus contrasted high- and low-drive groups.

The experimental design of the first in this series of studies[23] used a total of 120 Ss equally divided into high-drive and low-drive groups. These were in turn subdivided into a long-practice group (48 10 s trials, equal to 8 min of practice) and a short-practice group (18 10 s trials, equal to 3 min of practice). Massed practice for both groups was followed by a 6 min rest period, and this in turn by 4 min of massed practice (24 10 s trials). The reminiscence score used was first postrest trial − last prerest trial. Figures 4.5 and 4.6 show the results.

Reminiscence scores for the groups were as follows: short practice–high drive, 0.80: short practice–low drive, 0.54; long practice–high drive, 1.51; long practice–low drive, 0.51. These are the data plotted in Figure 4.7; the diagram was of course drawn to fit the data, i.e. the numbers on the abscissa and the ordinate were put in after the data had been collected. The general shape of the curves which make up the body of the diagram was of course predicted from the theory. Main effects and interaction were all significant, as expected.

Differences in prerest performance between high-drive and low-drive Ss are poor or nonexistent; they are non-significant for the short practice group, and only barely significant (at the 5% level) for the terminal portion of the curves for the long-practice groups. This is hardly in accord with Hullian theory, according to which D should multiply with $_sH_R$, giving the high-drive group

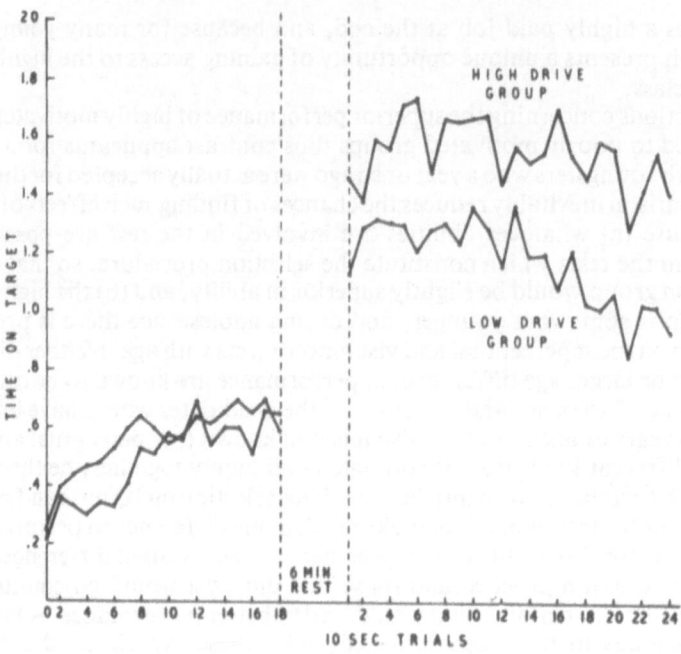

*Figure 4.5    Reminiscence for high- and low-drive groups after 3-min practice on the pursuit rotor. Taken with permission from Eysenck and Maxwell[23]*

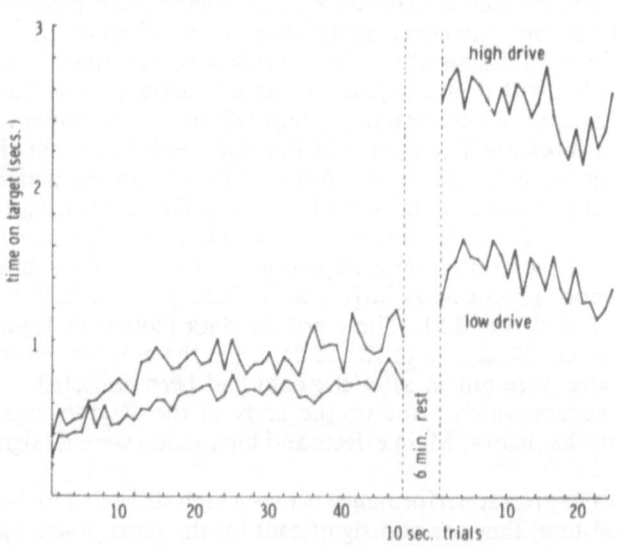

*Figure 4.6    Reminiscence for high- and low-drive groups after 8-min practice on the pursuit rotor. Taken with permission from Eysenck and Maxwell[23]*

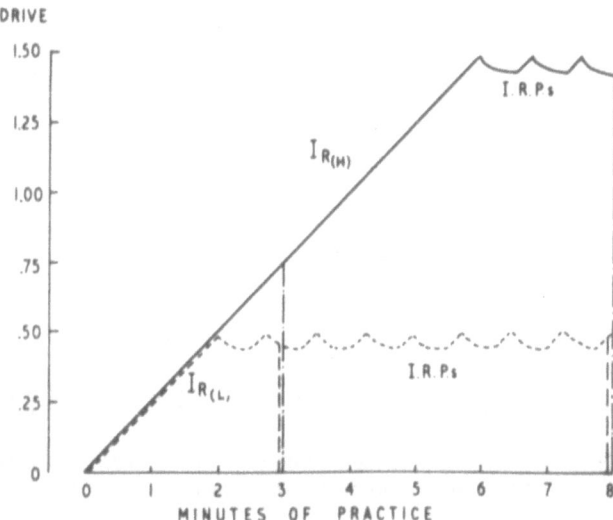

*Figure 4.7   Theoretical representation of Hullian drive theory applied to pursuit-rotor reminiscence. Ordinate shows drive indexed in terms of reminiscence. Taken with permission from Eysenck and Maxwell[23]*

much better performance. It might be argued that the high-drive group suffers from greater $I_R$, once the critical level had been reached, but this argument would simply suggest that differences should be apparent near the beginning of the learning curves, and then decline as both groups reach the critical level of $I_R$. These facts argue against an inhibition theory.

The Eysenck and Maxwell experiment was replicated by Eysenck and Willett[24], but with two changes. As Figure 4.7 suggests, there should be no difference in reminiscence between the high-drive and low-drive groups after 2 min of practice, and maximum reminiscence should have been reached after 6 min of practice (assuming zero values for $I_R$ at the beginning of practice). Consequently, the 6 min rest pause was introduced in this experiment either after 2 min or after 6 min of practice, and the results are shown in Figure 4.8 which also incorporates, for the sake of comparison, the reminiscence data from the previous experiment. It will be seen that for low drive the prediction is supported, in that length of prerest practice makes no difference between the limits of 2 and 8 min; allowing for random variations, the data fit a straight line reasonably well. For the high-drive group the 2 min practice group is also found where it should be, i.e. coinciding with the low-drive group. The 6 min practice group, however, shows less reminiscence than the 8 min practice group. The difference is of doubtful statistical significance, but the fact that the four points lie on a straight line must make us wary of dismissing the finding as unimportant and a statistical artifact. Clearly more evidence is required. If this straight line relationship is correct, then it must become curvilinear at values of less than 2 min prerest practice, as otherwise the line would cut the ordinate at a point other than zero, which is absurd.

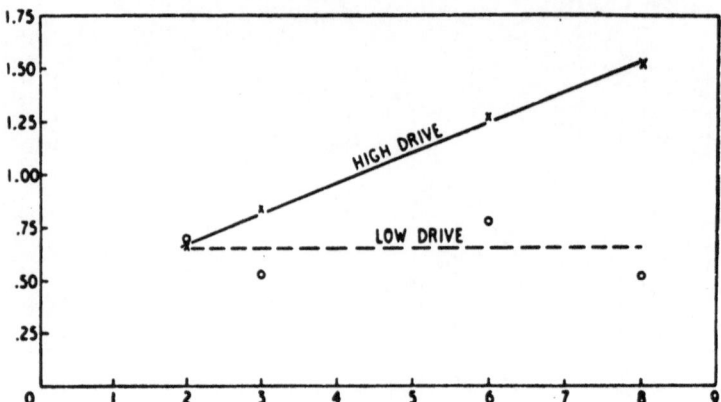

*Figure 4.8   Reminiscence for high- and low-drive groups after different periods of practice (abscissa). Taken with permission from Eysenck and Willett*[24]

If we accept the probability of a curvilinear instead of a linear relationship between length of prerest practice and reminiscence for the high-drive group, then clearly there is no reason to assume that this group has reached an asymptote at 8 min of practice, and longer periods may give even larger reminiscence scores. Willett and Eysenck[25] replicated the Eysenck and Maxwell study again, this time using practice periods of 12 and 15 min. A summary of the results is given in Figure 4.9 which shows the results in graphic form. All three experiments are combined in the figure, and it will be seen that a very regular negatively accelerated curve results for the high-drive group. When we plot reminiscence against the log of prerest practice, a straight line results which shows no evidence of an asymptote having been reached (Willett and Eysenck[25], Figure 2). The data for the low-drive groups do not deviate significantly from a straight line. As regards prerest performance, the low-drive groups are superior, but not significantly so; taking all our data together we find only random variations, with the high-drive groups sometimes superior, sometimes inferior, sometimes quite indistinguishable from the low-drive groups. We clearly cannot reject the null hypothesis with respect to the influence of drive on performance, as far as the pursuit rotor is concerned.

One important comparison was made by Willett and Eysenck[25], in answer to the objection that the low-drive group might have appeared superior because they had been selected on the basis of motor skills, and hence not comparable in ability with the high-drive group. Comparing Ss in the high-drive group who had been accepted and rejected, these authors found no difference in prerest performance; clearly the criteria of selection were irrelevant to ability on this test.

Willett and Eysenck make one further point which appears to be novel. The plotted data for the high-drive groups are more clearly lawful than those for the low-drive groups, and it might seem that this could be due to the lower reliability of single trial scores for the latter groups. Accordingly, product-moment correlations were calculated for the last and last but one prerest trials,

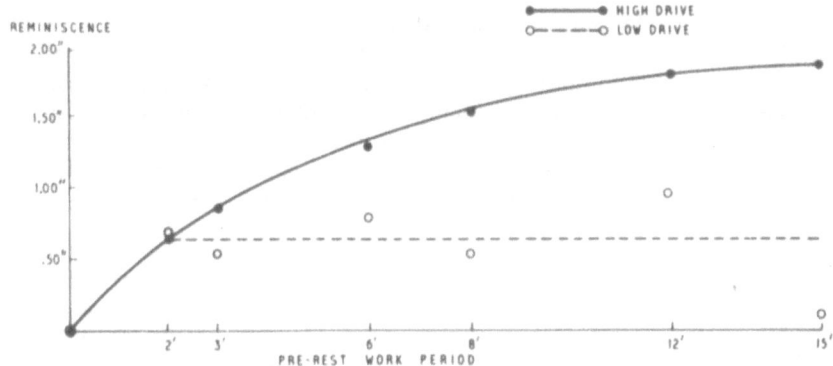

*Figure 4.9   Reminiscence on the pursuit rotor as a function of prerest work period, for high- and low-drive groups. Taken with permission from Willett and Eysenck[25]*

and the first and second postrest trials. These were 0.62 and 0.76 for the low- and high-drive groups, respectively, prerest, and 0.62 and 0.74 postrest. High drive clearly produces more reliable (less variable) performance.

The results of these experiments, as shown in Figure 4.9, are clearly lawful, but perhaps too much so; it is rare in psychology that predictions are borne out in such precise fashion. Consequently, a replication of the whole research seemed advisable, particularly as the high- and low-drive groups in the Eysenck and Willett studies had been less clearly separated in overall postrest performance than had the Eysenck and Maxwell ones. Reminiscence data, depending on just one 10 s period for their calculation, may not give an adequate picture of what is happening. Consequently, a large-scale replication of these studies was undertaken by Feldman[26] using high- and low-drive Ss selected along similar lines to those in the studies already reviewed. A total of 600 Ss were tested, half in each condition; Ss were randomly assigned to one of ten prerest practice periods, 0.5, 1, 2, 3.5, 5, 7, 9, 11, 13 and 15 min, followed by 15 min of rest and 4 min of postrest practice. Additional groups were tested later on, to clarify various points of interest; the results of the experiment, shown in Figure 4.10, include one such pair of additional groups which worked for a prerest period of 20 min. In the main, the results of the Eysenck, Maxwell and Willett studies are replicated. The low-drive group shows an increase in reminiscence up to 2 min, followed by a roughly straight plateau up to 15 min of prerest practice. The high-drive group shows an increase in reminiscence up to 11 min of prerest practice, followed by a decline. This decline is statistically somewhat doubtful if we do not include the 20 min prerest practice period; it was added to the original experiment precisely in order to clarify this point. The data are highly significant, and evidence for a decline in reminiscence late in learning is also apparent in the work of Adams[27], Kimble and Shatel[28] and Ammons[13]. We cannot doubt that there is an inversion of the regular pattern which governs reminiscence up to about 12 min of prerest practice. To make assurance doubly sure, Feldman tested two further sets of high-drive Ss for 20 min practice periods. One was compared with a set of high-drive Ss tested for 11 min, using a 15 min rest pause; there was a definite decline in reminiscence with increasing length of prerest practice. The other group was given a 6 min rest pause and compared with the various high-drive groups tested by Eysenck and his colleagues. Again there was a decline in reminiscence with such very long prerest practice periods. It is doubtful that inhibition theory can furnish us with a theoretical explanation of this phenomenon; Feldman discusses two possibilities, but neither can be said to emerge with much credit.

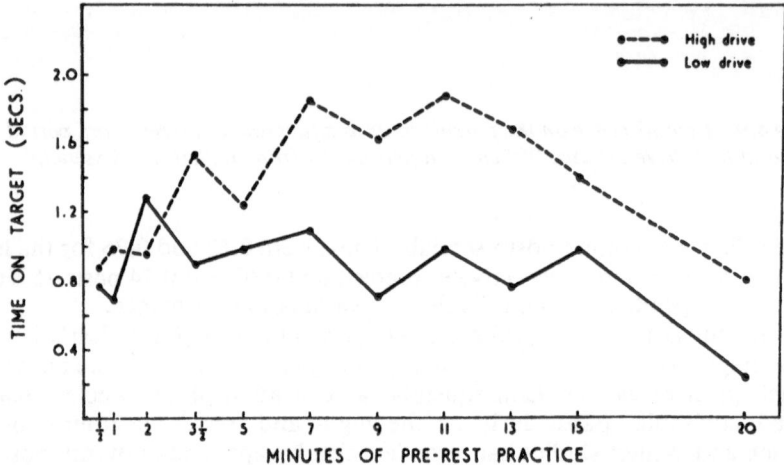

Figure 4.10 *Reminiscence on the pursuit rotor as a function of prerest work period, for high- and low-drive groups. Taken with permission from Feldman*[26]

## REMINISCENCE AND PERSONALITY

In addition to differences in motivation, differences in personality have also been studied. The major effort in this direction has been that of Eysenck, whose theories and many different empirical studies are reviewed in Eysenck and Frith[2]. The basis of his original theory was derived from the hypothesis that introverts are characterized by higher degrees of cortical arousal than extraverts[29]. This theory, which has been well supported by many physiological and psychological experiments[30], makes possible certain predictions in terms of the rival theories under consideration. Both would predict greater reminiscence for extraverts. The inhibition theory would suggest that extraverts would accumulate more inhibition, and hence would show greater reminiscence due to the dissipation of a larger amount of inhibition. The consolidation theory would suggest a great amount of consolidation in introverts, leading to a greater reminiscence effect. The two theories, however, differ decisively in just how this greater reminiscence of extraverts would show itself. On an inhibition theory, we would expect extraverts to show depressed scores at the end of the initial practice period, due to the greater inhibition characteristic of them; the greater reminiscence would appear due to their catching up after the rest pause, i.e. dissipating a greater amount of inhibition. This hypothesis has been clearly disproved by a number of studies in which it was shown that extraverts and introverts do not differ at the end of the initial practice period, but at the beginning of the postrest period. Figure 4.11 illustrates this phenomenon clearly[31]. The consolidation hypothesis taken in conjunction with Walker's action decrement hypothesis already discussed can explain these phenomena and indeed predict the precise nature of the curves shown, by suggesting that the greater cortical arousal of the introverts would lead to a longer consolidation period. The rest pause is too short to allow complete consolidation, and hence when practice is resumed, the action decrement hypothesis decrees that continuing consolidation interferes with performance and hence depresses the scores of the introverted group. The evidence is by no means conclusive that this is the correct theory, and an alternative will be discussed presently.

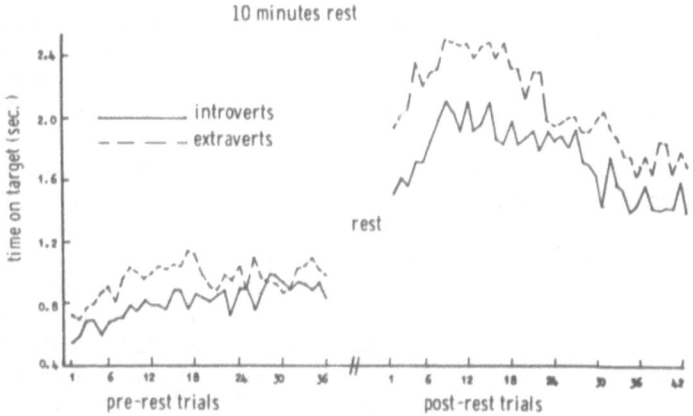

Figure 4.11  *Performance of extraverts and introverts pre- and post-rest, with rest interval of 10 min. taken with permission from Gray*[31]

This alternative theory relates to *strategies* of performance. Using a more diagnostic performance task, Eysenck and Frith[2] found marked differences in strategy between extraverts and introverts. It would take us too far to discuss these differences on strategy in detail, and the reader is referred to the Eysenck and Frith book. Let us note merely that according to this theory, and the work supporting it, differences in reminiscence between extraverts and introverts are not to be explained in terms of the general theory of reminiscence.

## THE EYSENCK–FRITH MODEL

We have so far only indicated very briefly the nature of consolidation theory, because in its original form it was clearly insufficient to account for all the phenomena of reminiscence. Eysenck and Frith[2] have contributed a revised version of consolidation theory, and it may be useful to close our account with a more detailed statement of this new version of the consolidation theory. In constructing this new theory of reminiscence we have tried to take account of all the problems and criticisms that have arisen in relation to previous theories. Recognizing the need for simplification we have abandoned all the inhibition concepts and tried to account for reminiscence entirely in terms of a consolidation process. Furthermore, we have not tried to account for all pursuit-rotor phenomena with this one theory. Postrest upswing we accept provisionally as a manifestation of 'set' reinstatement relating it to a rather different body of evidence which has been discussed in a previous chapter. Differences between introverts and extraverts are, we suggest, related to different strategies adopted in the performance of the task.

The facts left for our theory to explain are therefore those relating to reminiscence, downswing, and the effects of various rest and practice lengths. These facts can be summarized as follows: a small, but steady, amount of learning is manifested during prerest practice; after 15 min rest there is a considerable amount of reminiscence; however, a downswing in performance follows which eventually reaches the same level as a group having no rest. After a very long rest there is less downswing and final performance remains above that of a group with no rest.

To these facts must be wedded what we know about the consolidation process. Consolidation has two functions as a result of which before the consolidation process is complete, (a) learning cannot be fully manifested in performance and (b) learning can be destroyed.

To apply such a consolidation process to pursuit-rotor learning it is necessary to specify the nature of these two functions in more detail. It is convenient to imagine the learning and consolidation process passing through three stages. In the first stage the learning is neither available for improving performance nor is it protected against destruction. In the second stage the learning is available for improving performance, but is not protected against destruction. In the third stage the learning is available for improving performance and is protected against destruction. This specific ordering of the consolidation stages is clearly open to empirical testing. However, it is, of course, possible that this account of the consolidation process may only apply to the learning of motor skills.

In order to explain pursuit-rotor learning in terms of consolidation, we must specify more precisely the agents that can destroy the partially consolidated learning. It can be shown that there is ample experimental evidence that this learning can be destroyed by major disturbances of the CNS such as convulsions[2]. It is suggested that in addition the *partially consolidated learning can be destroyed by performance of the task being learned*. This would be plausible in physiological terms (not that such plausibility is necessary to our model) if the performance of the task involved precisely the same area of the CNS. However, major disturbances affecting the whole of the CNS would interfere with all consolidating traces.

In the chapter on interference and transfer Eysenck and Frith[2] presented evidence that pursuit-rotor learning is extremely specific. Activities carried on between sessions of pursuit-rotor performance have very little effect on pursuit-rotor learning, unless they are tasks very similar to the pursuit rotor. Such tasks would include performance on a pursuit rotor going backwards or at a different speed. A task only slightly more different from the standard pursuit rotor than these will interfere little with pursuit-rotor learning. The interpolated task which inferferes most with pursuit-rotor learning in these terms is clearly performance on the pursuit rotor itself. Indeed this is really what the phenomenon of reminiscence is all about.

Figure 4.12 shows how this hypothetical consolidation process can explain many phenomena appearing in pursuit-rotor performance. During a period of uninterrupted practice little learning can get through to the latter stages of the consolidation process since the consolidating traces are destroyed by the continuing performance. Thus only a slight and slow improvement in performance appears. During a short rest some of the learning passes into the second stage of the consolidation process where it is available for improving performance, but is also destroyed by that performance. Thus, immediately after the rest (and after the postrest upswing), there is a marked improvement in performance due to the partially consolidated learning. However, the performance also destroys that partially consolidated learning causing a downswing in performance. Eventually all the consolidated learning is destroyed and performance returns to the level that would have been achieved if no rest had been interpolated.

If the rest is longer more learning is partially consolidated and hence there is more reminiscence, but also more downswing since there is more learned material to be destroyed by the performance. Only after a relatively long rest does any learning become fully consolidated, i.e. it is both available for performance and immune from destruction. After such a rest what partially consolidated material still remains will be destroyed by the performance, causing downswing, but the performance will remain at a higher level than would have occurred without rest, because the fully consolidated material is not destroyed. The greater the proportion of the learned material that becomes fully consolidated the less downswing there will be. If all the material is fully consolidated there should be no downswing.

The amount of material consolidated during a rest (both temporary and permanent) is indicated by the difference between the last prerest trials and the maximum postrest trials (i.e. performance after postrest upswing). This was the measure used by Gray[31] and labelled rem. max. The amount of material permanently consolidated as a result of rest is indicated by the difference between performance after postrest downswing is complete and performance at an equivalent time in a group which had no interpolated rest. These measures are illustrated in Figure 4.12.

As we have seen, a good deal of work has been done on reminiscence, particularly in relation to the pursuit-rotor, and there are well established theories to account for many of the facts. It is equally obvious that the last word has not yet been spoken on the topic, and in particular the two major theories (inhibition versus consolidation) are still in the field, and no final decision can

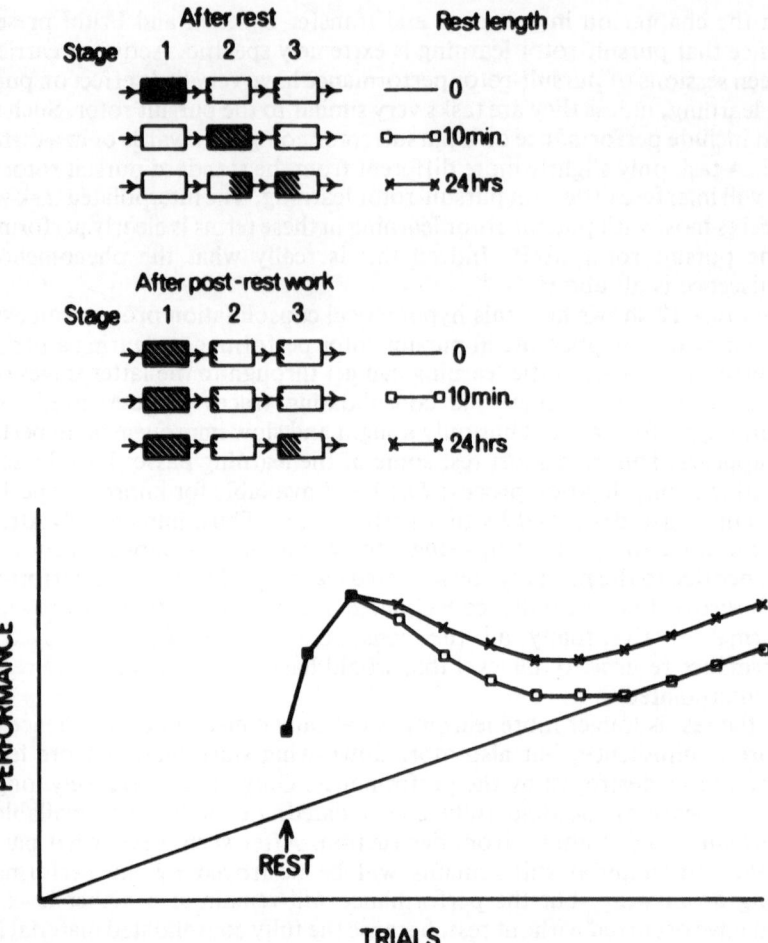

*Figure 4.12 The hypothetical course of pursuit-rotor performance based on a three-stage model of consolidation. With continuous work very little learning passes beyond stage 1. After a short rest learning has passed to stage 2 improving performance; however, postrest work destroys this learning causing downswing. Only after a long rest when learning has passed to stage 3 is learning retained permanently*

be made as to their adequacy. The topic is an important and an exciting one, and very relevant to the question of the learning of motor responses. As such it will no doubt soon come back into popularity, and we will hopefully expect to see the resolution of problems still found at the moment in this field.

# References

1. Eysenck, H. J., Nias, D. K. B. and Cox, D. V. (1982). Sport and personality. *Adv. Behav. Res. Ther.*, **4**, 1–56
2. Eysenck, H. J. and Frith, C. D. (1977). *Reminiscence, Motivation and Personality.* (New York: Plenum Press)
3. Ballard, P. B. (1913). Obliviscence and reminiscence. *Br. J. Psychol.,* Monogr., Suppl., **1**, No. 2
4. Oehrn, A. (1896). Experimentelle Studien zur Individual psychologie. *Psychol. Arb.,* **1**, 92–151
5. Hovland, C. I. (1951). Human learning and retention. In Stevens, S. S. (ed.) *Handbook of Experimental Psychology.* pp. 653–6. (New York: Wiley)
6. Osgood, C. E. (1953). *Method and Theory in Experimental Pysychology.* p. 509. (New York: Oxford University Press)
7. Denny, M. R. (1951). The shape of the post-rest performance curve for the continuous rotary pursuit task. *Mot. Skills Res. Exch.,* **3**, 103–5
8. Hoch, S. and Kraepelin, E. (1896). Ueber die Wirkung der Theebestandtheile auf koerperliche und geistige Arbeit. *Psychol. Arb.,* **1**, 378–488
9. Thorndike, E. L. (1914). Mental work and fatigue. *Educ. Psychol.,* **3**, 66–8
10. Ammons, R. B. (1947). Acquisition of motor skills. I. Quantitative analysis and theoretical formulation. *Psychol. Rev.,* **54**, 263–81
11. Eysenck, H. J. and Cookson, D. (1974). Unpublished manuscript
12. Hull, C. L. (1943). *Principles of Behaviour.* (New York: Appleton-Century-Crofts)
13. Ammons, R. B. (1947). Acquisition of motor skill. II. Rotary pursuit performance with continuous practice before and after a single rest. *J. Gen. Psychol.,* **37**, 393–411
14. Ammons, R. B. (1950). Acquisition of motor skill. III. Effects of initially distributed practice on rotary pursuit performance. *J. Exp. Psychol.,* **40**, 777–87
15. Mueller, G. E. and Pilzecker, A. (1900). Experimentelle Beitraege zur Lehre vom Gedaechtnis. *Z. Psychol., Ergbd.,* **1**, 1–300
16. Walker, E. L. (1956). The course and duration of the reaction decrement and the influence of reward. *J. Comp. Psychol.,* **49**, 167–76
17. Eysenck, H. J. (1956). 'Warm-up' in pursuit rotor learning as a function of the extinction of conditioned inhibition. *Acta Psychol.,* **12**, 349–70
18. Kimble, G. A. (1949). An experimental test of a two-factor theory of inhibition. *J. Exp. Psychol.,* **39**, 15–23
19. Kimble, G. A. (1950). Evidence for the role of motivation in determining the amount of reminiscence in pursuit rotor learning. *J. Exp. Psychol.,* **40**, 248–53
20. Kimble, G. A. (1952). Transfer of work inhibition in motor learning. *J. Exp. Psychol.,* **43**, 391–2
21. Eysenck, H. J. (ed.) (1964). *Experiments in Motivation.* (London: Pergamon Press)
22. Eysenck, H. J. (1964). An experimental test of the 'inhibition' and 'consolidation' theories of reminiscence. *Life Sci.,* **3**, 175–88
23. Eysenck, H. J. and Maxwell, A. E. (1961). Reminiscence as function of drive. *Br. J. Psychol.,* **52**, 43–52
24. Eysenck, H. J. and Willett, R. (1961). The measurement of motivation through the use of objective indices. *J. Ment. Sci.,* **107**, 961–8
25. Willett, R. A. and Eysenck, H. J. (1962). An experimental study of human motivation. *Life Sci.,* **4**, 119–27
26. Feldman, M. P. (1964). Pursuit rotor performance and reminiscence as a function of drive level. In Eysenck, H. J. (ed.) *Experiments in Motivation.* (London: Pergamon Press)
27. Adams, J. A. (1952). Warm-up decrement in performance on the pursuit-rotor. *Am. J. Psychol.,* **65**, 404–14
28. Kimble, G. A. and Shatel, R. B. (1952). The relationship between two kinds of inhibition and the amount of practice. *J. Exp. Psychol.,* **44**, 355–9
29. Eysenck, H. J. (1967). *The Biological Basis of Personality.* (Springfield: C. C. Thomas)
30. Eysenck, H. J. (ed.) (1981). *A Model for Personality.* (New York: Springer)
31. Gray, J. E. (1968). *Levels of arousal and length of rest as determinants of pursuit rotor performance. Unpublished PhD Thesis,* University of London

References

# 5

# Anxiety, stress and performance

## *Peter Glanzmann*

---

ANXIETY AS AN ENERGIZING DRIVE

Research on human anxiety and performance has been conducted within the framework of a narrowly defined paradigm: high and low anxious persons are selected on the basis of their scores on self-reports and then subjected to various experimental treatments designed to elicit situational anxiety. Dependent measures cover indices of autonomic and central-nervous activity, subjective feelings of anxiety, and a variety of performance parameters. This strategy combining quasi-experimental and experimental research turned out to be useful in elaborating and testing hypotheses concerning the relationships between the variables under study and has led to a vast body of relevant findings. In early research on anxiety and performance[1], anxiety was conceptualized as an energizing drive as specified in Hullian learning theory[2]. Observable behaviour was conceived of as an immediate consequence of the interaction between two theoretical constructs, *habit* (designating the degree of previous learning of specific S–R connections) and *drive* (as an index of the sum of momentary needs). Habit and drive jointly determine the strength of excitatory potential which manifests itself in observable behaviour in instances of a hypothetical response threshold being exceeded. It was postulated that habit and drive should be related multiplicatively, implying that the value of both variables had to be greater than zero in order to render observable responses possible.

In this theoretical context, drive was assumed to vary as a function of individual differences in emotional responsiveness as assessed by means of the Taylor Manifest Anxiety Scale[3], and as a function of situationally induced anxiety. Basically, the operationalization of habit strength in complex learning tasks followed two different strategies. On the one hand, verbal learning material was selected which differed in familiarity, association value, or intraserial similarity[4]; on the other hand, habit strength was determined *post hoc* on the basis of empirical item difficulty[5].

Two major kinds of learning tasks were employed, classical eyelid conditioning and paired associates or serial verbal learning. Each stimulus in these tasks was considered to activate a hierarchically structured habit family which, in the case of classical eyelid conditioning, consisted of a single habit only (the lid closure following an air puff to the cornea of the eye). In verbal learning tasks, competing habits differing in strength were assumed to be involved. In relatively easy tasks, in which subjects were asked to respond by 'roof' to the stimulus 'house', for example, high anxiety should facilitate performance, since the response 'roof' possesses high initial habit strength. In relatively difficult tasks, in which subjects were required to learn the more difficult response 'pen' to the stimulus word 'house', high anxiety should debilitate performance, because initial habit hierarchies associated with the stimulus 'house' will typically not include the response 'pen'. Therefore, anxiety will tend to activate those response tendencies in the hierarchy which have high initial habit strength (such as the response 'roof') and which are defined as inappropriate by the experimenter in the case of the difficult task. The latter relationship, however, is only postulated for the initial stages of learning, since the response to be learned ('pen') increases in habit strength during the course of learning, so that at a certain point of the learning process, high anxiety should again facilitate performance. This should happen when the response 'pen' has become the dominant habit in the 'house'-family as a result of learning. The change of relative positions of habits in 'difficult' tasks leads to an intersection of learning curves for high and low anxious subjects.

## ANXIETY AS AN INTERFERING EMOTION

While in this early stage of theorizing[6, 7] observable behaviour was assumed to be completely determined by the interaction of habits and drive, later studies demonstrated that high anxiety led to decrements in performance that were no longer commensurate with the simple notion of anxiety as an energizing drive[8]. As a result, drive theory was modified and extended in order to account for these findings[9]. This was accomplished by adapting a theoretical viewpoint originally put forth by Mandler and Sarason[10] in the field of test anxiety research. To explain performance decrements of high anxious persons on comparatively easy learning tasks another hypothetical mechanism of Hullian learning theory, namely the concept of *drive stimuli* ($S_D$), was integrated into drive theory. Drive as well as drive stimuli were now considered to vary as a function of anxiety or emotional responsiveness. As drive increases, the intensity and number of $S_D$ increase accordingly and elicit responses that can be described as 'task-irrelevant, e.g. heightened autonomic reactions or covert verbalizations reflecting self-depreciation, anger, desire to escape, etc.' (p.308)[9].

While it was acknowledged that drive stimuli may be elicited even in neutral situations at least in high anxious persons, it was especially the introduction of stress into the situation that was considered to increase drive and $S_D$. Increasing $S_D$ should be detrimental to performance only if the responses elicited by drive stimuli were incompatible with the responses to be learned on a specific task. While there should be a facilitation of performance following the introduction of mild stress as a consequence of increases in drive ($S_D$ not being very effective when stress intensity is low), further stress should be detrimental to performance by the increment of $S_D$. Adding the anxiety variable to this mechanism, the detrimental effects of increasing both strength and number of drive stimuli should deteriorate performance of high anxious subjects earlier on the stress continuum and deterioration should be much more pronounced in high anxious subjects than in low anxious subjects once it occurs.

$S_D$ was not considered a relevant variable in classical aversive conditioning, because $S_D$-related responses were not assumed to interfere with a relatively simple response such as the lid closure in the conditioning situation. Therefore, classical eyelid conditioning was considered separately from more complex learning phenomena. With regard to complex learning, neutral situations, in which no specific stressors were introduced, were distinguished from stress situations, the latter being further classified as psychological stress situations and situations involving noxious stimulation. The *psychological stress* continuum ranges from ego-involving instructions (relating subjects' performance to their intelligence) to failure feedback. While ego-involving instructions are considered to produce mild psychological stress, failure experiences pose considerable stress to self-esteem. The main theoretical assumption here is that psychological stress increases the number and intensity of $S_D$ which, in turn, activate responses that are incompatible with performance on more complex learning tasks. The evaluation of experimental evidence concerning the effects of *noxious stimulation* led Spence and Spence[9] to this conclusion: 'It is quite clear that with respect to the effects of shock *per se* the data from these studies are not adequately explained by either a hypothesis that assumes that shock acts primarily to raise Ss' drive level or a hypothesis that states its major effect is to elicit competing response tendencies that interfere with performance' (p.320).

A major problem within Spence–Taylor drive theory of anxiety[6, 7, 9] was the discussion of the *chronic* versus the *situational* hypothesis of emotional responsiveness. The chronic hypothesis states that individuals differ in their actual anxiety levels irrespective of the experimental situation they are in. Following this hypothesis, differences in the performance of high and low anxious persons were to be expected in any situation, including neutral situations. The situational hypothesis posits that emotional responsiveness may be considered a latent trait that manifests itself in behaviour only if the situation is threatening. The discussion of these alternatives arose within the context of Spence–Taylor drive theory since actual anxiety levels were hypothetically derived from individual differences in trait anxiety and from the belief in the effectiveness of experimental manipulations designed to induce situational anxiety. Differences in actual anxiety level were said to have occurred whenever differences in performance emerged.

The results of two experiments finally led Spence and Spence to decide in favour of the situational hypothesis[9]. Mednick[11] found anxiety-related performance differences only in subjects who were experimentally naive, and not in experienced subjects. Bindra, Paterson and Strzelecki[12] did not find any differences between high and low anxious subjects in salivary conditioning, i.e. in a situation which did not contain any threatening elements. Differences in performance of high and low anxious subjects in neutral situations were then attributed to the threatening effects of the novel laboratory situation.

## STATE ANXIETY AND TRAIT ANXIETY

The factorial distinction of anxiety as a trait and anxiety as a state on the basis of self-report data goes back to Cattell and Scheier[13] (and not to Marcus Tullius Cicero[14]). Utilizing this distinction, Spielberger, Gorsuch and Lushene[15] developed a carefully constructed questionnaire that contains two separate scales for the measurement of state anxiety and trait anxiety. Both measures consist of 20 items each, which are responded to on a four-point rating scale. The measures differ with respect to specific item content, dimensionality of the rating scales and instructions. The trait anxiety measure is set up of adjectives mainly describing stable personality characteristics which are responded to on a frequency scale and administered with the instruction to indicate how one generally feels. The state anxiety measure mainly consists of adjectives describing fluctuating feeling states which are scored on an intensity scale and administered with the instruction to indicate one's momentary feelings. Item overlap between the scales is minimal (four items).

State anxiety is defined as a transitory emotional condition characterized by subjective, consciously perceived feelings of tension and apprehension, and activation of the autonomic nervous system. Trait anxiety, on the other hand, refers to relatively stable individual differences in the disposition to perceive a

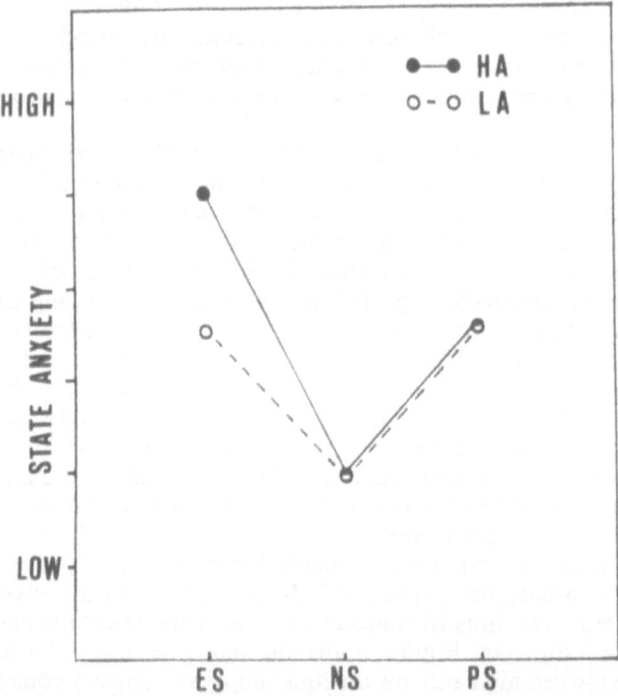

Figure 5.1  Predictions of the trait–state anxiety relationship in different stress situations according to Trait State Anxiety Theory (HA = high trait anxiety; LA = low trait anxiety; NS = neutral situation; ES = ego stress; PS = pain stress)

wide range of stimulus situations as dangerous or threatening, and in the tendency to respond to such threats with state anxiety increases[16]. It is evident from these definitions, that the state anxiety scale represents a more adequate measure of the Hullian concept of drive than trait anxiety scales[15].

In his Trait–State Anxiety Theory, Spielberger[16] specifies the relationship between trait anxiety and state anxiety. High trait anxiety should be predictive of higher increases in state anxiety only if the situation is characterized by threat to self-esteem, but there should be no relationship of trait anxiety and state anxiety increases if the situation involves physical danger. The theoretical predictions of Spielberger's Trait–State Anxiety Theory are depicted in Figure 5.1. With regard to the predicted differential *increases* dependent upon the specific type of stress situation, the experimental evidence appears rather unambiguous[17-20]: high trait anxious persons display higher increases in state anxiety than low anxious persons when confronted with ego threat, while increases in pain threat situations are unrelated to trait anxiety (see Figure 5.2).

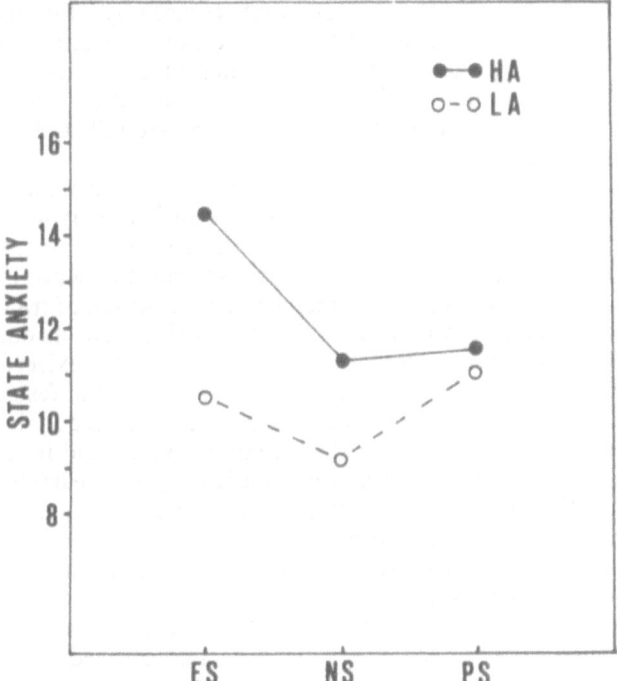

*Figure 5.2 Empirical trait–state anxiety relationship in different stress situations. The figure is based on data reported by Hodges[19]*

A closer inspection of the means obtained in these studies, however, reveals that there is a consistent tendency towards higher increases of low anxious as compared to high anxious persons in pain threat situations. In a recent field study in which pain threat was operationalized as a painful medical diagnostic procedure (hysterosalpingography), low trait anxious persons displayed anxiety increases nearly twice as high as those of high anxious persons, although this difference remained below conventional statistical significance levels[21]. Finally, in a study by Terasaki[22], low anxious persons showed a significant increase in state anxiety when confronted with 95 dB white noise, while high anxious persons' state anxiety levels remained unchanged.

These results clearly demonstrate that high and low anxious individuals react differently to different sources of stress. By ignoring most of these studies, it is hardly surprising that Watson and Clark[23] reach what appears to be an unjustified claim that existing data do not demonstrate differential sensitivity of high and low anxious subjects to different types of stressors. Watson and Clark discuss their review of selected data in terms of a broad theoretical construct which they labelled 'negative affectivity'. Negative affectivity is operationalized in terms of highly intercorrelated trait measures of anxiety, neuroticism, depressiveness, social desirability, repression-sensitization and the like. While it is true indeed that these constructs appear to be different labels for the same basic dimension when their intercorrelations are considered as the only source of information, it is also true that research based on median-split or extreme groups utilizing these constructs need not necessarily lead to comparable results. With regard to measures of general trait anxiety, at least, the existing evidence is definitely in favour of an interpretation that emphasizes situational factors in the determination of the trait–state[16] and the anxiety-performance relationship[9, 63].

Another aspect of the trait–state relationship in different situations concerns state anxiety *levels* of high and low trait anxious persons. In the vast majority of investigations, state anxiety is positively related to trait anxiety, irrespective of the specific situation. This is also true for neutral situations. These findings are in agreement with Spielberger's definition of trait anxiety as a disposition to perceive a wide range of stimulus situations as dangerous or threatening but they are at odds with the notion of trait anxiety as a latent variable requiring adequate situational triggers to be manifested in overt behaviour. Quite recently, further evidence has been presented in that high and low anxious persons would differ in their anxiety levels[24] and in the levels of anxiety-related states such as excitability, sensitivity, and fearfulness among others[25], even if the situation does not contain threatening cues. As a matter of fact, exceptions to this rule seem fairly rare: comparable anxiety levels for groups differing in trait anxiety were either found in situations involving pain threat[19, 21, 26] or in neutral situations[27–29].

Summarizing the results concerning the trait–state relationship, it seems obvious that high trait anxious persons are characterized by chronically heightened state anxiety levels. Differences in state anxiety levels between high and low anxious persons are large in the presence of ego threat, less marked in neutral situations and often negligible in the presence of pain threat. Differential increases in state anxiety in response to stress situations are only found in ego-threatening situations and there is usually no difference in response to pain threat. With regard to the drive theory notion of anxiety these results are well in favour of the chronic hypothesis of emotional responsiveness. Furthermore, high trait anxious persons display higher increases in state anxiety than low trait anxious persons if the situation designed to elicit situational anxiety is characterized by ego threat, as would be expected from Trait–State Anxiety Theory[16].

## MODES OF MEASUREMENT IN THE ASSESSMENT OF STATE ANXIETY

The instruction for the trait anxiety scale of the STAI is always the standard instruction printed on the questionnaire. The instruction for the state anxiety scale, on the other hand, may be modified in order to assess state anxiety levels in a variety of past and future situations[15]. Therefore, at least two separate classes of state anxiety measures may be distinguished from each other, measures of *momentary* and *non-momentary* anxiety states. Momentary anxiety states are assessed by means of the standard instruction of the state anxiety scale. They are usually conceived of as pre- or post-stressor baselines or as anticipatory stress reactions. Anxiety reactions to stressors are usually measured by retrospective self-reports immediately after the confrontation with the stressor, since assessment in the confrontation phase would often interfere with ongoing task performance. These self-reports therefore represent non-momentary anxiety states, which may be classified with regard to the temporal perspective (retrospective, prospective) and the temporal distance to the stressor (close, remote).

When studies of the relationship between trait anxiety and state anxiety in different stress situations are evaluated according to these distinctions[30], quite an interesting picture of results emerges. The interaction of trait anxiety and type of stressor predicted by Trait–State Anxiety Theory is found only if state anxiety is assessed retrospectively immediately after the confrontation with the stressor[17-20]. At that point in time no performance feedback had yet been given to the subjects in these studies. There is only one study in which momentary state anxiety reactions to different stressors were assessed in the confrontation phase. In this study[31], no interaction of trait anxiety and type of stressor was found. In another study[32], momentary state anxiety was measured in the confrontation phase of an ego-threatening situation, and no differential increases were found in high and low trait anxious persons. Finally, Schwenkmezger[33] reviewed a series of studies of the trait–state relationship in ego-threatening sport situations, showing that high and low anxious persons displayed comparable increases in momentary state anxiety assessed in the anticipation phase of the threatening event. If, however, the retrospective measurement mode was utilized, high anxious persons displayed higher increases than low anxious persons.

In sum, high and low anxious persons only display differential increases in state anxiety in an ego-threatening situation if state anxiety is assessed retrospectively after confrontation with the threatening event. This might indicate that self-reports of state anxiety are related to the way in which persons deal with specific threatening situations. In line with the hypothesis that reports of high levels of anxiety may be a result of 'plus-getting' tendencies[34], anxious persons may be characterized by a need to co-operate and not to disappoint the experimenter. Thus, high levels of state anxiety expressed by high trait anxious persons after the confrontation with ego threat might be interpreted as instrumental to the prevention of blame. The specific line of reasoning in a high anxious person might be as follows: 'It is possible that the experimenter will be disappointed by the way I have performed on this task. Therefore, I'll show him how miserable I felt. This will explain why I didn't do very well.' Providing for an explanation of anticipated failure might lead to an overestimation of anxiety levels in high anxious persons, especially if stress instructions are designed to emphasize the importance of one's own performance. Low anxious persons, on the other hand, might give a more realistic estimation of their anxiety levels, as they are not particularly concerned with pleasing the experimenter.

Similarly, Snyder and Smith[35] have argued that complaints of anxiety can be used as a strategy for discounting the image-related implications of poor performance in tests and examinations. More recently, Laux[36] has discussed anxiety reports in terms of self-presentation. He arrives at the conclusion that *self-handicapped strategies* are employed by those high anxious individuals who are highly concerned about their abilities and who report arousal-related anxiety symptoms as a strategy to deflect from an imagined or real deficit of abilities.

The fact that the trait–state relationship is modified by the way state anxiety reactions to stressors are assessed, requires a specification of Trait–State Anxiety Theory as well. The view that ego-threatening situations appear more threatening to high anxious subjects than they do to low anxious subjects has to be qualified. While the actual confrontation with ego threat does not appear to be differentially threatening to subjects differing in trait anxiety[31, 32], differences arise when feeling states are recalled immediately after the confrontation. This effect, however, does not seem to be very lasting: when high and low anxious subjects are asked to indicate how they had felt in a more remote stress situation ('indicate how you felt the last time you were in an examination for which you were inadequately prepared'), comparable increases in state anxiety are reported[30]. Therefore, it is probably not the ego-threatening situation *per se* that is perceived as differentially threatening by high and low anxious persons, but rather the additional ambiguity of a situation that is either open to interpretations of the adequacy of one's own performance or to the experimenter's evaluation of one's own performance.


## WORRY AND EMOTIONALITY

Self-reports of worry and emotionality have been identified as functionally distinct components of anxiety[37]. While the worry concept refers to any cognitive expression of concern about one's own performance, emotionality labels the perception of autonomic reactions. The worry–emotionality distinction has proven especially useful in the analysis of the anxiety–performance relationship. While performance and performance expectancy are negatively related to subjectively perceived worry cognitions, there is usually no relationship to the emotionality component of anxiety[38-43]. Occasionally, however, positive correlations of emotionality and performance are reported[44]. Although the componential view of anxiety has been largely exclusive to the domain of test anxiety research, promising attempts have been made to utilize the worry-emotionality distinction in research on general anxiety[39, 40].

It appears rather tempting to discuss the findings obtained with worry and emotionality scales on the background of drive theory terminology. Since worry cognitions should invariably have a negative effect on performance, they may be closely associated with $S_D$-responses which are elicited whenever there is an increase in drive level. These responses lead to a distraction from the main task and presumably exert their negative influence on performance by the consumption of task time[41]. The emotionality component, on the other hand, may be regarded as the equivalent of the absolute drive level which should have positive effects on performance whenever the task is relatively easy and psychological stress intensity is moderate.

The two components of anxiety have been conceptualized as either state[31, 37] or trait variables[43, 45]. Correlations between the state measures[46] usually range from $r = 0.55$ to $r = 0.62$; they are slightly lower than the intercorrelations of the trait measures[40, 43] which range from $r = 0.64$ to $r = 0.71$. It is evident from these correlation coefficients that worry and emotionality are highly inter-related concepts not to be easily disentangled by means of self-reports alone. Nevertheless, evidence concerning their differential functional properties is convincing. Unfortunately, there is no study published to date in which trait and state measures have been employed in different stress situations. Research efforts in this direction seem highly desirable, especially since existing data suggest that the worry dimension appears to be more stable over time than the emotionality component[42] and that different categories of stressors affect the two components in different ways[31].

## GENERAL AND SITUATION SPECIFIC ANXIETY TRAITS

General trait anxiety may be defined as a disposition to respond to threatening situations with elevations of state anxiety. This view assumes a broad generality of situations evoking differences in state anxiety reactions. General trait anxiety has been assessed by means of self-reports that specify a variety of feelings or behaviours assumed to be related to the concept of anxiety. No reference to specific situations is made in these questionnaires[3, 15]. Subjects are asked to indicate how they generally or normally feel. Despite the obvious lack of situational specificity, these anxiety measures display predictive validity merely or primarily in ego-threatening situations[16]. Although there is no apparent logical reason for this restriction, it seems to rest on a sound empirical basis. One may speculate that student samples who have mainly contributed to the existing data base establish an implicit situational definition in terms of situations they have already experienced in everyday school and university life. These exist mainly of written or oral examinations, and social evaluation situations in a still little known, new and strange university environment. This hypothesis implies that subjects are able to somehow identify the items of these scales as being related to anxiety, although the scales are usually introduced as 'self-evaluation' or 'self-description' questionnaires and reference to anxiety is avoided in the instructions.

In a recent experiment carried out at Mainz University, an introductory psychology class was divided into two groups. Both groups were administered the German version of the STAI[47]. One group ($n = 28$) received standard instructions printed on the questionnaires. The other group ($n = 29$) was told that the questionnaires were designed to measure state anxiety and trait anxiety, respectively. The groups neither differed in their trait nor in their state anxiety levels. These results seem in accord with the hypothesis that student subjects are able to recognize anxiety-specific item contents without being told the basic intention of measurement.

Besides the notion of anxiety as a general trait, situation-specific conceptions of trait anxiety were employed as early as 1952 by Mandler and Sarason[10]. In early research on human anxiety, however, situation-specific trait measures were almost exclusively restricted to the field of test anxiety. It was not until the publication of a study by Endler, Hunt and Rosenstein[48] that further facets of trait anxiety received consideration. Endler's interactional approach to anxiety rests on the assumption that behaviour is determined by dispositional and situational factors as well as by the interaction of these variables. Situation-specific anxiety traits that have received attention within this framework are social evaluation, physical danger, interpersonal, ambiguous, and daily routine anxiety traits[49].

Apart from the estimation of separate variance components related to either dispositional, situational or interactional influences, this area of research has been demonstrating that situation-specific trait anxiety measures are usually better predictors of actual behaviour in a trait congruent situation than either general trait anxiety measures or situation-specific measures related to incongruent situations. Although there are noticeable exceptions from these findings[50, 51], it has been accepted as a rule that the more specific the anxiety traits are, the more accurate is the prediction of actual behaviour in trait congruent situations[52].

Criticism of the interactional approach has mainly focused on methodological issues. It deals with the use of hypothetical situations in the study of anxiety, psychometric inadequacies of the employed scales and misemployed factor analytical techniques[53] and the use of the analysis of variance model to decide between dispositional, situational and interactional positions[54]. Despite some methodological weaknesses, the interactional approach has pointed out the complexities one has to expect when trying to relate individual differences in anxiety proneness to actual behaviour in different situations.

While situation-specific anxiety traits usually refer to a more or less restricted range of situations in which they are predictive of actual behaviour, the concept of general trait anxiety disregards situational references in its definition. The advantage of the general as opposed to the situation-specific approach seems to be that general trait anxiety is defined independent of the situation. Therefore, an a priori confounding of dispositional and situational variables is avoided and the whole variety of possible stress situations may be studied in the context of a general approach. The situation-specific approach, on the other hand, is often in danger of dealing with a series of rather trivial findings (for instance, persons who state that they would not touch snakes really do not touch snakes), which remain unrelated to each other and defy theoretical integration. If, however, the situation-specific approach is utilized to discover types of situations that may be meaningfully grouped together, it would serve as a valuable supplement to the general approach.

## PERFORMANCE AND TASK DIFFICULTY

It is widely accepted that performance varies as an inverted-U function of arousal, activation, anxiety or the like[55]. Increasing task difficulty moves the point of arousal necessary for optimal performance towards the lower end of the arousal continuum. While this description of the anxiety–performance relationship is shared by nearly all theorists, there has been considerable diversity in attempts to explain this relationship. In most theories, two or more variables are assumed that affect performance adversely. Both variables are considered to be monotonically related to performance but differentially effective at different points of the arousal continuum.

But there are also single variable explanations, the most influential of which has been Easterbrook's hypothesis of attentional narrowing[56]. Easterbrook assumes that task performance requires the utilization of cues that may either be relevant to the task or not. Increasing arousal or activation leads to a reduction of the range of cue utilization. At low levels of arousal the range of cue utilization is maximal, i.e. relevant as well as irrelevant cues are processed, thus leading to a relatively low level of performance. Additional increases in arousal lead to the exclusion of task-irrelevant cues from processing, thus increasing performance until the point of optimal arousal is reached. At that point, the full range of relevant cues is utilized. When arousal is further increased, relevant cues are also excluded from the attentional range, which leads to performance decrements. This hypothesis has an immediate appeal because of its simplicity. In its re-interpretation by Wine[41] it remains a valuable contribution especially to the understanding of test anxiety phenomena. Nevertheless, some of its basic assumptions appear rather arbitrary and may hardly be subjected to empirical testing[57].

The problems associated with the drive theory interpretation of the anxiety–task difficulty relationship are similarly severe[58]. According to drive theory, the probability of a specific response not only depends on drive level, but also on two further independent variables, first the number of habits involved in a specific habit hierarchy, and second the relative habit strength of this specific response. Therefore, the difficulty of any S–R connection is not only a function of the absolute strength of the corresponding habit; it is also dependent on the specific task context in which it is embedded. This implies that the difficulty of a specific response can only be reliably determined empirically and that its difficulty varies from one task to the other. But if response difficulty is determined empirically, both drive and habit factors may have influenced the result and there is no possibility of deciding between the relative contribution of these two groups of variables.

A solution to this dilemma might be achieved by the use of procedures from sentence–picture comparison research[59, 60]. Sentence–picture comparison tasks require decisions about the match or mismatch of two simultaneously or successively presented complex stimuli, where decision latencies characteristically vary as a function of the specific type of comparison. Current sentence–picture comparison models have reached a degree of sophistication allowing the *a priori* determination of difficulty of a specific comparison. More stringent tests of drive theory predictions may be performed by using this method, since the intervals between different tasks can be predetermined numerically on logical grounds.

Within the framework of drive theory, task difficulty (or task complexity) was conceptualized as a pure task variable, i.e. the only effect of variations in task difficulty was assumed to be related to the number and strength of the involved habits. But there is still another effect of task difficulty: difficult tasks result in higher increases in state anxiety than easy tasks[32, 61, 62]. These differential increases show that task difficulty is not only to be conceived of as a task variable, but also as a stressing agent[34, 63].

A further problem in the drive theory interpretation of the anxiety–performance relationship refers to the assumption of a hypothetical response threshold. As Weiner[64, 65] has pointed out, this assumption may lead to contradictory predictions with regard to anxiety-related performance differences. To remedy this inconsistency, the notion of a hypothetical response threshold has to be discarded.

Assuming a multiplicative relationship of drive level and habit strength and further assuming that number and strength of task-related habits are independent of drive level, it then follows that differences in the performance of high and low trait anxious persons would appear only when these persons differ in actual state anxiety level, which they usually do. Abandoning the concept of a response threshold would lead to the seemingly paradoxical drive theory prediction of increased probabilities of correct as well as incorrect responses in high anxious as compared to low anxious persons. If, however, the additional plausible assumption is made, that performance differences will mainly emerge from those response tendencies that dominate a specific habit hierarchy, these predictions can be derived from drive theory: in easy tasks, when correct responses are dominant, high anxious persons should show more correct responses than low anxious persons. In difficult tasks, when incorrect responses are dominant, high anxious persons should show more incorrect responses than low anxious persons. Thus, the renunciation of the assumption of a hypothetical response threshold leads to a greater precision of drive theory predictions. The point where the learning curves of high and low anxious persons intersect when performing on difficult tasks would then be specified as that stage of learning where correct and incorrect response tendencies balance.

## COPING WITH ANXIETY

The concept of coping with anxiety has been widely neglected in drive theory. Early criticism of the theory refers to this aspect of the anxiety–performance relationship. Eriksen[66] suggests that high and low trait anxious persons might differ in the way they deal with the arousal of situational anxiety. While high anxious persons habitually prefer strategies such as rationalization and intellectualization, low anxious persons prefer avoidance. Eriksen and Davids[67] draw this conclusion from high correlations of the Taylor Manifest Anxiety Scale and the hysteria–psychasthenia dimension of the MMPI. According to Eriksen, avoidance is an effective strategy in situations that are characterized by threats to self-esteem, but it is ineffective in situations involving physical danger. Rationalization and intellectualization, on the other hand, should be effective when dealing with physical danger and ineffective when threat to self-esteem is implied. Thus, the type of stress situation determines the anxiety–performance relationship, where high anxious persons should perform worse than low anxious persons in stress situations characterized by ego threat and better than low anxious persons in situations characterized by pain threat.

This type of reasoning was further developed by Eriksen[68] and more recently by Krohne[69] who arrives at the same predictions regarding the anxiety–performance relationship by relating trait anxiety to the repression–sensitization dimension: high trait anxious persons prefer sensitization and low anxious persons prefer repression when stress-related cues have to be processed. In a similar manner, the interaction of trait anxiety and task difficulty is explained[70]. Sensitive coping is associated with an extreme appreciation of those situational aspects that might imply threat to self-esteem, while repressive coping is characterized by the denial of these aspects. Since threat to self-esteem is more likely to occur when task difficulty is high, learning difficult material should be disadvantageous to high anxious persons. When the task is comparatively easy, performance of low anxious subjects should be negatively affected, since threat to self-esteem is minimal which leads to a reduction of effort as a consequence of the repressive coping strategy.

The results of a study reported by Houston[71] seem quite instructive with regard to these interpretations. Houston investigated the relationship of trait anxiety to self-report coping strategies in an ego-threatening and a pain threat situation. In the pain threat situation, small but significant correlations with lack of strategy ($r = +0.16$) and intellectualization ($r = -0.18$) emerged. Contrary to expectation, high anxiety was associated with *less* intellectualization. In the ego-threatening situation, only the correlation with preoccupation ($r = +0.27$) reached statistical significance. Denial and rationalization did not correlate with trait anxiety. Because of strong relationships between those strategies that were related to trait anxiety and measures of situational anxiety (self-reports and pulse rate), Houston concluded that the strategies employed by high trait anxious persons were generally ineffective in reducing anxiety. These results show that trait anxiety is not associated with trans-situationally consistent coping strategies but that it may co-vary with different strategies dependent on the specific type of stress situation.

Coping processes have played an important role in cognitive stress research[72]. If coping is conceptualized as dealing with arousal of situational anxiety, two functionally different situations may be considered. In the first case, the arousal of situational anxiety can be reduced or inhibited by the use of psychological defence mechanisms. In the second case, it is the arousal of situational anxiety that leads to the initiation of coping behaviour. While the first case may not very easily be studied, as the phenomenon under investigation (the elicitation of situational anxiety) is not supposed to occur, there are also several conceptual problems associated with the second case. Experimental laboratory investigations are restricted to the use of comparatively mild stressors. Therefore, the very same situation may often elicit feelings of anxiety in one person and opposite effects such as amusement, relaxation or even joy in another person. Because of the extreme variability of individual reactions to laboratory situations the concept of subjective appraisal becomes extremely important[16, 72]. To demonstrate the effectiveness of some sort of coping behaviour, it therefore seems necessary to at least fulfil the following requirements:

(1) It must be shown that a specific stress situation leads to the elicitation of situational anxiety.

(2) It must be shown that changes of affective, motivational, cognitive or behavioural variables which correspond to anxiety increases are effective in either reducing anxiety level or in counteracting actual or anticipated negative consequences of threat.

Coping with anxiety may be considered a palliative strategy in the terminology of Lazarus and Launier[73], i.e. it aims at the reduction of unpleasant feelings, which have to be subjectively perceived before they can be dealt with. Since individuals differ widely in their 'normal' anxiety levels, it seems plausible that the initiation of coping behaviour is not a function of the absolute anxiety level, but of changes, and specifically, increases of anxiety levels relative to intra-individual baselines. Increases in state anxiety require the appraisal of a situation as threatening[16]. A situation is perceived as threatening if the evaluation of available resources and options leads to the conclusion that these would not suffice to deal with the situation[74]. Once an anxiety reaction is elicited coping habits are activated similar to the way in which task-related response hierarchies are activated when persons deal with learning tasks. The process of the activation of task-related and coping response tendencies is summarized in Table 5.1.

Applying drive theory terminology[9], an observable response would then not only be a function of task-specific correct and incorrect response tendencies but also of task-irrelevant coping response tendencies, so that

$$p(\text{Hc}) + p(\text{Hi}) + p(\text{Ha}) = 1,$$

where the probabilities ($p$) for correct (Hc), incorrect (Hi) and coping response tendencies (Ha) add up to unity. The amount and intensity of coping responses would then be a direct function of $S_{\Delta D}$ (drive stimuli associated with increments of drive), because it may be assumed that the experience of one's 'normal' anxiety level will not necessitate the activation of coping responses. This view has several implications. First, at a certain point in time, any of these three response classes has a certain probability of occurrence. With regard to task-related responses, either correct or incorrect responses will occur. By definition, any other response will have to be a coping response. In the anticipation interval of a paired associate learning task, for example, even responses that are not

*Table 5.1    Processes associated with the activation of task-related and coping response tendencies*

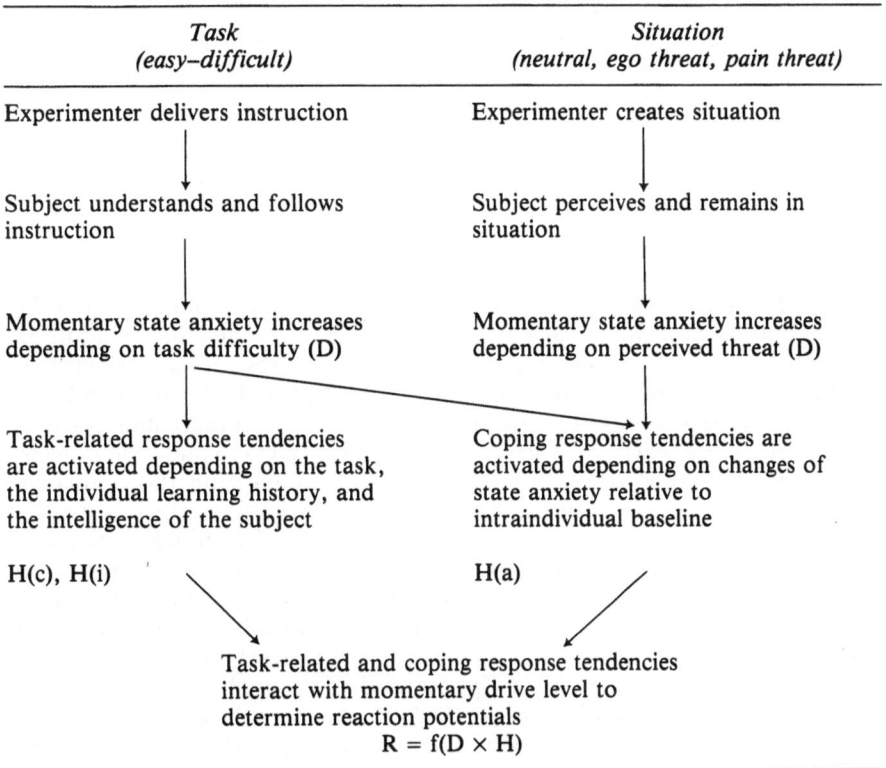

| Task (easy–difficult) | Situation (neutral, ego threat, pain threat) |
|---|---|
| Experimenter delivers instruction | Experimenter creates situation |
| Subject understands and follows instruction | Subject perceives and remains in situation |
| Momentary state anxiety increases depending on task difficulty (D) | Momentary state anxiety increases depending on perceived threat (D) |
| Task-related response tendencies are activated depending on the task, the individual learning history, and the intelligence of the subject | Coping response tendencies are activated depending on changes of state anxiety relative to intraindividual baseline |
| H(c), H(i) | H(a) |

Task-related and coping response tendencies interact with momentary drive level to determine reaction potentials
$$R = f(D \times H)$$

observable may be considered as representing covert coping responses. Although the proposed tripartition of response tendencies is definitely not the only conceivable classification, it seems sufficient for the present analysis. Second, to explain the anxiety–performance relationship only those coping responses are of interest that may occur simultaneously with or instead of task-related responses. This implies that the activation of coping response tendencies will always lead to a decrement of task performance whenever they occur[75]. Third, for the explanation of the anxiety–performance relationship it is irrelevant what specific kinds of coping responses are initiated. It is only the number and strength of coping responses that will exert an influence on performance. This view bears much similarity to a suggestion put forth by Eysenck[57]. He assumes that the arousal of situational anxiety (primarily the arousal of the worry component of anxiety) puts persons into a dual-task situation, in which attention has to be shared between task requirements and anxiety-related cognitions. This should lead to performance decrements by the reduction of working memory capacity. Finally, it is assumed that all the habits which are activated in a performance situation will interact with drive level to determine what specific type of response will be elicited at a certain point in time. In accordance with these assumptions, Morris and Engle[76] found that all coping strategies that were related to performance in a testing situation correlated negatively with performance. Furthermore, none of the six strategies they investigated (denial, intellectualization, isolation, preoccupation, rationalization, resignation) was related to changes of anxiety level.


## PERFORMANCE IN STRESS SITUATIONS

Early research on stress and anxiety in human subjects rested on the assumption that any kind of stressor would increase anxiety levels. The rapid growth of the experimental literature in the early 1950s nevertheless suggested that, in addition to an increase in situational anxiety, different kinds of stressors have effects that are specific to the concrete operationalization employed. A prominent distinction is the one between psychological stress (ego threat) and noxious stimulation (pain threat)[9, 16, 63]. Psychological stress refers to manipulations or events that pose some threat to self-esteem by emphasizing the evaluative character of the situation. In the laboratory, psychological stress is usually induced by the announcement of an intelligence test[5] or by failure feedback[77]. Real life situations considered to induce psychological stress are tests and examinations in school or university. The common denominator of these situations is the evaluation of the self or one's performance in a socially relevant context[42]. Noxious stimulation (physical harm, pain stress) is usually produced in the laboratory by utilizing the anticipation and/or the application of electrical shocks. Further manipulations used in the laboratory are the cold pressor test, accident films or loud noise. Field situations supposed to induce physical threat are medical surgery, painful medical diagnostic procedures or dental treatment.

McGrath[78], in addition to these two types of stress situations, considers a third class of situations, viz., interpersonal stress situations. According to McGrath, the stressing agent in all three of these situations is some form of constraint or deprivation of either psychological, physical or interpersonal needs. In another classification attempt[79] different stress situations were described and subjects were asked to indicate their 'inner reactions' to each of these situations on a five-point rating scale. A two-factor solution emerging from the analysis of 11 subscales clearly favours an interpretation in terms of physical and ego threat, the latter factor being composed of two subscales only, labelled personal failure in performance situations and personal failure in interpersonal situations.

While there may be many different ways to classify stress situations, it seems evident from studies concerning the relationship between trait anxiety and performance[63] or trait anxiety and state anxiety[57] and from factor analytic classification attempts[79] that at least two classes of situations emerge that possess clearly distinguishable characteristics. While a common feature of these situations is their potential to elicit increases of state anxiety in the majority of people, they most likely differ with regard to their specific impact: ego threat implies dangers related to personal integrity, pain threat poses danger to physical well-being. Both aspects, however, may be jointly present in some situations, hindering the interpretation of their respective effects. Thus, in designing experiments, extreme care should be taken for the sake of conceptual clarity and precision not to confound ego threat and pain threat in one specific manipulation.

In a review of studies concerning the relationship between trait anxiety and performance in different stress situations, Saltz[63] has provided strong evidence for the fact that whereas ego stress is likely to debilitate high anxious subjects' performance, pain stress is especially detrimental to low anxious subjects' performance in complex learning tasks. Therefore, Saltz suggested labelling persons at the extremes of general trait anxiety scales 'failure-disrupted' and 'pain-disrupted', respectively. Saltz arrives at these conclusions solely on the basis of performance decrements, but he remains theoretically vague with regard to the mediating mechanisms being responsible for these decrements. Since Houston's study[71] demonstrates that habitual differences in coping strategies can hardly account for the differential performance decrements, other variables might be better candidates.

There are three groups of variables deserving particular consideration: subjective feelings of anxiety, autonomic and central-nervous activity. With regard to subjective feelings of anxiety, levels have to be distinguished from increases. In ego-threatening situations, high anxious persons display higher levels of actual anxiety and in addition, higher increases in state anxiety if retrospective reports immediately after the confrontation with the stressor are considered. In pain threat situations, on the other hand, differences in anxiety levels of high and low anxious persons appear to be minimal, whereas low anxious persons seem to respond with tendentiously higher increases than high anxious persons. When autonomic variables such as heart rate or skin conductance reactions are considered, there seems to be no consistent relationship to anxiety, either as a trait or as a state[81], at least in healthy, non-patient populations.

A more promising approach seems to be the study of central-nervous activity. It is especially the contingent negative variation (CNV), a surface-negative slow potential[82] that arises in constant foreperiod reaction time tasks in anticipation of the imperative stimulus, which has proven a useful measure. When the situation is characterized by ego threat, consistent reductions in CNV magnitude are reported for high anxious as compared to low anxious persons[83–85]. When the situation is characterized by pain threat, the anxiety–CNV relationship is modified by the intensity of the stressor. Mild pain threat leads to a marked reduction of CNV magnitude in low anxious persons[83, 86–88]. Painful electrical shocks, on the other hand, lead to a clear reduction of CNV magnitude in high anxious persons[86, 88–90]. These results show that there is a definite dependency of the anxiety–CNV relationship on the specific type of stress situation. It is yet unclear whether reductions in CNV magnitude reflect deficits in motor preparation[80], or attention towards the imperative stimulus[91, 92], or in task-specific effort expenditure[58]. Nevertheless, these deficits correspond to the performance decrements in ego-threatening situations and in pain threat situations of low intensity as specified by Saltz's hypothesis.

The Effects of Ego Threat

Reviews of studies concerning the relationship between trait anxiety, ego threat and complex learning[9, 63, 93] are easily summarized. If task complexity or task difficulty is relatively high, persons high in trait anxiety show performance decrements relative to persons low in trait anxiety. If task complexity or task difficulty is relatively low, high anxious persons may either perform better or worse than their low anxious counterparts or at a comparable level. The results of more recent studies not included in these reviews are largely consistent with these generalizations[17, 18, 94–96].

These results can be predicted from the revised drive theory model[9]. They also largely agree with expectations formulated by Heinrich and Spielberger[93] who supplement drive theory by notions of Spielberger's Trait–State Anxiety Theory. Nevertheless, it seems necessary to specify some of these theoretical notions to achieve (a) logical consistency within the theory to avoid conflicting predictions, (b) a better fit of the drive theory model to existing data, and (c) the integration of coping behaviour into the drive theory model.

The fact that high and low anxious persons differ in state anxiety levels even in neutral situations[24, 25] demonstrates that high state anxiety levels do not require the immediate experience of threat. It is nevertheless plausible that persons who freely admit to experiencing symptoms of anxiety (as specified in the trait scale of the STAI) rather often possess higher 'rest' levels of anxiety than persons who state that they experience anxiety states rather infrequently. Therefore, stressor effects are not so much reflected in absolute state anxiety levels, but rather in the amount of change they elicit relative to intraindividual base levels. Consequently, the amount and intensity of coping response tendencies depend on the amount of change in anxiety level as a response to stress situations. Once activated, it is nevertheless the absolute level of drive that energizes coping response tendencies in the same way it energizes task-related response tendencies.

Given a neutral situation, the activation of coping response tendencies is highly improbable since there is no necessity to cope with one's 'normal' anxiety level. Therefore, performance differences between high and low anxious individuals in neutral situations will mainly depend on state anxiety levels. Since high trait anxious persons usually display higher levels of state anxiety they should produce more correct responses than low trait anxious persons on easy tasks and more incorrect responses on difficult tasks. Task difficulty or task complexity, in addition, leads to state anxiety increases so that coping response tendencies are activated. Since these increases are approximately the same for high and low trait anxious individuals[32, 61, 62], it will again depend on absolute drive level as to what extent they will lead to observable behavioural manifestations.

If ego stress is introduced into the situation, high anxious persons will respond with higher state anxiety increases than low anxious persons. Although this finding is restricted to a specific mode of measurement (retrospective report immediately after confrontation with an actual stressor), it may reflect, at least to a certain extent, actual differences in the perception of ego threat. The following predictions, nevertheless, can be made whether one assumes differential state anxiety increases of high and low anxious persons or not. The essential qualification is that high and low anxious persons will differ in state anxiety levels in ego-threatening situations, which, in fact, they do.

On *easy tasks,* ego stress of low intensity should not affect the performance superiority of high anxious persons because the activation of coping response tendencies remains negligible relative to the activated task-related response tendencies. Increasing the intensity of ego stress will continually impair high anxious subjects' performance since coping response tendencies are activated more frequently and more intensely in high anxious persons than in low anxious persons. This effect may be a result of either higher state anxiety *increases* or higher state anxiety *levels* of high anxious persons or both. When ego stress intensity is extremely high, so that coping responses dominate over task-related responses, high anxious subjects' performance will eventually be inferior to performance of low anxious subjects, even on comparatively easy tasks. On *difficult tasks,* on the other hand, the introduction of ego stress will continually impair performance of high anxious relative to low anxious subjects. This impairment will be primarily due to the dominance of incorrect task-related responses when ego stress intensity is low, and it will be increasingly due to the dominance of coping responses as stress intensity increases.

## The Effects of Pain Threat

Reviews of studies concerning the relationship between trait anxiety, pain threat and complex learning[9, 63, 97] convincingly demonstrate inferior performance of low anxious subjects relative to high anxious subjects. This difference can be found consistently and it seems to be independent of the task difficulty variable. Furthermore, increases in state anxiety are tendentiously higher for low anxious as compared to high anxious persons, while state anxiety levels scarcely differ. Assuming that high and low anxious persons display comparable levels of state anxiety in pain threat situations, performance differences cannot be attributed to task-related response tendencies. But since low anxious persons show somewhat higher increases in state anxiety, coping responses should be elicited more frequently and more intensely in low anxious as compared to high anxious persons, thus leading to a performance decrement. Furthermore, it is possible that scales designed to measure state anxiety possess a differential sensitivity for high and low anxious persons. Specifically, deviations from intraindividual base levels may be perceived as more aggravating when these base levels are relatively low, thus necessitating an intensified employment of coping behaviour.

In most of the recent attempts to provide for explanations of the anxiety-performance relationship in pain threat situations, person-specific modes of coping with impending stress are postulated[58, 69]. Quite recently, a dual emotion explanation has been proposed by Laux and Spielberger[98]. They argue that pain threat is especially likely to elicit the emotion of anger in addition to the emotion of anxiety. While high anxious persons are hindered from expressing anger because of their high fear of failure and their need to please the experimenter, low anxious persons freely express their feelings of anger which lead to a

107

reduction of their co-operation with the experimenter and thus to performance decrements. None of these explanations has received direct empirical support to date. Further considerations are readily added. It even seems plausible that pain threat exerts a 'therapeutical' effect on high anxious persons. In a study reported by Glover and Cravens[18], high anxious persons displayed a minimal *reduction* of state anxiety levels when unpleasant electrical shocks were administered; low anxious subjects responded with minimal increases.

If the existing evidence concerning the anxiety–performance relationship in different stress situations is viewed together, it seems that there is one basic distinction between ego threat and pain threat. Under ego threat, the importance of one's own performance is emphasized, while under pain threat, a situation is created that distracts from task performance and thus from the aspect of performance evaluation[99].

## CURRENT DEVELOPMENTS IN THEORY AND METHODOLOGY

While there have been few attempts to explain anxiety phenomena within the framework of a more general theory of personality[100], a large portion of current approaches to anxiety is specifically concerned with anxiety-related attentional changes in stress situations. These changes may either be reflected in electrocortical indices[58,92], or in processing effectiveness[57]. Still another line of research emphasizes the importance of coping behaviour in understanding anxiety phenomena[101]. Regarding attentional changes in anxiety, the worry component seems to be of prime importance[42]. To further knowledge about its functional properties is the aim of the test anxiety approach by Sarason[43], who proposes a decomposition of anxiety in tension, worry, test-irrelevant thinking, and bodily symptoms. Within a more general approach to anxiety, Schönpflug[102] argues that the analysis of worry cognitions with regard to their semantic content and their logical structure will reveal valuable information about the impact of the worry component on behaviour. Finally, when different components of anxiety are investigated, it seems highly desirable to look at these components from a trait–state point of view[103].

As is evident from the discrepancy in findings concerning the trait–state relationship depending on the specific mode of measurement, issues relating to the validity of self-report measures of anxiety deserve further research. A better understanding of self-reports seems to be possible, if temporal patterns of anxiety are analysed in sufficient detail[104], especially when self-reports and physiological measures are considered conjointly[105]. Quite recently, Laux[36] has described applications of video-reconstruction techniques in the field of stress research. By means of these techniques self-report measures can be directly related to behavioural indices of anxiety.

Although there are a number of unresolved issues in anxiety research, it is suggested that the proposed modifications of drive theory can account for a variety of findings pertinent to the relationship between trait anxiety, state anxiety, and performance in different stress situations. Obviously, the theory is restricted to the prediction of those processes that occur at the response stage of learning performance. But this does not necessarily preclude the possibility that anxiety may also be an important variable in determining intake and storage of information. Although the present status of the theory does not yet allow for an application of its basic principles on these learning stages, future elaborations may remedy this situation. Drive theory predictions do not often deviate from predictions derived from alternative approaches; but drive theory is formulated on a comparatively high level of abstraction. Thus, it seems especially apt to integrate research from rather diverse fields. Current theorizing on anxiety usually does not explicitly refer to drive theory notions, although noticeable exceptions[93, 106] exist. The neglect of these notions may be partly due to the fact that they have erroneously been judged as not providing for valid concepts in the prediction of behavior. But drive theory remains a sound theory of anxiety, if recent developments in the refinement of anxiety- and stress-related concepts are utilized to modify and supplement the theory.

# References

1. Taylor, J. A. (1951). The relationship of anxiety to the conditioned eyelid response. *J. Exp. Psychol.*, **41**, 81–92
2. Hull, C. L. (1943). *Principles of Behavior.* (New York: Appleton-Century-Crofts)
3. Taylor, J. A. (1953). A personality scale of manifest anxiety. *J. Abnorm. Soc. Psychol.*, **48**, 285–90
4. Spence, K. W., Farber, I. E. and McFann, H. H. (1956). The relation of anxiety (drive) level to performance in competitional and non-competitional paired-associates learning. *J. Exp. Psychol.*, **52**, 296–305
5. Spielberger, C. D. and Smith, L. H. (1966). Anxiety (drive), stress, and serial-position effects in serial-verbal learning. *J. Exp. Psychol.*, **72**, 589–95
6. Spence, K. W. (1958). A theory of emotionally based drive (D) and its relation to performance in simple learning situations. *Am. Psychol.*, **13**, 131–41
7. Taylor, J. A. (1956). Drive theory and manifest anxiety. *Psychol. Bull.*, **53**, 303–20
8. Nicholson, W. M. (1958). The influence of anxiety upon learning: interference or drive increment? *J. Pers.*, **26**, 303–19
9. Spence, J. T. and Spence, K. W. (1966). The motivational components of manifest anxiety: drive and drive stimuli. In Spielberger, C. D. (ed.) *Anxiety and Behaviour.* pp. 291–326. (New York: Academic Press)
10. Mandler, G. and Sarason, S. B. (1952). A study of anxiety and learning. *J. Abnorm. Soc. Psychol.*, **47**, 166–73
11. Mednick, S. A. (1957). Generalization as a function of manifest anxiety and adaptation to psychological experiments. *J. Consult. Psychol.*, **21**, 491–4
12. Bindra, D., Paterson, A. L. and Strzelecki, J. (1955). On the relation between anxiety and conditioning. *Can. J. Psychol.*, **9**, 1–6
13. Cattell, R. B. and Scheier, I. H. (1961). *The Meaning and Measurement of Neuroticism and Anxiety.* (New York: Ronald)
14. Eysenck, H. J. (1983). Cicero and the state–trait theory of anxiety: another case of delayed recognition. *Am. Psychol.*, **38**, 114–15
15. Spielberger, C. D., Gorsuch, R. L. and Lushene, R. E. (1970). *Manual for the State–Trait Anxiety Inventory.* (Palo Alto, CA: Consulting Psychologists Press)
16. Spielberger, C. D. (1972). Anxiety as an emotional state. In Spielberger, C. D. (ed.) *Anxiety: Current Trends in Theory and Research.* Vol. 1, pp. 23–49. (New York: Academic Press)
17. Glanzmann, P. and Laux, L (1978). The effects of trait anxiety and two kinds of stressors on state anxiety and performance. In Spielberger, C. D. and Sarason, I. G. (eds.) *Stress and Anxiety.* Vol. 5, pp. 145–64. (Washington, DC: Hemisphere)

18. Glover, C. B. and Cravens, R. R. (1974). Trait anxiety, stress, and learning: a test of Saltz's hypothesis. *J. Res. Pers.*, **8**, 243–53
19. Hodges, W. F. (1968). Effects of ego threat and threat of pain on state anxiety. *J. Pers. Soc. Psychol.*, **8**, 364–72
20. Lamb, D. H. (1973). The effects of two stressors on state anxiety for students who differ in trait anxiety. *J. Res. Pers.*, **7**, 116–26
21. Margalit, C., Teichman, Y. and Levitt, R. (1980). Emotional reaction to physical threat: re-exaination with female subjects. *J. Consult. Clin. Psychol.*, **48**, 403–4
22. Terasaki, M. (1981). Manifest anxiety, noise, and serial reaction performance. *Jap. J. Psychol.*, **52**, 53–6
23. Watson, D. and Clark, L. A. (1984). Negative affectivity: the disposition to experience aversive emotional states. *Psychol. Bull.*, **96**, 465–90
24. Lazarus-Mainka, G. (1984). Ängstlichkeit – auch ein Sprachstil. Presented at the *26th Meeting of Experimental Psychologists*, April 15–19, Nürnberg
25. Kirkcaldy, B. D. (1984). The interrelationship between state and trait variables. *J. Pers. Individ. Differences*, **5**, 141–9
26. Kendall, P. C., Finch, A. J., Auerbach, S. M., Hooke, J. F. and Mikulka, P. J. (1976). The State–Trait Anxiety Inventory: a systematic evaluation. *J. Consult. Clin. Psychol.*, **44**, 406–12
27. Schönpflug, W. and Wieland, R. (1982). *Untersuchungen zur Äquivalenz schwankender Schallpegel: Schwankende Schallpegel, Leistungshandeln und der Wechsel von Arbeit und Erholung.* Forschungsbericht Nr. 82 - 10501204. (Berlin: Umweltforschungsplan des Bundesministers des Innern)
28. Fröhlich, W. D. and Glanzmann, P. (1983). Kortikale Aufmerksamkeitsregulation, Angstneigung und subjektive Erwartung. In Lüer, G. (ed.) *Bericht über den 33. Kongreß der Deutschen Gesellschaft für Psychologie in Mainz 1982.* Vol. 1, pp. 232–6. (Göttingen: Hogrefe)
29. Lazarus-Mainka, G., Friebel, U. and Unshelm, S. (1982). Ängstlichkeit und das Vorstellen bedrohlicher Situationen. *Psychol. Beiträge*, **24**, 356–69
30. Glanzmann, P. (1985). Zusammenhänge zwischen Angstneigung und Zustandsangst in unterschiedlichen Stress-Situationen. *Zeitschrift für Differentielle und Diagnostische Psychologie.* (In press)
31. Morris, L. W. and Liebert, R. M. (1973). Effects of negative feedback, threat of shock, and level of trait anxiety on the arousal of two components of anxiety. *J. Counsel. Psychol.*, **20**, 321–6
32. O'Neil, H. F., Spielberger, C. D. and Hansen, D. N. (1969). Effects of state anxiety and task difficulty on computer-assisted learning. *J. Educ. Psychol.*, **60**, 343–50
33. Schwenkmezger, P. (1985). *Modelle der Eigenschafts- und Zustandsangst: Theoretische Analysen und empirische Untersuchungen zur Angsttheorie Spielbergers.* (Weinheim: Beltz)
34. Sarason, I. G. (1960). Empirical findings and theoretical problems in the use of anxiety scales. *Psychol. Bull.*, **57**, 403–15
35. Snyder, C. R. and Smith, T. W. (1982). Symptoms of self-handicapping strategies: the virtues of old wine in a new bottle. In Weary, G. and Mirels, H. L. (eds.) *Integrations of Clinical and Social Psychology.* (New York: Oxford University Pres)
36. Laux, L. (1985). A self-presentational view of coping with stress. In Appley, M. H. and Trumbull, R. (eds.) *Advances in Stress Theory.* (In press)
37. Liebert, R. M. and Morris, L. W. (1967). Cognitive and emotional components of test anxiety: a distinction and some initial data. *Psychol. Rep.*, **20**, 975–8
38. Heckhausen, H. (1982). Task-irrelevant cognitions during an exam: incidence and effects. In Krohne, H. W. and Laux, L. (eds.) *Achievement, Stress, and Anxiety.* pp. 247–74. (Washington, DC: Hemisphere)
39. Spielberger, C. D., Anton, W. D. and Bedell, J. (1976). The nature and treatment of test anxiety. In Zuckerman, M. and Spielberger, C. D. (eds.) *Emotions and Anxiety: New Concepts, Methods, and Applications.* pp. 317–45. (Hillsdale, NJ: Erlbaum)
40. Spielberger, C. D., Gonzales, H. P., Taylor, C. J., Algaze, B. and Anton, W. D. (1978). Examination stress and test anxiety. In Spielberger, C. D. and Sarason, I. G. (eds.) *Stress and Anxiety.* Vol. 5, pp. 167–91. (Washington, DC: Hemisphere)
41. Wine, J. (1971). Test anxiety and the direction of attention. *Psychol. Bull.*, **76**, 92–104

42. Wine, J. D. (1982). Evaluation anxiety: a cognitive attentional construct. In Krohne, H. W. and Laux, L. (eds.) *Achievement, Stress, and Anxiety*. pp. 207–19. (Washington, DC: Hemisphere)

43. Sarason, I. G. (1984). Stress, anxiety, and cognitive interference: reactions to tests. *J. Pers. Soc. Psychol.*, **46**, 929–38

44. Hodapp, V. (1982). Causal inference from nonexperimental research on anxiety and educational achievement. In Krohne, H. W. and Laux, L. (eds.) *Achievement, Stress, and Anxiety*. pp. 355–72. (Washington, DC: Hemisphere)

45. Spielberger, C. D. (1980). *Test Anxiety Inventory ('Test Attitude Inventory')*. (Palo Alto, CA: Consulting Psychologists Press)

46. Morris, L. W. and Liebert, R. M. (1970). Relationship of cognitive and emotional components of test anxiety to physiological arousal and academic performance. *J. Consulting Clin. Psychol.*, **35**, 332–7

47. Laux, L., Glanzmann, P., Schaffner, P. and Spielberger, C. D. (1981). *Das State-Trait-Angstinventar (STAI). Theoretische Grundlagen und Handanweisung*. (Weinheim: Beltz)

48. Endler, N. S., Hunt, J. M. and Rosenstein, A. J. (1962). An S–R inventory of anxiousness. *Psychol. Monogr.*, **536**, 1–31

49. Endler, N. S. (1980). Person–situation interaction and anxiety. In Kutash, I. L. and Schlesinger, L. B. (eds.) *Handbook on Stress and Anxiety*. pp. 249–66. (San Francisco: Jossey-Bass)

50. Mellstrom, M., Cicala, G. A. and Zuckerman, M. (1976). General versus specific trait anxiety measures in the prediction of fear of snakes, heights, and darkness. *J. Consulting Clin. Psychol.*, **44**, 83–91

51. Mellstrom, M., Zuckerman, M. and Cicala, G. A. (1978). General versus specific tests in the assessment of anxiety. *J. Consulting Clin. Psychol.*, **46**, 423–31

52. Laux, L., Glanzmann, P. and Schaffner, P. (1985). General vs. situation-specific traits as related to anxiety in ego-threatening situations. In Spielberger, C. D., Sarason, I. G. and Defares, P. B. (eds.) *Stress and Anxiety*. Vol. 9, pp. 121–8. (Washington, DC: Hemisphere)

53. Cooper, C. (1981). The utility of a general anxiety trait: some methodological considerations. *Br. J. Soc. Psychol.*, **20**, 135–9

54. Furnham, A. and Jaspars, J. (1983). The evidence for interactionism in psychology: a critical analysis of the situation-response inventories. *Pers. Individ. Differences*, **4**, 627–44

55. Yerkes, R. M. and Dodson, J. D. (1908). The relation of strength of stimulus to rapidity of habit-formation. *J. Comp. Neurol. Psychol.*, **18**, 459–82

56. Easterbrook, J. A. (1959). The effect of emotion on cue utilization and the organization of behavior. *Psychol. Rev.*, **66**, 183–201

57. Eysenck, M. W. (1982). *Attention and Arousal: Cognition and Performance*. (Berlin: Springer-Verlag)

58. Fröhlich, W. D. (1983). Perspektiven der Angstforschung. In Thomae, H. (ed.) *Enzyklopädie der Psychologie. Serie Motivation and Emotion*. Vol. 2, pp. 110–320. (Göttingen: Hogrefe)

59. Carpenter, P. A. and Just, M. A. (1975). Sentence comprehension: a psycholinguistic processing model of verification. *Psychol. Rev.*, **82**, 45–73

60. Shoben, E. J. (1978). Choosing a model of sentence–picture comparisons: a reply to Catlin and Jones. *Psychol. Rev.*, **85**, 131–7

61. Head, L. Q. and Lindsey, J. D. (1983). The effects of trait anxiety and test difficulty on undergraduates' state anxiety. *J. Psychol.*, **113**, 289–93

62. Tennyson, R. D. and Wooley, F. R. (1971). Interaction of anxiety with performance on two levels of task difficulty. *J. Educ. Psychol.*, **62**, 463–7

63. Saltz, E. (1970). Manifest anxiety: have we misread the data? *Psychol. Rev.*, **77**, 568–73

64. Weiner, B. (1966). Role of success and failure in the learning of easy and complex tasks. *J. Pers. Soc. Psychol.*, **3**, 339–44

65. Weiner, B. (1972). *Theories of Motivation*. (Chicago: Markham)

66. Eriksen, C. W. (1954). Some personality correlates of stimulus generalization under stress. *J. Abnorm. Soc. Psychol.*, **49**, 561–5

67. Eriksen, C. W. and Davids, A. (1955). The meaning and clinical validity of the Taylor Anxiety Scale and the hysteria-psychasthenia scales from the MMPI. *J. Abnorm. Soc. Psychol.*, **50**, 135–7

68. Eriksen, C. W. (1966). Cognitive responses to internally cued anxiety. In Spielberger, C. D. (ed.) *Anxiety and Behavior*. pp. 327–60. (New York: Academic Press)
69. Krohne, H. W. (1980). Angsttheorie: Vom mechanistischen zum kognitiven Ansatz. *Psychol. Rundschau*, **31**, 12–29
70. Krohne, H. W. and Rogner, J. (1982). Repression–sensitization as a central construct in coping research. In Krohne, H. W. and Laux, L. (eds.) *Achievement, Stress, and Anxiety*. pp. 167–93. (Washington, DC: Hemisphere)
71. Houston, B. K. (1982). Trait anxiety and cognitive coping behavior. In Krohne, H. W. and Laux, L. (eds.) *Achievement, Stress, and Anxiety*. pp. 195–206. (Washington, DC: Hemisphere)
72. Lazarus, R. S. (1966). *Psychological Stress and the Coping Process*. (New York: McGraw-Hill)
73. Lazarus, R. S. and Launier, R. (1978). Stress-related transactions between person and environment. In Pervin, L. A. and Lewis, M. (eds.) *Perspectives in Interactional Psychology*. pp. 287–327. (New York: Plenum)
74. Folkman, S., Schaefer, C. and Lazarus, R. S. (1979). Cognitive processes as mediators of stress and coping. In Hamilton, V. and Warburton, D. M. (eds.) *Human Stress and Cognition: An Information-processing Approach*. pp. 265–98. (Chichester: John Wiley & Sons)
75. Grzegołowska-Klarkowska, H. J. (1980). Use of defense mechanisms as determined by reactivity and situational level of activation. *Polish Psychol. Bull.*, **11**, 155–68
76. Morris, L. W. and Engle, W. B. (1981). Assessing various coping strategies and their effects on test performance and anxiety. *J. Clin. Psychol.*, **37**, 165–71
77. Lucas, J. D. (1952). The interactive effects of anxiety, failure, and intraserial duplication. *Am. J. Psychol.*, **65**, 59–66
78. McGrath, J. E. (1982). Methodological problems in stress research. In Krohne, H. W. and Laux, L. (eds.) *Achievement, Stress and Anxiety*. pp. 19–48. (Washington, DC: Hemisphere)
79. Boucsein, W., Erdmann, G., Janke, W. and Albrecht, D. (1982). Die Erfassung der individuellen Reaktionsbereitschaft auf verschiedene Klassen von Stressoren. I Konstruktion, Aufgabenanalyse und Normierung des Belastungsfragebogens BELA. *Z. Differentielle Diagnostische Psychol.*, **3**, 185–200
80. Rohrbaugh, J. W., Syndulko, K. and Lindsley, D. B. (1976). Brain wave components of the contingent negative variation in humans. *Science*, **191**, 1055–7
81. Hodges, W. F. (1976). The psychophysiology of anxiety. In Zuckerman, M. and Spielberger, C. D. (eds.) *Emotions and Anxiety: New Concepts, Methods, and Applications*. pp. 175–94. (Hillsdale, NJ: Erlbaum)
82. Walter, W. G., Cooper, R., Aldridge, V. J., McCallum, W. C. and Winter, A. L. (1964). Contingent negative variation: an electric sign of sensori-motor association and expectancy in the human brain. *Nature*, **203**, 380–4
83. Glanzmann, P. and Froehlich, W. D. (1984). Anxiety, stress, and contingent negative variation reconsidered. *Ann. NY Acad. Sci.*, **425**, 578–84
84. Low, M. D. and Swift, S. J. (1971). The contingent negative variation and the 'resting' D. C. potential of the human brain: effects of situational anxiety. *Neuropsychologia*, **9**, 179–85
85. McCallum, W. C. and Papakostopoulos, D. (1973). The CNV and reaction time in situations of increasing complexity. *Electroencephalogr. Clin. Neurophysiol. Suppl.*, **33**, 179–85
86. Knott, J. R., Van Veen, W. J., Miller, L. H., Peters, J. F. and Cohen, S. I. (1973). Perceptual mode, anxiety, sex, and the contingent negative variation. *Biol. Psychiatry*, **7**, 43–52.
87. Proulx, G. S. and Picton, T. W. (1984). The effects of anxiety and expectancy on the CNV. *Ann. NY Acad. Sci.*, **425**, 617–22
88. Van Veen, W. J., Peters, J. F., Knott, J. R., Miller, L. H. and Cohen, S. I. (1973). Temporal characteristics of the contingent negative variation: relationships with anxiety, perceptual mode, sex, and stress. *Biol. Psychiatry*, **7**, 101–11
89. Knott, J. R. and Irwin, D. A. (1973). Anxiety, stress, and the contingent negative variation. *Arch. Gen. Psychiatry*, **29**, 538–41
90. Rizzo, P. A., Caporali, M., Pierelli, F., Spadaro, M., Zanasi, M., Morocutti, C. and Albani, G. (1984). Pain influence on brain preparatory sets. *Ann. NY Acad. Sci.*, **425**, 676–80
91. Tecce, J. J. (1972). Contingent negative variation (CNV) and psychological processes in man. *Psychol. Bull.*, **77**, 73–108

92. Tecce, J. J. and Cole, J. O. (1976). The distraction–arousal hypothesis, CNV, and schizophrenia. In Mostofsky, D. I. (ed.) *Behavior Control and Modification of Physiological Activity*. pp. 162–219. (Englewood Cliffs, NJ: Prentice-Hall)

93. Heinrich, D. L. and Spielberger, C. D. (1982). Anxiety and complex learning. In Krohne, H. W. and Laux, L. (eds.) *Achievement, Stress, and Anxiety*. pp. 145–65. (Washington, DC: Hemisphere)

94. Shearer, E. and Fulkerson, F. E. (1973). The effects of physical and psychological stress on the performance of high- and low-anxious Ss on a difficult verbal discrimination task. *Bull. Psychonomic Soc.*, 1, 255–6

95. Reeves, R. A. and May, W. M. (1977). Effects of state–trait anxiety and task difficulty on paired associate learning. *Psychol. Rep.*, 41, 179–85

96. Anson, O., Bernstein, J. and Hobfoll, S. E. (1984). Anxiety and performance in two ego threatening situations. *J. Pers. Assess.*, 48, 168–72

97. Eysenck, M. W. (1979). Anxiety, learning, and memory: a reconceptualization. *J. Res. Pers.*, 13, 363–85

98. Laux, L. and Spielberger, C. D. (1983). Stress, trait–state anxiety, and learning: two competing models. In Spielberger, C. D. and Diaz-Guerrero, R. (eds.) *Cross-cultural Anxiety*. Vol. 2, pp. 145–54. (Washington, DC: Hemisphere)

99. Dunn, J. A. (1968). Anxiety, stress, and the performance of complex intellectual tasks: a new look at an old question. *J. Consult. Clin. Psychol.*, 32, 669–73

100. Humphreys, M. S. and Revelle, W. (1984). Personality, motivation, and performance: a theory of the relationship between individual differences and information processing. *Psychol. Rev.*, 91, 153–84

101. Krohne, H. W. (1985). Das Konzept der Angstbewältigung. In Krohne, H. W. (ed.) *Angstbewältigung in Leistungssituationen*. pp. 1–13. (Weinheim: edition psychologie)

102. Schönpflug, W. (1985). Anxiety, worry, prospective orientation, and prevention. In Spielberger, C. D. and Sarason, I. G. (eds.) *Stress and Anxiety*. Vol. 12, in press. (Washington, DC: Hemisphere)

103. Morris, L. W., Franklin, M. S. and Ponath, P. (1983). The relationship between trait and state indices of worry and emotionality. In van der Ploeg, H. M., Schwarzer, R. and Spielberger, C. D. (eds.) *Advances in Test Anxiety Research*. Vol. 2, pp. 3–13. (Lisse: Swets and Zeitlinger SV)

104. Wieland, R. (1984). Temporal patterns of anxiety: towards a process analysis of anxiety and performance. In Schwarzer, R. (ed.) *The Self in Anxiety, Stress, and Depression*. pp. 133–50. (Amsterdam: North Holland)

105. Otto, J. and Bösel, R. (1978). Angstverarbeitung und die Diskrepanz zwischen Selfreport und physiologischem Stressindikator: eine gelungene Replikation der Weinstein-Analyse. *Schweiz. Z. Psychol. und ihre Anwendungen*, 37, 321–30

106. Albert, D. (1980). Anxiety and learning-performance. *Arch. Psychol.*, 132, 139–63.

# SECTION 2

# PHYSIOLOGICAL AND CLINICAL STUDIES

# 6
# Mental chronometry.
# I. Behavioural and
# physiological techniques

## *Kenneth B. Campbell*

---

Investigations into the speed of 'decision-making' are amongst the oldest in the area of experimental psychology. The dependent measure that has dominated this field is the subject's reaction time (RT). Precisely which brain processes RT indexes remains nevertheless very much an issue of debate.

In this article, the term, 'mental chronometry' will be used to refer to the timing and duration of information processing activities. Since the pioneering work of Donders in 1868 (translated by Koster[1]), researchers have attempted to divide RT into a number of mediating components or stages. Donders' procedure consisted of measuring RT under two different conditions. One required the involvement of a proposed stage, the other did not. The difference between the RTs collected under the two different conditions was the estimate of the time required for that stage to be processed. Ironically, the very success of the method was to lead to its downfall. Wundt adopted the method as a means of quantifying the results from the data obtained from introspection. The procedure (reporting exactly when a mental event occurred) produced results that were highly variable. While it is now clear that in fact the method of introspection was the guilty party and not the RT paradigm, quite the reverse was held to be true. Indeed, the method of introspection was employed to discredit the utility of Donders' subtraction procedures – a turnaround if ever there was one! Even today the method of subtraction is still not widely accepted in spite of the fact that some authors (cf. Taylor[2]) claim that it has never been disproven on any basis other than introspection.

## STAGES OF INFORMATION PROCESSING

The component analysis of RT regained credit only recently[3]. Even then, perhaps because of the fact that the stage analysis was derived on the basis of mathematical models and not empirical data, the subject matter did not gain much attention until the late 1960s. This was largely due to the

117

innovative and creative methods of Sternberg[4]. He also ran a series of ingenious experiments to support his model. Since its introduction, the very powerful 'method of additive factors' has been widely accepted, although it too has had its share of distractors.

Several other models have subsequently been developed. In virtually all of them, it is assumed that a series of processes intervene between the stimulus event and the later overt response. These include sensory encoding, stimulus storage, perceptual encoding, memory comparison and response selection, to name just the most common often cited by cognitive psychologists[5-8]. Individual differences in performance may reflect deficits in one or more of these stages. It should be noted that much controversy exists – several researchers have reviewed on the dimensions for which the processing of a stage can be determined[7, 9-11]. Taylor[2] uses the term 'element' to refer to the things that are being processed. In general, the element is identified as the smallest unit of information processed in a particular stage. Two fundamentally distinctive stage models concerning the manner in which elements are processed have been suggested. These are the serial and parallel models (Miller[8]). In the serial model, the elements are processed one at a time. The processing of one element must be completed before the processing of the next element is initiated. In the parallel model, the processing of all elements is initiated simultaneously. It is also possible to combine both models. For example, the processing of elements may be initiated serially but some or even a considerable degree of overlap between the elements is permitted. There are, of course, other possibilities. In a fairly flexible or plastic model, processing of the various elements might begin simultaneously, but priority is given to particular elements in a serial manner to speed the completion of their processing before 'attention' is paid to elements having lower priority.

Parallel models, while attractive conceptually, have received little experimental validation. The simple matter is that it is extremely difficult to design studies to test out the models. Thus, most authors, either explicitly or implicitly, have adopted some form of a serial model. In the most simple of serial models, the decomposition of RT into stages is based on the assumption that the reaction process is a linear sequence of discrete stages. RT is therefore the sum of the stage times. An additional assumption is also usually made – the times required by each stage are independent of one another. Let us assume that a reaction process consists of four stages, labelled a, b, c and d. Thus $RT = T_a + T_b + T_c + T_d$, where T is a random variable describing the time required by a particular stage. Even though $T_c$ might be very long, this will have no influence on the later $T_d$, nor does its unusually high value depend on either $T_a$ or $T_b$. The Sternberg 'additive' model cast serious doubt on the assumption of the independence of stages. Thus, some authors believe that in many cases the time required to process a particular stage may well depend on the time required to process previous stages. As an example, if the processes of one stage are mimicked in part by subsequent stages (i.e. the stages are not independent), then its contribution to the overall reaction time is exaggerated. One could also think of an opposite effect – the duration of one stage compensates for that of another. More recently even the Sternberg model has become an issue of debate[2].

Let us turn to the very crux of the serial stage model of information processing – the stages themselves. It is generally accepted that the identification of particular stages of processing is a tenuous business. To prove the existence of a particular stage, experimental manipulations must be designed that affect that stage and no others. However, even given the assumption that such vastly complex and creative experiments could be designed and further assuming that the duration of a stage could be estimated, it is critical that no other stage be influenced by the manipulations. If there is overlap, the assumption of a serial and independent stage of processing is violated. To make matters worse, there is no means of determining the degree of overlap (or confounding with previous or subsequent stages). The methodological limit of most behavioural RT studies is that the existence of a particular stage of processing must be inferred through a subtraction, or additive or interactive process. It can never be directly observed! The harsh reality is that many so-called 'stages' of information processing have often been determined by inference (if not speculation), and not on the basis of hard data.

For the sake of this discussion, let us assume for the moment that there are at least two distinctive and independent stages of information processing: stimulus evaluation and response production. These occur serially and with durations that can be manipulated separately[12-14]. Stimulus evaluation refers to the general class of processes for obtaining information about stimuli, permitting the discrimination of one stimulus from another. Response processes refer to the general class of processes for choosing overt responses, based not only on current perceptual information but also on the subject's prior expectancies for the occurrence of the various stimuli and of the anticipated outcome contingencies of the reponse to these stimuli[14]. The terms 'the speed of information processing' or 'decision-making' time, often employed in the studies of individual differences are ambiguous. What is probably meant is the duration of stimulus evaluation processes. What, in fact, is being measured by the behavioural reaction time is, at least in part, the duration of stimulus evaluation, but also summed to it, the duration of response production. As will be pointed out in later sections, in many studies purporting to show group differences in the speed of information processing, what is actually being shown to differ is the speed of response production.

The problem with behavioural measures such as RT is that they have access to the cognitive state only after the response has occurred. For this reason, a number of authors have turned to physiological measures, in particular the averaged evoked potential, to obtain information before, during and after the actual decision-making process. This advantage has not escaped researchers interested in the study of individual differences. There are of course a number of methodological limitations to the use of 'biological' measures. Many of these are unique to the evoked potential technique. Unfortunately, in many cases, those employing the evoked potential technique have not respected the methodological rigour required for their use and proper interpretation. Because many readers may not be familiar with evoked potential methods, a brief overview of the technique will be presented.

## THE COMPONENT STRUCTURE OF THE HUMAN EVOKED POTENTIAL

Evoked potentials (EP) are the changes in the electrical activity of the nervous system that are elicited by some physical stimulus or psychological event[15]. The evoked potential is usually, but not always, swamped by the massive ongoing electroencephalographic (EEG) activity. Through the application of techniques such as signal averaging, the EP can be extracted from the EEG. Several excellent reviews have pointed out the usefulness and the limitations of the technique (see, for example Vaughan[16] and Glaser and Ruchkin[17]).

### The Stimulus

We can begin with the stimulus itself. The physiologist must pay obsessive attention to the stimulus. It must be exactly controlled and reproducible since the nature of the averaging process assumes its constant and consistent repetition. Fluctuations in the intensity, duration or location of the stimulus can markedly alter the response. Many of these same parameters can affect RT. While some of these points may seem obvious and trivial, it is surprising to see how many studies still neglect (or fail to report) stimulus parameters.

Whenever possible, auditory stimuli should be presented through calibrated earphones. Constancy of stimulus input cannot be assured with loudspeakers. The intensity of the stimulus should be reported. This is expressed in dB relative to a standard reference. Unfortunately, the 'standard reference' is not always reported. Common reference scales include the subject's own threshold or SL (thus intensity is expressed in terms of dB above subjective threshold), the international standard adult threshold (or ISO), the general threshold for the particular group or sample of subjects being studied (or HL). The ISO and HL references assure that physical energy of the auditory stimulus for a particular frequency is constant across all subjects. The subjective threshold (SL) assures that the perceived or psychological stimulus is equated across subjects although the level of physical energy may vary. The problem with the various threshold references is that the amount of physical energy required to reach the threshold of the human ear varies across frequencies. The ear is most sensitive in the 1–2000 Hz range and least sensitive to extremely high or low frequencies. For this reason, many laboratories prefer to calibrate the auditory stimulus relative to a known reference, usually 20 $\mu$Pa (SPL) – the minimum audible intensity for the most sensitive of human ears. This assures a constant physical intensity across all frequencies. However, the perceived loudness may well vary. Thus, although the voltage that is applied to the headphones to produce a 100 dB SPL 1000 Hz signal and a 100 dB SPL 10 000 Hz signal may be very similar; the former will sound very loud, the latter barely audible.

Reaction times for visual stimuli are typically 50–100 ms longer than for auditory. Most of this time can be explained by the differences in transmission time to the cortex. However, depending on the visual stimulus employed, at least a few ms of the RT can be explained by the physical qualities of the stimulus itself. Tungsten light bulbs require several ms before reaching maximum intensity. Short duration tachistoscopic stimuli will obviate these effects as will the use of light emitting diodes. Many modern laboratories present visual stimuli on a television-type monitor. The time taken to change the pattern will be some percentage of the scanning cycle (16.7 ms in North America and 20 ms in Europe). There appears to be no standard or laboratory norm for luminence, intensity or contrast although each of these will affect the response. When different groups are being compared, it is essential that pupillary gaze be controlled. This is particularly the case with children and patients who are either unwilling or unable to comply to the experimenter's instructions.

## The Averaging Process

In order to separate the evoked potential from the ongoing electrical activity of the brain, the process of signal averaging is used. This involves the repeated presentation of the same stimulus to the subject. Each time the stimulus is presented, the EEG, consisting of the signal embedded in the background 'noise', is converted into numbers by the analogue-to-digital converter of the computer and stored in addresses of the computer's memory. The digitized waveforms are then averaged together and plotted as the 'average evoked potential'. Because noise by definition is random, with summation, it tends to cancel itself out. Sometimes it is negative, sometimes it is positive – on averaging, it becomes a straight line. The evoked potential or 'signal' is constant. On averaging therefore, it remains the same.

The background noise decreases during averaging by the square root of the number of samples in the average. Thus if the evoked potential waveform is not clear enough after the initial averaging, to make it twice as clear will require four times as many trials. In theory, if one were to average an infinite number of trials, the background noise would disappear altogether. In practice, compromise is usually required. There is always therefore some degree of background noise remaining in any evoked potential average. This being the case, one can never be certain that the averaged waveform represents a true cerebral evoked potential or the residual random background activity. It is always advisable to repeat the recording session a second time. If the waveform is reproducible, one can be confident that it was true response. Figure 6.1 provides an example of the averaging process. A subject was presented with an 80 dB 1000 Hz tone pip presented at a fairly slow rate (every 5 s). The e.e.g. was digitized 300 times over a 900 ms period beginning 150 ms prior to stimulus onset (in principle, there should be no change in the EEG prior to stimulus onset). The 'raw' EEG is presented in trials 1–8. A relatively constant negative polarity response beginning at approximately 80 ms may be observed in these single trials. These responses are embedded in random high amplitude background noise. When trials 1–4, 5–8, 9–12 and 13–16 are averaged, the background noise begins to diminish in amplitude, but the response remains constant. As the composite average becomes based on 8, 16, 32 and finally, 64 trials, the signal gradually begins to become much more clear in the increasingly diminished background noise. Note that after 32 trials, the two separate averages are essentially identical. The waveform is therefore reproducible. The signal-to-noise ratio is hardly altered by continuing the averaging process out to 64 trials.

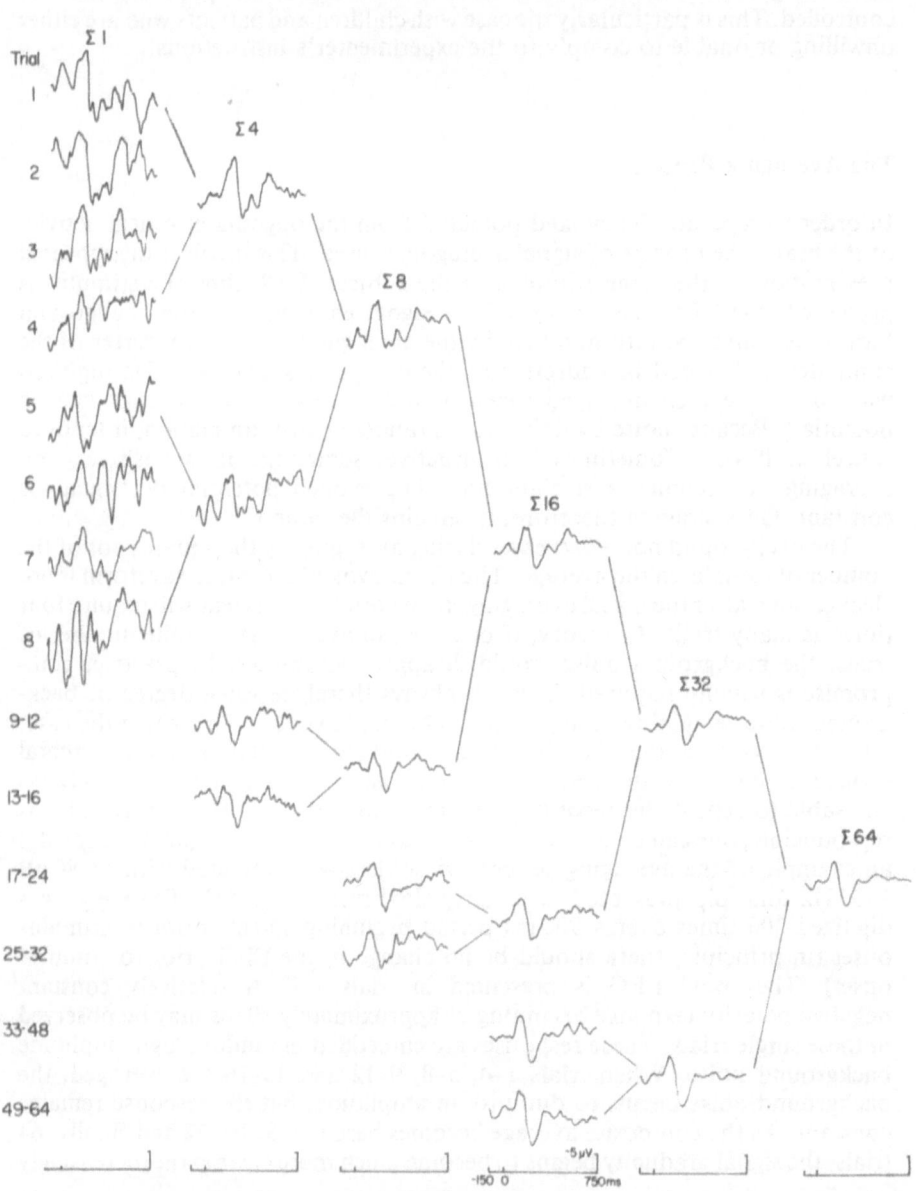

## EEG Recording

In general, most clinical EEG recording techniques work well in the experimental laboratory. With the exception of long-lasting or slow potentials, such as the CNV, electrodes constructed of almost any precious metal will suffice. In the case of the slow potentials, reversible electrodes such as those with silver–silver chloride coatings are preferred in order to reduce bias and polarization potentials. It is essential that the electrodes be affixed securely. This usually implies that the electrodes be cemented to the scalp with collodion.

## Electrode Montage

The origins of the various components of the evoked potential are widespread. For example, in the auditory evoked potential, N1 appears to be maximum over frontal regions of the scalp, while a later positive wave, P3, is maximum over parietal zones. In general monopolar recordings (as opposed to bipolar) dominate the literature. The inactive or reference electrode must be located in an area that is electrically neutral. The mastoid process is often employed. Yet it is active during the very early evoked potentials. Moreover artifacts from

---

*Figure 6.1   The averaging process. Auditory evoked potentials were recorded to 80 dB SPL tone pips, presented at a rate of one every 5 s. Electrodes were placed at the vertex and mastoid process. Trials with excessive artifact ( ± 100 μV) were rejected. Negativity at the vertex in this and other figures is represented by an upward deflection. In the far left column, individual responses to the first eight stimuli are shown. Although a response appears to be evident in the 100-200 ms following the stimulus (the sweep was initiated 150 ms prior to stimulus onset), random background 'noise' makes it difficult to discern. In the second column, the average of the first four trials is illustrated as is the average of trials 5-8, 9-12, and 13-16. Note that the averages based on four trials are now beginning to reveal a much clearer response in the 100-200 ms range and that the background noise is becoming reduced in amplitude. The third column represents the 'grand average' of the average of trials 1-4 and 5-8 and 9-12 and 13-16 (i.e. the average is based on eight stimulus presentations). The average of trials 17-24 and 25-32 is also illustrated. Although the four different averages reveal a distinctive N1-P2, there is still a relatively large amount of noise remaining in the average. Note also that the signal-to-noise ratio is not twice as good as one moves from an average based on four to an average based on eight trials. However, when 16 trials are averaged, the evoked potential is clearly superior to that obtained after four trials, in keeping with the tenets of the theory of signal averaging. The first and last 32 trials were also averaged. These could serve as replicate averages - as such, both averages are almost identical. Therefore, very little background noise remains in the composite average. The grand average, based on 64 stimulus presentations indicates a definite negative–positive deflection beginning at about 100 ms. The remaining smaller deflections might be true cerebral responses or they might be residual background noise. Only after considerably more stimulus presentations could this be resolved*

muscle reflexes and skin potentials are quite prominent here. Whenever possible, multiple channel recordings should be used. An evoked potential derived from only a single pair of electrodes gives only a restricted view of the brain's activities. Frequently, eight and often 16 channels are employed. Figure 6.2 illustrates evoked potentials recorded from 22 different channels. As may be observed, the morphology of the response varies across the scalp location.

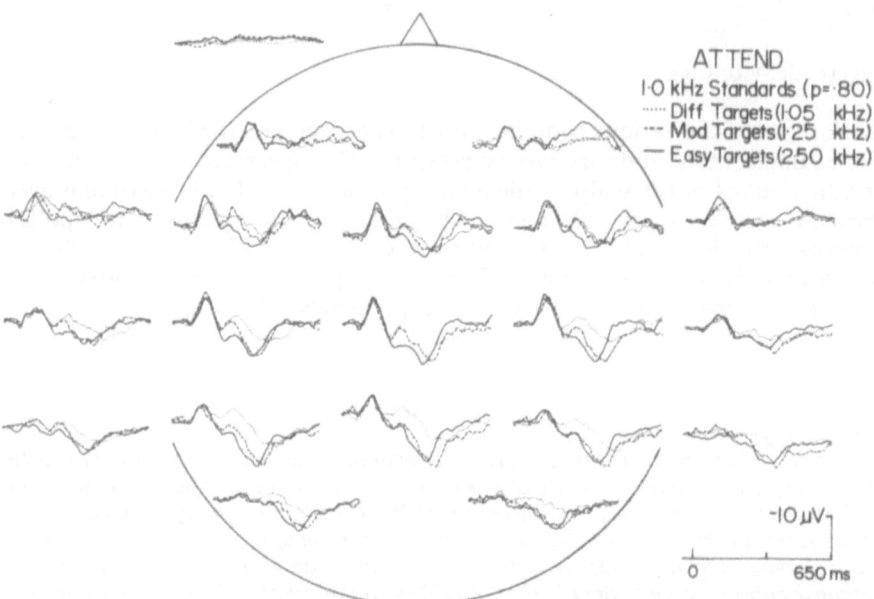

ATTEND

1·0 kHz Standards (p=·80)
······ Diff Targets (1·05 kHz)
--- Mod Targets (1·25 kHz)
— Easy Targets (2·50 kHz)

-10 μV

0    650 ms

*Figure 6.2   Multiple channel-recording of event-related potentials. In this example, 22 electrodes were placed on the scalp of six different subjects. The waveforms that are illustrated represent the grand average of the target evoked potentials at the various sites for these six subjects. Subjects were asked to detect the occurrence of a rare 'target' (0.20 probability of occurrence) amongst a train of 1000 Hz 'standard' tone pips. In different conditions, the ease of target detection was varied, being either difficult or easy to detect or between the two extremes (target frequency being either 1050, 2500 or 1250 Hz respectively). In the upper left-hand portion of the map, EOG activity is clearly 'flat'. The deflections that are apparent in the other channels are therefore not due to artifact from eye movements or blinking. Note that an early negative wave is largest in frontal regions and decreases in amplitude in posterior zones. The auditory stimuli were presented to the right ear. In the most lateral regions, particularly at the left central side, its morphology changes (perhaps due to the fact that the electrode is placed over the temporal lobe – the primary auditory cortex). A late positive wave, with a peak latency around 325 ms (although this is variable, depending on ease of target discriminability), manifests a widespread scalp distribution although it is largest in parietal sites. Because the early negative and late positive waves show differing scalp distributions, it is assumed that they have different intracranial generators*

Measurements of scalp-distribution are used to demonstrate that different components are generated in different areas of the brain. In the example mentioned above, N1 is probably generated by a different source than P3. More recently, however, scalp distribution studies have been employed to distinguish the various subcomponents of what appears to be a single waveform. The N1 peak of the auditory evoked potential as mentioned is maximally recorded in frontocentral regions of the scalp. As may be observed in Figure 6.2, when it is simultaneously recorded from temporal electrodes, earlier and later subcomponents appear. These may be related to the sensory qualities of the stimulus, such as its ear of presentation[18].

Artifact

One of the greatest methodological concerns of the evoked potential researcher is for artifact originating from non-cerebral sources. The scalp-recorded EEG can often be contaminated by a variety of types of artifact. These may be electrical or physiological. Such non-cerebral artifacts can markedly distort the evoked potential waveform. Electrical artifacts result from electrostatic or electromagnetic fields which are generated by the equipment (stimulators or other electrical instruments) or connections. This problem can be reduced by ensuring low impedance connections between the electrodes and the scalp and where possible, by recording in electrically quiet areas. Physiological artifact originates from a variety of sources including scalp and neck muscles, eye movements and blinks, skin potentials and the EKG. To make matters worse, the artifact may not even be visible in the ongoing EEG. If the artifact is time-locked to the stimulus, the averaging process will make the previously invisible artifact visible. Debriefing of the subject is almost always required. It must be explained that they must not do anything that is time-locked to the stimulus. They cannot blink, gulp, move, or frown regardless of how startling or unexpected the stimulus. When subjects are asked to behaviourally respond by, for example, button pressing, the researcher must be certain that the evoked potential waveforms occurring at the time of the button press are not artificial in nature. Frequently, as a control, in a separate condition subjects are asked to keep a running count of the behavioural events rather than making a physical movement. The evoked potential waveforms generated under the two conditions are then compared – if they are not different, then the waveform in question was probably generated by a true cerebral source and not by the non-cerebral muscle artifact. When semantic stimuli are being employed, the experimenter should be aware that touching the tip of the tongue to the roof of the mouth can cause a potential of up to $100\,\mu$V at the vertex. By comparison, the cerebral EP thus recorded might not exceed $5\,\mu$V. Subjects must avoid even the smallest of subvocalizations. The most prominent contaminants often encountered in the evoked potential laboratory are eyeblinks and eye movements. The artifact so caused by these sources can be as high as several millivolts.

The methodological concern becomes an obsession for those attempting to make inferences about group differences on the basis of averaged evoked potentials. Can we be absolutely certain that the group differences were not due to artifact? Certain groups co-operate less than others. Others may not completely understand the instructions. Children are especially prone to movement. If visual stimuli are used, can it be proven that the gaze of all the subjects was fixated on the stimulus? In many instances, group differences tend to be very small. Thus, even very minute artifact contaminating the EEG could account for group differences.

In the light of this rather lengthy foreword, a good conservative rule to follow is: assume that any evoked potential is due to artifact unless proven otherwise. The onus is thus on the researcher to demonstrate that a potential is cerebral in origin and that non-cerebral sources could not possibly have evoked it.

The effects of artifact therefore must be completely removed. As mentioned, subjects should be told to reduce movements and eye blinking to a minimum. In principle, if the artifact is not time-locked, it should average out. Given the fact that the amplitude of many sources of artifact greatly exceeds that of the actual evoked potential, this may require the presentation of several additional trials, hence markedly prolonging the experiment.

There are several methods available to remove the effects of artifact (see Picton et al.[19], for a review). Many of these involve complex mathematical operations requiring sophisticated computer routines. A fairly simple and common approach is to remove those trials containing artifact from the average. In spite of instructions to the contrary, subjects do blink and move and swallow and persist in doing whatever the experimenter does not want them to do. The use of the artifact rejection technique should assure that trials containing high-level noise do not contribute to the overall averaged evoked potential. This usually implies that sources of artifact must be recorded simultaneously with the EEG. To prove that the averaged evoked potential was not contaminated by sources of artifact, it is critical that both the averaged EEG and artifact channels be displayed. If the artifact channels are flat, the changes in the polarity of the EEG channels are independent of non-cerebral sources.

In some studies, authors devote as many channels to sources of artifact as they do to the EEG. Within the last few years, a group of Ottawa colleagues[20] have been studying the neurophysiology of the naming process. Evoked potential studies of language had been plagued by methodological problems. When word or picture stimuli are presented, one must be especially concerned about artifact. In the Stuss et al. experiment[20], seven of 15 polygraph channels were devoted solely to the monitoring of artifact. In addition to the usual blinking (vertical EOG) and movement contaminants, there is the possibility that subjects might subvocalize, perhaps more on one side of the mouth than the other. Therefore, facial and tongue movements were monitored by electrodes placed on the left and right cheeks. The English language is read from left to right. Since eye movements contribute positivity to those areas of the scalp towards which the eyes move, differences in polarity between left and right cerebral hemispheres may have been affected by these non-cerebral sources. Thus, horizontal eye movements were also monitored. Finally, to insure that the evoked potentials were not influenced by respiration, it was monitored using a strain gauge respirometer. The authors wisely included sample recordings from their artifact monitors in their publication indicating quite clearly and convincingly that all such sources were 'flat'. Therefore the evoked potential waveforms that were recorded were most likely of cerebral origin.

## Component Structure of the Averaged Evoked Potential

There are many different evoked potentials that can be recorded from the human scalp. Davis[21] has classified the evoked potentials on the basis of their peak latency into 'fast', 'middle', 'slow' and 'late'. In general, the earlier or faster the component, the more it is dependent on the qualities of the stimulus, such as its modality, intensity, frequency and rate of presentation. On the other hand, the later the component, the more the component depends on factors that are independent of the physical quality of the stimulus, such as its meaningfulness, task relevance, etc. Because the later components are dependent on psychological 'events' and not the stimulus *per se*, they are often termed 'event-related' potentials or ERPs.

An alternative system of classification identifies specific components that signify the operation of serial stages of information processing, using designs borrowed from experimental and cognitive psychology. Thus 'exogenous' components vary as a function of the physical stimulus and are relatively insensitive to psychological manipulations. The fast and middle components fit neatly into this category. At the other extreme, 'endogenous' components only appear when the stimulus demands perceptual or cognitive processing. As such, these components are minimally affected by the physical characteristics of the stimulus itself. These are, of course, the ERPs or the late components. In between the two extremes lie the so-called 'mesogenous' components. These waves are affected by both the physical parameters of the stimulus and the psychological state of the subject[22]. It is possible that in a parallel system, the mesogenous components may be composed of overlapping exogenous and endogenous components. The physiological laboratory, like the behavioural discussed earlier, has encountered difficulties in designing experiments to test this possibility.

Different systems for establishing the nomenclature of the components of the evoked potential have also developed. Figure 6.3 illustrates the system most commonly used in the auditory modality. In this system, the early positive components are designated by Roman numerals I–VI. The middle and later components are designated by their polarity P or N and followed by a lower case letter or number (Na, N1, P3, etc.). Another means of identifying the component is to name its polarity and usual latency in milliseconds. Thus, wave V of the early components becomes P6. P3 of the slow components becomes P300. The problem with the former system is that there are often subcomponents, forcing complication on the original nomenclature. N2, for example, is often labelled as N2a and N2b to distinguish subcomponents of the N2 wave. The problem with the second method is that the component's latency may vary dependent on experimental manipulation. The P3 wave can have a peak latency as short as 275 ms and as long as 875 ms[23] depending on task requirements.

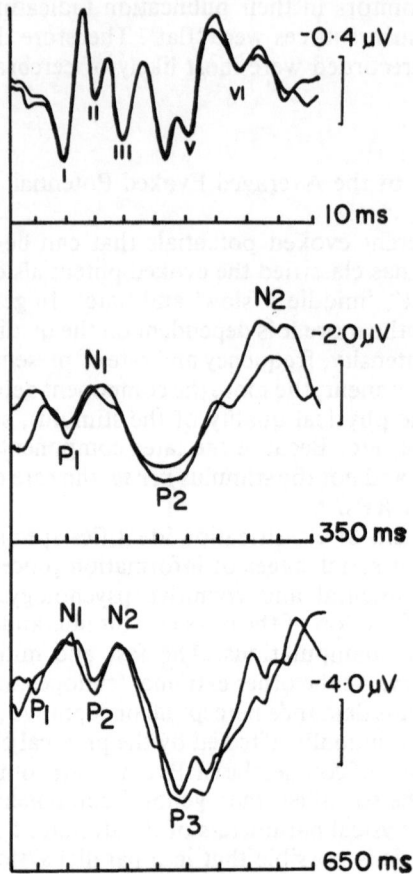

*Figure 6.3 Components of the human auditory evoked potential. Responses were averaged over 2000, 150 and 50 trials in the upper, middle and lower portions of the figure. The EEG was recorded from Cz and referenced to the mastoid. Note the different time base for each of the tracings. Note also the different amplitude calibration signals. The lower responses are of a much higher amplitude than the upper responses. The endogenous components were recorded during a signal detection task in which the subject was asked to detect a rare target occurring amongst the more frequently presented standards*

The parallel to cognitive psychology, 'cognitive psychophysiology'[24], has as its goal the identification of particular ERP components in relation to specific stages of information processing. The task has been arduous. Experimental manipulations must be designed to establish the independence of the various components. As mentioned, components often overlap in time. In spite of the many difficulties that have been encountered, the progress that has been made is impressive.

## Exogenous Components

The earliest components originate in specific subcortical brainstem centres (auditory) or primary cortical receiving areas (somatosensory). The auditory brainstem evoked potential has proven to be of immense value in neurology and audiology. Because peak I represents activity in the auditory nerve and peak V, activity in the midbrain region, the latency difference between peaks I and V provides an index of the speed of neuronal conduction from the peripheral to the central nervous systems. This time on average is about 4 ms.

For the cognitive psychologist, the exogenous components have important implications from a negative point of view. The exogenous components are relatively independent of psychological processes. Click-evoked brainstem potentials remain invariant regardless of the subject's level of attention[25, 26]. Indeed, Campbell and Bartoli[27] have found that they are stable even during an 8 h period of sleep. Salamy and McKean[28] have indicated that the exogenous components do not habituate. On the other hand, Lukas[29] has reported that waves I and V of the tone-evoked potential increase in amplitude and/or reduced in latency when the tones were attended. We have not been able to replicate these findings using essentially identical methods[30]. Desmedt and Robertson[31] noted that the early primary cortical components of the somatosensory evoked potential were independent of the manipulation of the subject's level of attention.

On the interpretive level, the exogenous components have implications which differ from those of the later components. Individual differences in 'higher mental' or cognitive functioning should affect the endogenous components, but presumably should have little effect on the exogenous components. A number of authors, for example, believe that ageing results in a slowing of cognitive processes that is independent of sensory impairment. Others believe that the apparent slowing is due to a decrement in motivation. If either theory is true, one would not predict an alteration of the exogenous components in the aged (again, assuming normal sensory processing). Most studies (see for example Harkins and Lenhardt[32]) agree that although the latency of wave V is somewhat later (from 0.0 to 0.2 ms) in the aged, this is probably due to a high frequency hearing loss rather than a slowing of 'information processing' *per se*. There appears to be a slight, but very small decrease in peak V amplitude (perhaps 0.05 $\mu$V). By contrast, as we shall point out in later sections, the endogenous components are much more susceptible to the effects of ageing.

## Mesogenous Components

A distinct negative–positive complex, commonly called N1-P2, is recorded maximally from the frontocentral areas of the scalp at typical peak latencies of 100 and 200 ms following an auditory stimulus (middle portion of Figure 6.3). A response of similar morphology occurs following stimuli in the visual or somatosensory modalities[33]. These waves are affected by the physical parameters of the stimulus, such as its intensity, frequency and rate of presentation.

In the 1970s, Hillyard *et al.*[34] and Picton and Hillyard[25] noted that during dichotic listening tasks, attended auditory stimuli delivered at rapid rates elicited a broad negative ERP which began as early as 60–80 ms and produced an increase in the amplitude of the N1 component compared to conditions in which the stimuli were ignored. Initially, this early attention effect was interpreted as an augmentation of the N1 component in the attended channel. More recent studies[35, 36] have noted that the negativity extends well beyond the time course of N1, and is primarily endogenous in nature. This attention-related component was termed 'processing negativity' by Naatanen and his colleagues. Hansen and Hillyard employ the term negative 'difference wave' (Nd), Nd being the difference between the attended and unattended channels. The Nd effect has been interpreted as being an early mode of stimulus selection, analogous to Broadbent's[37] 'stimulus set' or 'filter' or Treisman's[38] 'input selector'.

In summary, a series of components (N1–P2) in the 75–250 ms latency range are primarily affected by the physical qualities of the stimulus. They are thus exogenous in nature. Overlapping or summed to these waveforms is a long-lasting negativity that appears to be endogenous in nature.

Studies of individual and group differences occurring at the time of N1–P2 must take the mesogenous nature of these components into account. Few, in fact, have done so. Examples of such studies are reported in the second article of this series.

Endogenous Components

The evoked potential to a detected, highly informative signal or 'target' contains a series of late components, the most studied of which are N2, P3 and the Slow Wave (SW) – (lower portion of Figure 6.3). N2 appears to be modality-specific (and thus is not a 'pure' endogenous component). It has been associated with sensory discrimination[39] and mismatch detection[40]. The P3 component has been an area of far more study (see Donchin *et al.*[41] and Pritchard[42] for reviews). The P3 component varies in amplitudes as a function of stimulus probability[43–45]. P3 is largest in parietocentral regions of the scalp, regardless of the modality of the stimulus, or for that matter any other physical characteristic of the stimulus.

In recent years, the latency of the P3 wave has come to complement behavioural RT by allowing measurement of the timing and duration of some of the component structures that underlie RT. As we have mentioned previously, RT reflects the duration of at least two stages: stimulus evaluation and response production. The two terms are used to distinguish those operations required to evaluate a stimulus (including cognitive operations involved in the encoding, identification and categorization of a stimulus) from those required to select and execute a response. In contrast to RT, processes involved in response selection and execution have little effect on P3 latency.

The evidence for such a claim is now quite convincing. McCarthy and Donchin[46] manipulated stimulus discriminability and stimulus–response compatibility. Subjects were asked to respond with the right or left hand to the words LEFT or RIGHT. Stimulus discriminability was varied by embedding these words in a matrix of ' # ' signs or in a matrix of letters chosen randomly from the alphabet. Response compatibility was manipulated by having subjects respond with either the left or right hand indicated by the word (e.g. LEFT signalled a left hand response) or with the opposite hand (e.g. LEFT signalled a right hand response). The more difficult signal detection task and having to make an incompatible response increased RT. In contrast, P3 latency increased during the difficult signal detection task but was unaffected by the need to make an incompatible response. Thus, processes that are involved in response selection and execution have little effect on P3 latency. These data have subsequently been replicated in a separate study[23] designed to determine that the late positive wave observed by McCarthy and Donchin was indeed a true 'P3'.

Duncan-Johnson and Kopell[47] employed the Stroop Colour–Word Interference Test to compare its effects on both P3 and RT latency. In the standard Stroop test, the time required to name the ink colour in which a word is printed is increased if the word spells a conflicting colour name (e.g. the word 'green' printed in red ink). The source of the delay in RT could either be due to stimulus encoding or response production. The 'perceptual conflict' theory used to explain the Stroop effect assumes that reading the colour of the word, which is unavoidable, disrupts or delays identification of the ink colour. The 'response competition' hypothesis, on the other hand, assumes that interference occurs *after* stimulus evaluation has already occurred. If the first hypothesis is true, the latency of P3 should be longer in trials in which the colour of the stimulus and the stimulus word are incongruous, paralleling the changes in RT. If the 'response competition' hypothesis is true, then regardless of category of stimuli, the latency of P3 would be invariant. In this instance, RT and P3 latencies would be disassociated. The results supported the 'response competition' theory. P3 latency was unaltered by the different categories of stimuli whereas RT was much longer when the colour of the stimulus and its meaning were incongruous. The Stroop effect is therefore primarily an output, rather than an input, phenomenon.

Duncan-Johnson and Donchin[48] have used a similar line of logic to determine the processes underlying a well-known phenomenon: RT increases as the probability of the stimulus decreases. The goal in this case was to determine the stage or stages at which stimulus probability operates. Many authors propose that a perceptual bias in favour of the more likely event is established, with the consequence that the subject is more prepared to receive the frequent stimulus[49, 50]. Others argue that the response to the more frequent stimulus is more readied or 'primed' although this may be additive or in parallel to an already existing perceptual bias[51, 52]. Still other investigators have maintained that a response bias is almost entirely responsible for the effect[13, 53].

Duncan-Johnson and Donchin[48] employed both macro- and micro-analyses of their data. Not only did they examine the overall mean data but also the manner in which a response depends on the preceding sequence of stimuli (trial ... n − 2, n − 1, and n). No attempt will be made here to summarize the entire results of what was a magnificently elegant and elaborate study. The relation of RT to P3 latency suggests that both stimulus and response processes affect RT. In certain conditions – when a stimulus is highly probable – RT may actually precede P3 (which itself is speeded), indicating response processes were initiated before stimulus evaluation was complete. In other conditions, when strong expectancy is violated, then the close relationship of RT to P3 latency suggests that response selection is more contingent on stimulus-evaluation processes. Inevitably, as the relationship would suggest, P3 almost always precedes RT.

In studies concerned with the speed of information processing, it should be fairly obvious that I consider P3 to be a powerful complement to the much more commonly used behavioural measure, RT. It should be understood that my claim is not that P3 is essential for an accurate interpretation of RT. As explained in the next section, through careful measurement and sophisticated analysis of RT in and by itself, very precise and specific interpretations can be made. These analyses are not without a cost. To meet the statistical assumptions of many of the more sophisticated analyses, a large number of trials and/or conditions will have to be run. One of the very real benefits of P3 is that due to its relatively large amplitude in most subjects, it can usually be observed in the ongoing averaged EEG waveform after a small number of trials.

## METHODOLOGICAL CONSIDERATIONS OF REACTION TIME MEASURES

It should now be apparent that the total duration of overt, behavioural responses (RT) is fraught with methodological difficulties. The use of RT as a measure of 'processing time' must take methodological precision into account. Some very clever suggestions that provide for a thorough and complete analysis of the data contained in the typical RT experiment have been offered. Again, the present article will limit itself to a brief overview.

A serial stage analysis of human information analysis has thus far been assumed. Variation in RT can be due to alterations of virtually any one or combination of the hypothesized stages. The role of the behavioural researcher is to determine precisely how these various stages are being affected by his/her experimental manipulations.

Lappin and Disch[54] have pointed out that in most RT studies, subjects' decision processes are assumed to remain constant from one trial condition to another. Variation in RT is assumed to reflect the contributions of sensory, perceptual or cognitive processes, free from variation in decision strategies. This assumption is especially questionable in studies purporting to have demonstrated group differences in processing speed based on RT measures. In these instances, it is my opinion that what most researchers studying individual differences are measuring in terms of processing speed is, in fact, the latency to the completion of stimulus evaluation processes. Those processes involved in response selection generally fit poorly into these theories. It will be demonstrated, however, that in almost all cases in which group differences have been reported, processes related to response selection and execution cannot be ruled out as a possible alternative.

132

## Speed–accuracy Trade-off

In the usual paradigm, the instructions that are given to the subject are somewhat ambiguous. Often, subjects are asked to respond as quickly as possible, keeping errors to a minimum. Thus, it is expected that subjects will adopt a strategy wherein speed and accuracy will be traded off. As such, it has usually been found that very high levels of accuracy are generally associated with slower responding. Reductions in accuracy are associated with increasingly faster responding. As Figure 6.4 indicates, the relationship is far from linear. Pachella[55] has pointed out that very small changes in error rate at high levels of accuracy (i.e. error rates less than 10%) may be associated with large changes in RT. Unfortunately, this is precisely the region of the speed–accuracy trade-off function from which much of the data in 'error-free' experiments have been derived. For the study of individual differences, the distinction can be critical.

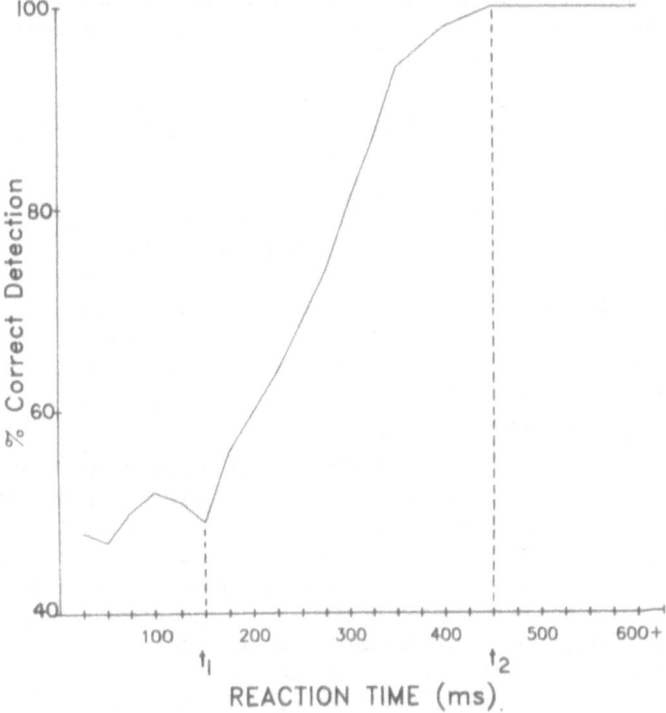

*Figure 6.4   Speed–accuracy trade-off function. A well-practised subject was presented with 1000 trials in a two-choice RT experiment. She was asked to maintain accuracy at approximately 0.75. RTs were ranked from fastest to slowest, then grouped in equal 25 ms blocks and finally, plotted as a function of accuracy. At the fastest rates of responding, performance is at chance levels (50% correct) until a certain critical value, $t_1$ (approximately 225 ms for this subject), is reached. Accuracy then increases in a more or less linear function of RT until another critical value, $t_2$ (approximately 450 ms with this subject), is reached, when accuracy is at a maximum*

Very small differences in high-accuracy conditions can lead to very large group differences in RT. In many instances, the very existence of erroneous responses has been treated as an embarassment rather than the result of a process that may occasionally generate errors. Although some authors report error rate, few also report mean error RT[56]. As will be noted in the discussion of the physiological measures that complement RT, the speed–accuracy trade-off affects principally processes underlying response production. In the case of individual differences, I have already suggested that most authors are either overtly or covertly attempting to examine processing underlying stimulus evaluation. Thus, unless the speed–accuracy trade-off function is taken into consideration and appropriate corrections made, serious errors of interpretation are inevitable. A number of methods providing an understanding of human information processing that is far more complete than the simple mean RT is able to provide have recently been developed. The mathematical computations and procedures are sometimes complex, as one might well expect given the nature of higher mental functioning. Common to each of the procedures is a concern for error responses.

Lappin and Disch[54] have proposed that the complete trade-off function between speed and accuracy be used as a measure of RT.

'This technique is based upon the proposition that a decision process determines the point in time at which perceptual processing is terminated and an overt response is selected. Thus, a given pair of RT and error rate values reflects performance under a specific decision criterion: but the complete trade-off function between RT and error rate is presumed to reflect performance under varying decision criteria applied to a constant perceptual process. The functional relation between the two dependent variables is thereby used to obtain a decision-free measure of the perceptual process. The same approach is used in signal detection theory: the functional relation between the hit rate and false-alarm rate, the receiver operating characteristic (ROC), is used as the decision-free measure of the decision, rather than any specific value of hit or false-alarm rate' (p. 420).

Wood and Jennings[57] have provided the computational details of the procedure. In brief, the accuracy $(A)$ of the subject (where $A$ ranges from 0 to 1) is plotted as a function of RT. Often the symbol '$A$' is replaced by '$h_t$' which represents, in a truer sense, the amount of information transmitted by the subject to the experimenter – for the sake of simplicity, I shall persist with '$A$'. $A$ is represented on the ordinate and RT on the abscissa. The complete speed–accuracy trade-off function can be divided into a minimum of three regions. (1) A period of time on the abscissa during which accuracy varies around chance. In Figure 6.4, this is when $RT < t_1$ and $A = 0$. Some authors (Edwards[58]) assume that the upper bound of this region, $t_1$, approximates the mean RT required for simple detection of the stimuli involved when no choice response is required. (2) A second phase during which accuracy rises as a linear function of RT such that $t_1 < RT < t_2$. (3) A final asymptotic phase such that $RT < t_2$ and $A = 1$. The third region includes those instances when subjects are error free (i.e. 100% accurate). In many studies, this is exactly what the experimenter's instructions specify. The only problem is that the resultant RT is essentially uninterpretable since an infinite number of RTs can result in zero errors[55].

Because the second phase is nearly linear ($A$ increasing as a function of RT), the relationship can be approximated by the linear equation

$$A = m(\mathrm{RT} - c)$$

where $A$ and RT represent measures of accuracy and reaction time respectively, $c$ corresponds to $t_1$ in Figure 6.4 (the intercept of the function with the RT axis at $A = 0$), and $m$ is the slope of the function representing the amount of increase in $A$ for each unit increase in RT. What is so very exciting about the speed–accuracy trade-off function is that the $x$-intercept and slope parameters can be employed as summary statistics to represent the effects of various independent variables.

'On the assumption that a decision process determines the point in time at which perceptual processing is terminated and a response is selected, the trade-off function is used to obtain a decision-free estimate of the perceptual process, in the same sense that the response operating characteristic function in signal detection experiments is employed as a decision-free measure of detection. Identical trade-off functions across experimental conditions imply that any systematic differences in either choice RT or accuracy were generated by changes in decision criteria. Trade-off functions that differ across experimental conditions, either in intercept or slope, imply differences in processing efficiency' (Rundell and Williams[59], p. 434).

In the usual signal detection paradigm, in order to trace the ROC curve, several different conditions must be run. In these, the subject is typically asked to vary their criterion for deciding signal presence or absence. In each, errors must occur in order for d' to be calculated. The same principles hold for the determination of the speed–accuracy trade-off function. Wood and Jennings[57] discuss two methods for the generation of these functions.

In the first, termed the 'speed–accuracy trade-off function' (SATF), a set of experimental conditions is established that manipulate the subjects' speed–accuracy criteria over a wide range. In one condition subjects might be asked to 'go as fast as possible without concern for error'. At the other extreme, subjects might be asked 'to be as accurate as possible, without concern for speed'. A third condition might ask the subject to balance the two. Other experiments might manipulate rewards and pay-offs, such that in one condition, subjects are rewarded for speed and only minimally penalized for error and vice versa in other conditions. In these examples, payment is usually dependent on RT falling within a certain range (or accuracy falling above a certain limit). In this multiple-condition design, a minimum of two conditions are required (although it is far more common to see many more) to develop the SATF.

The second major type of speed–accuracy trade-off function is called the 'conditional accuracy function' (CAF). This function is formally defined as the conditional probability of a correct response given that RT equals a particular value $t$, computed at all values of $t$. Usually within an experiment, the single-trial RTs are ranked from fastest to slowest, partitioning the data into equal-$N$ categories and plotting accuracy against mean RT for each RT category. Such a procedure requires only a single condition, the function being computed from a single RT distribution. In these instances, the experimenter's instructions usually inform the subject to maintain an error rate at some level well above chance (e.g. 75% accuracy). While the CAF offers the advantage that it is probably less time consuming than the SATF and is certainly less demanding in terms of experimental complexity, it has certain disadvantages. The CAF approximates the SATF-generated data only if the subject maintains a constant speed–accuracy criterion across the experimental trials. The problem with this assumption is that it is difficult to test empirically. Let us see how the use of the speed–accuracy trade-off function might radically alter our interpretation of our data.

## Alcohol and the Speed–accuracy Trade-off

Alcohol is a rather commonly used drug. It should produce a depressant effect on the CNS. A series of studies indicate, however, that at least under some conditions mean RT is unaffected by even quite high doses of alcohol. Tharp et al.[60] have replicated this finding but also noted that under the influence of alcohol, error rates increase. Rundell and Williams[59] reasoned that what might really be happening is that alcohol affects the speed–accuracy criterion of the subject. Under the influence of alcohol, subjects trade-off accuracy for speed. In their study, subjects were engaged in either an auditory pitch discrimination task or a side discrimination task (determine whether the auditory stimulus was delivered to the right or left ear). In different conditions subjects were asked to emphasize accuracy, speed or somewhere in between. On different days, dosage was varied. The results indicated that alcohol had no significant effect on mean RT, the difference between the placebo and the highest dose being about 4 ms for the side discrimination task and about 12 ms for the pitch discrimination task. Accuracy declined significantly from 0.88 in the placebo to 0.84 in the high dose condition. This is not a very large difference nor were the effects on RT particularly large. Yet when a sophisticated analysis of the speed–accuracy trade-off function is employed (Figure 6.5), the effect becomes much clearer. Alcohol significantly decreased the slope of the trade-off function but did not affect the intercept values at $H_t = 0$. Alcohol therefore appears to cause a deficit in processing efficiency. When speed is sacrificed at a cost of accuracy, alcohol has no effect. When relatively slow but accurate responding is required, RT will be noticeably slowed. We can be reasonably certain that since the $x$-intercept was unaffected, simple motor speed probably cannot account for the findings. Even granted the sophistication of this form of analysis, it is still quite difficult to determine at which stage of processing – stimulus evaluation or response production – alcohol has its effects.

## ERPs and the Speed–accuracy Trade-off

In 1977, Kutas, McCarthy and Donchin[61] manipulated the P3–RT latency relationship by requiring subjects to perform simple or complex semantic categorizations to detect target stimuli. In different conditions, instructions

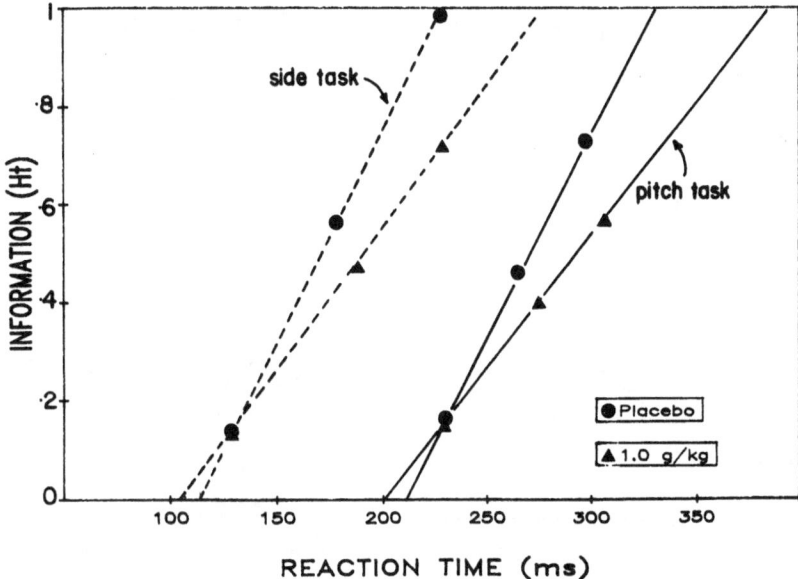

*Figure 6.5    Effects of alcohol and task on the speed–accuracy trade-off function (after Rundell and Williams[59]). The slopes of side and pitch tasks are indicated by dashed and solid lines respectively. Alcohol decreases the slope of the trade-off function in both tasks but has no effect on the intercept (where $H_t = 0$)*

were altered so as to put emphasis on speed or accuracy. Under speed conditions RT often occurred before the peak of P3. Inevitably, subjects made errors. Under accuracy conditions, both RT and P3 latency were delayed, but RT much more so than P3. Typically, RT was well after the peak of P3. In short, the speed–accuracy manipulation has its major effects on RT and had only a small effect on P3. We have obtained essentially the same results here in Ottawa. Figure 6.6 provides sample data from one subject in a speed–accuracy type experiment. The subject was presented with a 'standard' stimulus on 70% of the trials and at random on the other 30% of the trials, a 1500 Hz 'target'. She was asked to press one button in response to the presentation of the standard and press another button in response to the target. In different conditions, emphasis was placed on either speed ('go as fast as possible, having minimal concern for error') or accuracy ('be as accurate as possible, avoiding error'). In the accuracy conditions, detection rates were approximately 0.98, these falling to 0.60 in the speed conditions. Mean RT to the standard and target stimuli was 308 and 352 ms respectively when accuracy was stressed and 179 and 253 ms when speed was stressed. As may be noted P3 was only slightly affected by the experimental instructions, it being slightly earlier (295 ms) in the speed compared to the accuracy (322 ms) conditions. In these conditions, RT often occurred well before the peak of P3. When the emphasis was placed on accuracy, RT usually occurred at the peak of P3 or slightly later.

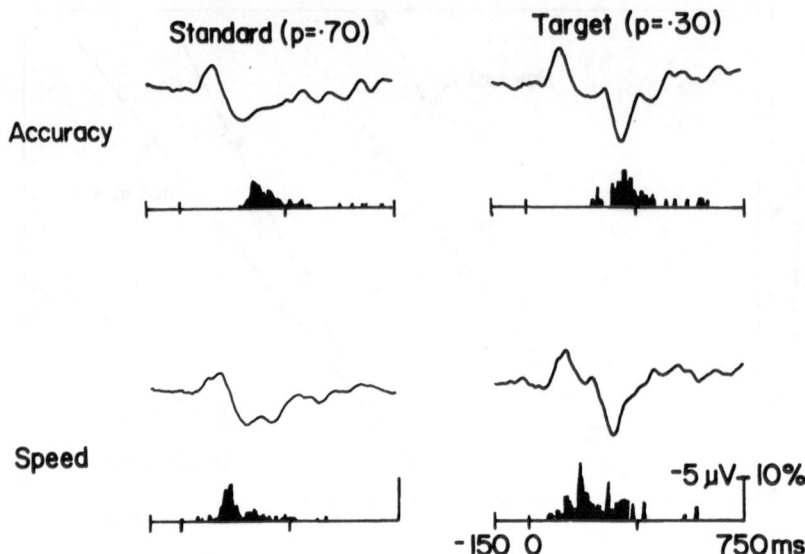

*Figure 6.6   Event-related potentials and the speed–accuracy trade-off. In an oddball task, subjects were asked to button press upon detection of either a frequent standard or a rare, target tone pip. In one condition, emphasis was on speed while in another on accuracy. Data are from one subject (NC). RT distributions (in 10 ms bins) to correctly detected stimuli are presented along the time base. The responses are much faster to the frequently presented standards and show a definite shift in the speed condition. By contrast the physiological data are only minimally affected by the manipulations*

Again, the evidence suggests that RT and P3 may be measuring very different aspects of cognitive processing. RT encompasses all the processes leading to a cognitive decision and behavioural response, whereas P3 latency is largely determined by the duration of stimulus evaluation processes, independent of response selection and execution. The implication of this study should not be overlooked: *while the speed–accuracy trade-off may have a very large effect on mean RT, its effect is almost entirely on processes mediating response production.* Thus, if the researcher is primarily interested in processes leading to and including stimulus evaluation, a very major constraint of the RT measure can be circumvented by the use of the physiological index, the latency to P3. The example of the ingestion of alcohol will again be employed to illustrate the point. As already observed, depending on the task at hand, alcohol may slow RT. This could be due to a slowing of either stimulus evaluation or response selection processes.

It has already been established that mean RT by itself is essentially an uninterpretable measure, without parallel measures of error rates. The calculation of the speed–accuracy trade-off function is cumbersome. It is also time-consuming . . . and in the end, the researcher is still not certain of the interpretation of the data. The physiological measure, P3, takes only a few minutes to obtain. It is minimally affected by subjective strategies favouring speed or accuracy. On the other hand, the response is complex and the cost to obtain the recording quite expensive. Roxane Marois, Lin Arcand and I[62] decided to examine the effects of alcohol on endogenous evoked potentials. To give credit where it is due, we were certainly not unique in this field. A good part of our rationale comes from the exploratory work of Pfefferbaum, Roth and their colleagues in Palo Alto, in California. Roth et al.[63] had noted that even though alcohol has been reported to decrease the subject's ability to sustain attention, the amplitude of N1 appeared to be unaffected. Their task was one that made rather heavy demands on the subject. In simpler tasks, the same laboratory did report an attenuation of N1 following ingestion of alcohol[64]. We decided to manipulate task difficulty and to determine its influence on the N1 and P3 waveforms. Subjects participated in the now familiar 'oddball' paradigm in which they were asked to detect a rare target occurring amongst a much more frequently occurring standard stimulus, a 1025 Hz tone pip. In the difficult task, the target was only slightly different from the standard, the target's frequency being 1100 Hz. In the easy task, target frequency was set at 2000 Hz. As Figure 6.7 indicates, we essentially replicated the Stanford group's data. During the difficult task, the amplitude of N1 was unaffected by even heavy doses of alcohol. In contrast, during easy detections, N1 was attenuated following ingestion. Performance, in terms of the number of correct detections, was unaffected. Therefore, if our N1 is a reflection of the subject's level of attention (and we admit that it may not be since we did not directly manipulate it, rather it was inferred on the basis of our results), the decline of N1 in easy tasks is probably without serious consequence. As the level of difficulty increases, it appears that subjects may be able to draw upon compensatory effort to maintain performance. With respect to P3, an interaction with task difficulty was again found, such that it was unaltered in difficult tasks and was significantly attenuated in easy ones following ingestion of alcohol. The amplitude of P3 may provide an index of certainty of the previously made decision[65]. The decline in its amplitude in the easy task may thus be an indication of the subjects' equivocation perhaps as a consequence of their inability to sustain attention. Now the key issue – the latency of P3. Although slight differences were noted in some conditions following the ingestion of alcohol, none were significant. This suggests that stimulus evaluation processes remain more or less unaffected by alcohol intoxication. We would agree with Tharp, Rundell, Lester and Williams[60] and Huntley[66] that alcohol probably impairs output of cognitive processes associated with response selection rather than input of processes involved with stimulus evaluation.

## ALTERNATE METHODS OF ANALYSIS OF RT DATA

Most authors that use speed–accuracy trade-off functions group correct and error RTs together. Other authors believe that the errors are by themselves extremely informative and should therefore be treated separately.

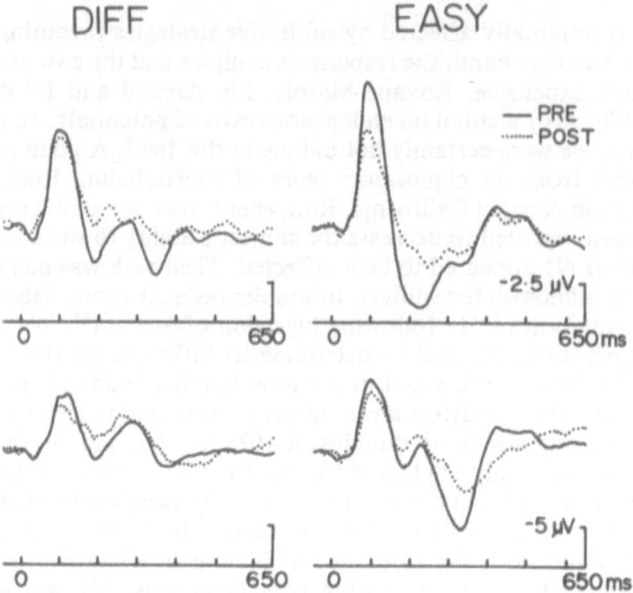

*Figure 6.7   Effects of alcohol on event-related potentials. Subjects were engaged in an oddball task in which the rarely presented target was either difficult or easy to detect. The grand average of the standard (upper portion) and target (lower portion) evoked potentials is illustrated prior to and following the ingestion of 1.1 ml/kg of pure ethanol. Note the different calibration signals. Alcohol appeared to have its largest effects during easy conditions. The standard N1 and the target P3 are attenuated following ingestion. There is, however, only a slight, non-significant shift in P3 latency*

Link in a series of articles[56, 67, 68] has discussed the importance of error to understand the strategy adopted by the subject. Indeed, any suitable experiment will be designed to allow errors to occur. A very elaborate method using the error RT to generate corrections that produce orderly data is described. Although the mathematical computations are beyond the scope of this chapter, it should be mentioned that Link, unlike most psychologists, does not believe errors are additive components of the measured response, but rather suggests they occur as a result of imperfect mental processing. Furthermore, they are not normally distributed. With detailed investigation of response–time distributions, a better view of the underlying psychological processes can be obtained. A very major practical consideration is that for the model to be adequately employed, several thousand trials are often required. Another obvious limitation to Link's models is their mathematical complexity. Link may, in fact, be a victim of his own making. Because the model is so complex, it remains largely untested. As such, there is little empirical evidence to support the model and until this evidence is furnished, it will probably not meet with common appeal.

A better known theorist, Rabbitt[69, 70], shares Link's concerns for error and, moreover, the consequence of error. Rabbitt has examined the mechanisms whereby subjects attain over long series of trials a balance between speed and accuracy. It is known that over time, with practice, RT becomes shorter. How is this possible if one assumes a rigid, invariant psychological system of processing? Rabbitt argues that if the subject is to comply with the ambiguous instructions provided by the experimenter ('Go as fast as possible, but avoid error'), and yet still improve speed, some form of trial-by-trial tracking mechanism must be operating. He suggests that subjects, in some instances, may respond faster and faster until they respond too quickly and an error occurs. After recognizing the error, on the next trial, subjects slow down but in the ensuing trials again pick up speed until another error is made. With practice, most subjects can 'learn' a safe, efficient region in which speed is at an optimum and error at a minimum. Thus, in any particular experiment, it is the commission, recognition and correction of errors which permits the efficient compromise between speed and accuracy. As should be obvious, the use of the overall mean RT statistic completely masks these operations. An overall slow mean RT could be due to a number of factors, including simple inefficiency even though the subject may be capable of responding much more rapidly. The study of individual differences must take into account the fact that certain, but not all, subjects are able to internally monitor the accuracy of their responses if they are to avoid making errors. As such, they must be able to detect their errors and recognize what response should have been made. Secondly, these subjects must be able to monitor their speed of responding if they are to discriminate between responses that differ in speed. Finally, these subjects must not only be able to monitor speed and accuracy, but be able to regulate or adjust speed of responding within relatively narrow RT limits, if high accuracy is to be maintained. It is indeed possible that different groups of subjects may be more efficient or inefficient in carrying out some or all of the steps implied by this sort of task.

The attraction of Rabbitt's model is that it allows an understanding of how, on a trial-to-trial basis, RT can be quite variable until individuals discover the fastest but safest bands. In this context, one is reminded of the Kutas et al. study[61]. Often RT occurred before P3. This suggests that response production was initiated before stimulus evaluation was complete. Thus, response processes can be based on minimum evidence. As such, the likelihood of error will be far greater than if response production begins after the completion of stimulus evaluation. To date, a physiological examination of Rabbitt's model has not been carried out. It is difficult therefore to determine whether the trial-to-trial fluctuation represents alterations in processes underlying stimulus evaluation or response production or perhaps a combination of both. I rather suspect that at least after a few trials when templates or referents of the stimuli have developed, stimulus evaluation processes will likely remain constant. Response production may, on the other hand, be quite variant.

The goal of this chapter was to present an overview of behavioural techniques that have been developed to provide for a full understanding of the data contained in a typical RT experiment. Certainly, measures of central tendency such as the mean or the median may obscure or distort the significance of the findings. In cases in which subjects make few errors, an accurate interpretation of the mean RT may be difficult if not impossible to provide. Trial-to-trial variation in RT may serve to skew the overall distribution. This is especially important for the consideration of group differences. One group's responses may be skewed in a direction completely opposite to that of a second group. The mean RT can offer very little in the way of an understanding of a stage analysis of information processing. RT may be affected by an almost infinite number of factors. It provides a composite measure of the time required for the completion of both stimulus evaluation and response production processes. The addition of event-related potentials to the battery of cognitive measures provides an additional source of information. Certain of these potentials (for example, Nd) appear to be affected by manipulations in the subject's level of attention. A late positive component, P3, appears to be related to the time required for the completion of stimulus evaluation processes. On the other hand, P3 appears to be far less dependent on processes related to response production. Thus, by combining the behavioural and physiological indices, RT and P3 respectively, it should be possible to obtain metrics of the time required for both stimulus evaluation and response production. Chapter 7 will demonstrate how the combined use of both RT and P3 can markedly alter the interpretation of between-group differences in the speed of information processing.

## References

1. Donders, F. C. (1969). On the speed of mental processes. In Koster, W. G. (ed.) *Attention and Performance II*. pp. 412–31. (Amsterdam: North-Holland)
2. Taylor, D. A. (1976). Stage analysis of reaction time. *Psychol. Bull.*, **83**, 161–91
3. Christie, L. S. and Luce, R. D. (1956). Decision structure and time relations in simple choice behavior. *Bull. Math. Biophys.*, **18**, 89–112
4. Sternberg, S. (1969). The discovery of processing stages: extension of Donders' method. In Koster, W. G. (ed.) *Attention and Performance II*. pp. 276–315. (Amsterdam: North-Holland)
5. Posner, M. I. (1978). *Chronometric Explorations of Mind*. (Hillsdale, NJ: Erlbaum)
6. McLelland, J. R. (1979). On time relations and mental processes: a framework for analyzing processes in cascade. *Psychol. Rev.*, **86**, 287–330
7. Grice, G. R., Nullmeyer, R. and Spiker, V. A. (1982). Human reaction time: toward a general theory. *J. Exp. Psychol.: Gen.*, **111**, 135–53
8. Miller, J. (1982). Discrete versus continuous stage models of human information processing: in search of partial output. *J. Exp. Psychol.: Hum. Percept. Perform.*, **8**, 273–96
9. Egeth, H. E. (1966). Parallel versus serial processes in multidimensional stimulus discrimination. *Percept. Psychophys.*, **1**, 674–98
10. Smith, E. E. (1968). Choice reaction time: an analysis of the major theoretical positions. *Psychol. Bull.*, **69**, 77–110
11. Townsend, J. T. (1974). Issues and models concerning the processing of a finite number of inputs. In Kantowitz, B. H. (ed.) *Human Information Processing: Tutorials in Performance and Cognition*. pp. 133–85. (Potomac, Md.: Erlbaum)
12. Welford, A. T. (1960). The measurement of sensory-motor performance. Survey and reappraisal of twelve years' progress. *Ergonomics*, **3**, 189–230
13. Theois, J. (1975). The components of response latency in simple human information processing tasks. In Rabbitt, P. M. A. and Dornic, S. (eds.) *Attention and Performance V*. pp. 418–40. (London: Academic)

14. Lappin, J. S. (1978). The relativity of choice behavior and the effect of prior knowledge on the speed and accuracy of recognition. In Castellan, Jr., N. J. and Restle, F. (eds.) *Cognitive Theory.* Vol. **3**, pp. 179–86. (Hillsdale, NJ: Erlbaum)
15. Picton, T. W. and Hink, R. F. (1974). Evoked potentials: How? What? and Why? *Am. J. EEG Technol.*, **14**, 9–44
16. Vaughan, H. G. (1974). The analysis of scalp-recorded brain potentials. In Thompson, R. F. and Patterson, M. M. (eds.) *Bioelectric Recording Techniques. Part B. Electroencephalography and Human Brain Potentials.* pp. 157–207. (New York: Academic)
17. Glaser, E. M. and Ruchkin, D. S. (1976). *Principles of Neurobiological Signal Analysis.* (New York: Academic)
18. McCallum, W. C. and Curry, S. H. (1981). Late slow wave components of auditory evoked potentials: their cognitive significance and interaction. *Electroenceph. Clin. Neurophysiol.,* **51**, 123–37
19. Picton, T. W., Linden, R. D., Hamel, G. and Maru, J. T. (1983). Aspects of averaging. *Sem. Hearing,* **4**, 327–41
20. Stuss, D. T., Sarazin, F. F., Leech, E. E. and Picton, T. W. (1983). Event-related potentials during naming and mental rotation. *Electroenceph. Clin. Neurophys.,* **56**, 133–46
21. Davis, H. (1976). Principles of electric response audiometry. *Ann. Oto. Supp.,* **28**, 4–96
22. Hillyard, S. A., Picton, T. W. and Regan, D. (1978). Sensation, perception and attention. In Callaway, E., Tueting, P. and Koslow, S. (eds.) *Event-Related Brain Potentials in Man.* pp. 223–321. (New York: Academic)
23. Magliero, A., Bashore, T. R., Coles, M. G. H. and Donchin, E. (1984). On the dependence of P300 latency on stimulus evaluation processes. *Psychopysiology,* **21**, 171–86
24. Donchin, E. (1981). Surprise! ... Surprise? *Psychophysiology,* **18**, 493–513
25. Picton, T. W. and Hillyard, S. A. (1974). Human auditory evoked potentials. II. Effects of attention. *Electroenceph. Clin. Neurophysiol.,* **36**, 191–9
26. Picton, T. W., Campbell, K. B., Baribeau-Braun, J. and Proulx, G. B. (1978). The neurophysiology of human attention: a tutorial review. In Requin, J. (ed.) *Attention and Performance VII.* pp. 429–67. (Hillsdale, NJ: Erlbaum)
27. Campbell, K. B. and Bartoli, E. A. (1986). Human auditory evoked potentials during natural sleep: the early components. *Electroenceph. Clin. Neurophysiol.* (In press)
28. Salamy, A. and McKean, C. M. (1977). Habituation and dishabituation of cortical and brainstem evoked potentials. *Int. J. Neurosci.,* **7**, 175–82
29. Lukas, J. H. (1981). Human auditory attention: the olivo-cochlear bundle may function as a peripheral filter. *Psychophysiology,* **17**, 444–52
30. Picton, T. W., Stapells, D. R. and Campbell, K. B. (1981). Auditory evoked potentials from the human cochlea and brainstem, *J. Otolaryngol.,* **10** (suppl. 9), 1–41
31. Desmedt, J. E. and Robertson, D. (1977). Differential enhancement of early and late components of the cerebral somatosensory evoked potentials during forced-paced cognitive tasks in man. *J. Physiol. (Lond.),* **271**, 761–82
32. Harkins, S. W. and Lenhardt, M. (1980). Brainstem auditory evoked potentials in the elderly. In Poon, L. W. (ed.) *Aging in the 1980s.* (Washington: American Psychological Association)
33. Goff, W. R., Matsumiya, Y., Allison, T. and Goff, G. D. (1969). Cross-modality comparisons of averaged evoked potentials. In Donchin, E. and Lindsley, D. B. (eds.) *Average Evoked Potentials. Methods, Results and Evaluations.* pp. 95–141. (Washington: NASA SP-191)
34. Hillyard, S. A., Hink, R. F., Schwent, V. L. and Picton, T. W. (1973). Electrical signs of selective attention in the human brain. *Science,* **182**, 177–80
35. Naatanen, R. and Mitchie, P. T. (1979). Early selective attention effects on the evoked potential: a critical review and reinterpretation. *Biol. Psychol.,* **8**, 81–136
36. Hansen, J. C. and Hillyard, S. A. (1980). Endogenous brain potentials associated with selective auditory attention. *Electroenceph. Clin. Neurophysiol.,* **49**, 277–80
37. Broadbent, D. E. (1970). Stimulus set and response set: two kinds of selective attention. In Mostofsky, D. I. (ed.) *Attention: Contemporary Theory and Analysis.* pp. 51–60. (New York: Appleton-Century-Crofts)
38. Treisman, A. M. (1969). Strategies and modes of selective attention. *Psychol. Rev.,* **76**, 282–99
39. Ritter, W., Simson, R. and Vaughan, Jr., H. G. (1979). A brain event related to the making of a sensory discrimination. *Science,* **203**, 1358–61

40. Naatanen, R., Simpson, M. and Loveless, N. M. (1982). Stimulus deviance and event-related brain potentials. *Biol. Psychol.*, **14**, 53–98
41. Donchin, E., Ritter, W. and McCallum, W. C. (1978). Cognitive psychophysiology: the endogenous components of the ERP. In Callaway, E., Tueting, P. and Koslow, S. (eds.) *Event-Related Brain Potentials in Man.* pp. 349–441. (New York: Academic)
42. Pritchard, W. S. (1981). Psychophysiology of P300. *Psychol. Bull.*, **89**, 506–40
43. Tueting, P., Sutton, S. and Zubin, S. (1971). Quantitative evoked potential correlates of the probability of events. *Psychophysiology*, **7**, 385–94
44. Duncan-Johnson, C. C. and Donchin, E. (1977). On quantifying surprise: the variation of event-related potentials with subjective probability. *Psychophysiology*, **14**, 456–67
45. Campbell, K. B., Courchesne, E., Picton, T. W. and Squires, K. C. (1979). Evoked potential correlates of human information processing. *Biol. Psychol.*, **8**, 45–68
46. McCarthy, G. and Donchin, E. (1981). A metric for thought: a comparison of P300 latency and reaction time. *Science*, **211**, 77–80
47. Duncan-Johnson, C. C. and Kopell, B. S. (1981). The Stroop effect: brain potentials localize the source of interference. *Science*, **214**, 938–40
48. Duncan-Johnson, C. C. and Donchin, E. The P300 component of the event-related brain potential as an index of information processing. *Biol. Psychol.*, **14**, 1–52
49. Biederman, I. and Zachary, R. A. (1970). Stimulus versus response probability effects in choice reaction time. *Percept. Psychophys.*, **7**, 189–92
50. Miller, J. O. and Pachella, R. G. (1973). Locus of the stimulus probability effect. *J. Exp. Psychol*, **101**, 227–31
51. Hinrichs, J. V. and Krainz, P. L. (1970). Expectancy in choice reaction time: anticipation of stimulus or response. *J. Exp. Psychol.*, **85**, 330–4
52. Miller, J. O. and Pachella, R. G. (1976). Encoding processes in memory scanning tasks. *Mem. Cognit.*, **4**, 29–34
53. Rabbitt, P. M. A. (1959). Effects of independent variations in stimulus and response probability. *Nature*, **183**, 1212
54. Lappin, J. S. and Disch, K. (1972). The latency operating characteristic: I. Effects of stimulus probability on choice reaction time. *J. Exp. Psychol.*, **92**, 419–27
55. Pachella, R. G. (1974). The interpretation of reaction time in information processing research. In Kantowitz, B. (ed.) *Human Information Processing: Tutorials in Performance and Cognition.* pp. 41–82. (New York: Erlbaum)
56. Link, S. W. (1975). The relative judgment theory of two-choice response time. *J. Math. Psychol.*, **12**, 114–35
57. Wood, C. C. and Jennings, J. R. (1976). Speed–accuracy tradeoff functions in choice reaction time: experimental designs and computational procedures. *Percept. Psychophys.*, **19**, 92–101
58. Edwards, W. (1965). Optimal strategies for seeking information: models for statistics, choice reaction times, and human information processing. *J. Math. Psychol.*, **2**, 312–29
59. Rundell, O. H. and Williams, H. L. (1979). Alcohol and speed–accuracy tradeoff. *Hum. Factors*, **21**, 433–43
60. Tharp, V. K., Rundell, O. H., Lester, B. K. and Williams, H. L. (1974). Alcohol and information processing. *Psychopharmacol. (Berlin)*, **40**, 33–52
61. Kutas, M., McCarthy, G. and Donchin, E. (1977). Augmenting mental chronometry: The P300 as a measure of stimulus evaluation time. *Science*, **197**, 792–5
62. Campbell, K. B., Marois, R. and Arcand, L. (1984). Ethanol and the event-related potentials: effects of rate of stimulus presentation and task difficulty. *Ann. NY Acad. Sci.*, **425**, 551–5
63. Roth, W. T., Tinklenberg, J. and Kopell, B. S. (1977). Ethanol and marijuana effects on event-related potentials in a memory retrieval paradigm. *Electroenceph. Clin. Neurophysiol.*, **42**, 381–8
64. Pfefferbaum, A., Roth, W. T., Tinklenberg, J., Rosenbloom, M. and Kopell, B. (1979). The effects of alcohol and meperidine on auditory evoked potentials. *Drug and Alcohol Dependence*, **4**, 371–80
65. Ruchkin, D. S. and Sutton, S. (1978). Equivocation and P300 amplitude. In Otto, D. (ed.) *Multidisciplinary Perspectives in Event-Related Brain Potential Research* pp. 175–8. (Washington: EPA-600/9-77-043)

66. Huntley, M. S. (1972). Influence of alcohol and S-R uncertainty upon spatial localization time. *Psychopharmacol. (Berlin)*, **27**, 131–40
67. Link, S. W. (1981). Correcting response measures for guessing and partial information. *Psychol. Bull.*, **92**, 469–86
68. Link, S. W. and Tindall, A. D. (1971). Speed and accuracy in comparative judgments of line length. *Percept. Psychophys.*, **9**, 284–8
69. Rabbitt, P. M. A. (1979). How young and old subjects monitor and control responses for accuracy and speed. *Br. J. Psychol.*, **70**, 305–11
70. Rabbitt, P. M. A. (1981). Sequential reactions. In Holding, D. H. (ed.) *Human Skills.* pp. 153–75. (London: Wiley)

# 7

# Mental chronometry.
# II. Individual differences

## *Kenneth B. Campbell and*
## *Nancy Noldy-Cullum*

The previous chapter examined problems in the interpretation of RT data purported to serve as an index of the speed of decision-making. Alternative methods of analysis and the possibility of the inclusion of recent developments in the physiological realm were stressed. The present chapter will examine the issue of group differences in RT. We shall draw upon a sampling of studies that have purported to have found group differences in 'speed of information processing'. The sampling of topics is anything but complete. They reflect areas of personal interest. Included in this discussion will be a review of RT as related to (a) intelligence, (b) extraversion, (c) hyperactivity, (d) brain trauma, and (e) ageing. As will become apparent, most researchers in these areas have at least given some consideration to 'non-cognitive' factors affecting RT. Many authors realize that part of the overall duration of RT is spent in making the overt motor response. To control for the time required for the motor reaction, a 'movement time' (MT) measure is often included in the analysis of RT. In the usual choice RT experiment, subjects are told to respond to one of a number of stimuli by pressing a corresponding button or lever. Their finger is often placed upon a 'home' button from which they move to the appropriate 'signal' button after presentation of the stimulus and once their decisions have been made. RT thus consists of the time required to decide which stimulus was presented – 'decision time' or DT and the time it takes to select the appropriate button and move to it – MT. On the other hand, few authors appear to make distinctions between stimulus evaluation and response selection processes or the effects of the speed–accuracy trade-off. Even basic assumptions such as equal group motivation, level of attention and sensory functioning are rarely considered.

## INTELLIGENCE

The idea that an individual's intelligence can be measured by his reaction time is one of the oldest and most controversial in psychology. From a common-sense, folklore point of view, it might be reasonable. Robert Sternberg[1], as part of his recent development of a theory of intelligence, asked people to list behaviours characteristic of intelligent persons. Behaviours such as 'learns rapidly', 'acts quickly', 'talks quickly' and 'makes judgements quickly' were commonly listed. This form of logic has proven to be the rationale for many of the RT studies of intelligence. More recently, as will be mentioned later in this section, a similar line of reasoning has been applied to the latency of various components of the evoked potential. Sternberg, however, questions this common, street assumption. Reflective rather than impulsive cognitive style tends to be associated with more intelligent problem-solving performance. In a study of planning behaviour in problem-solving, it was found that more intelligent persons tend to spend relatively more time on global (higher-order) planning and relatively less time on local (lower-order) planning. In contrast, the less intelligent seem to emphasize local rather than global planning. What matters, therefore, is not the total time spent, but rather distribution of this time across the various kinds of planning one can do.

Jensen[2], in the same article, provided a commentary to Sternberg. He points out that there is indeed a common belief that 'quick-witted' people are quite bright. On the other hand, some of the world's most creative individuals who undoubtedly would fall into the 'genius' category on today's IQ tests were apparently 'slow thinkers'. The examples of Darwin, Einstein and Beethoven are given. One could also cite Flaubert, the French writer who laboured over every word, phrase and sentence of his beautifully written (although some would say, incoherent) novels. Jensen points out that indeed in complex tasks such as items in Raven's Progressive Matrices, the correlation between individual differences in response latency to test items and psychometric intelligence is almost nil. On the other hand, in very simple cognitive tasks, there does appear to be some correlation with psychometric intelligence.

Behavioural Measures

In general, simple perceptual tasks have been employed within an information-processing framework. Many studies use timed measures (such as RT), rather than number correct, 'since the tasks are so simple or well practised that most can perform them without error'[3].

Galton[4] more than a century ago found only very low correlations between intelligence and keypress RT. Admittedly, this was a simple RT task (only one stimulus). With the advent of the theory of information processing and the increasing sophistication of experimental psychology, the issue returned. Jensen and Munro[5] provided subjects with 30 trials on one-, two-, four-, six- or eight-choice tasks. The correlations were reasonably high, particularly for choice RT. In the six-choice task, the correlation between DT and intelligence was $-0.49$. A later study[6] examined differences in DT and MT in almost 800 subjects, ranging from the retarded to university students. The correlations were mainly in the $-0.30$ to $-0.40$ range. A number of other investigators[7-9] have subsequently replicated these findings, the correlations running from $-0.30$ to $-0.80$.

148

One of the many problems with these studies is the use of individuals whose IQ is sufficiently low as to warrant a diagnosis of mental retardation. Such individuals are slower than non-retarded individuals on a number of tasks[10]. Nettelbeck and Kirby[11] tested choice RT in almost 200 subjects, including retarded, non-retarded and above-average non-retarded individuals. Their correlations were remarkably similar to those that had already been reported in the literature. However, when the extremely high or low IQ scorers were excluded, the correlations dropped significantly. Furthermore, when those with IQs below 85 were excluded, the correlations fell to near zero! In short, both in their work and in previous studies, the modest correlations that were found were, in any case, probably inflated due to the inclusion of retarded subjects.

Another serious methodological question arises from the finding that low IQ subjects generally have RT distributions that are much more variable than those with high IQs. What does this mean? In almost all studies errors are rare or virtually non-existent. As mentioned previously, this makes interpretation extremely difficult. It could be, for example, that low IQ subjects adopt a strategy for responding that is completely different from their colleagues. They may emphasize accuracy at a cost of speed. It might be that the less intelligent are less motivated by the boring and monotonous tasks given to them. Nettelbeck and Brewer[12] have suggested that the evidence points to mentally retarded individuals being characterized by a general attentional deficit, with impairment of those executive processes that direct attention to the different features of the processing operation. Therefore, is their RT slowed because they are less intelligent or because they are less attentive to the task at hand? Carlson, Jensen and Widaman[9] have tested this possibility. Their findings did indeed suggest that the less intelligent were also less attentive, perhaps explaining their longer RTs.

Brewer and Smith[13] recently conducted a Rabbitt-type trial-by-trial tracking experiment in an attempt to explain the slower and more varied performance of the retarded (illustrated in Figure 7.1). The retarded were able to discriminate errors, either overtly or covertly. On error + 1 trials, their RTs slowed significantly, indicative that an error had been recognized and corrective behaviour undertaken. On the other hand, the retarded were less efficient at constraining RTs within safe, fast RT bands. They were frequently observed to undershoot RT levels that should have been tracked on error + 1 trials and to also frequently overshoot RT levels that should have been tracked when making downward RT adjustments on subsequent posterior trials (i.e. error + 2 ... error + 5 ...). 'This combination of under- and over-shooting produced local regions of inaccurate responding prejudicial to the maintenance of low error rates. In compensating for these localized error regions, retarded subjects adjusted RT levels to track bands that allow sequences of error-free responding. In so doing, retarded subjects generally tracked relatively fast, safe RT bands' (p.89). There thus appear to be differences between retarded and non-retarded subjects in the way trial-to-trial RT adjustments are made. Once again, the evidence suggests that a simple measure of central tendency such as the mean or median RT would completely mask these differences. The point is not that the retarded cannot respond rapidly. Rather, they apparently fail to profit from past experience – rapid responding in even simple choice RT tasks demands that the subject

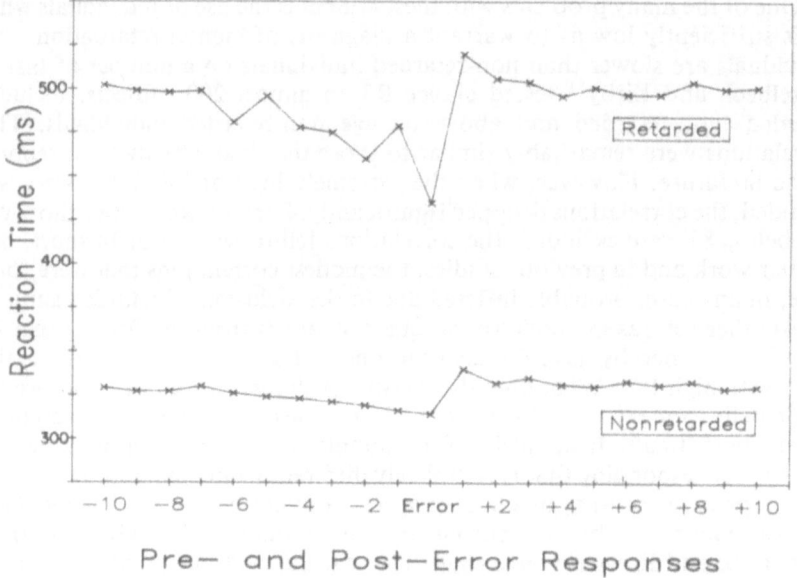

*Figure 7.1 Average median RT for correct responses of retarded (upper) and non-retarded (lower) subjects on the ten trials preceding and following error (after Brewer and Smith[13]). The RT pattern of both groups shows a gradual speeding of RT until an error is made. On the trial following the error, subjects tend to be much more cautious with a resultant slowing of RT. These data indicate that the retarded, either overtly or covertly, are able to recognize errors, and take compensatory action. Note, however, that prior to the error, the slope of the retarded group is steeper than that for the non-retarded, perhaps pointing to an inefficient mode of processing*

monitor both RT and accuracy of previous trials. Based on these and other findings in their studies, Brewer and Smith suggest that differences in intelligence reflect differences with respect to the availability, sophistication and proficiency of usage of information-processing strategies. In many ways, these notions are quite similar to Sternberg's belief that less intelligent behaviour is characterized by impulsive, lower-order responding whereas more intelligent behaviour is reflective, relying on higher-order planning.

In spite of the elegance (and necessity) of this form of analysis, it is difficult to identify where, in the flow of information processing, differences in intelligent behaviour begin to be manifested. It is, for example, not really possible to conclude whether there are differences at the level of stimulus evaluation or perhaps later, at the time of the organization of response processes. To date, there has been little attempt to apply cognitive evoked potentials (for example, P3) to this problem, although as discussed in the following paragraphs, earlier components have been used (perhaps inappropriately) for this purpose.

150

## Physiological Measures

One of the earliest and most controversial uses of the evoked potential technique has been as an attempt to demonstrate 'biological' causality in individuals varying in IQ. A major question that has arisen over the many years of intelligence testing is whether intelligence is genetically or culturally (environmentally) determined. Various psychometric tests have been devised to measure intelligence, but they are often culture bound. Even the so-called culture-free tests (such as Raven's Progressive Matrices) have been demonstrated to be influenced by environmental factors. The event-related potential would appear to provide a measure that is truly culture-free. In the early days of evoked potential research, Ertl[14] here at the University of Ottawa published the findings that the latency of the major components in the 100–250 ms range of the visual evoked potential correlated significantly ($r = -0.3$) with IQ. Ertl reasoned that the latency of a particular component served as an index of the speed of information processing – intelligent individuals are those who are able to solve problems quickly. As will become apparent in a later section, a similar sort of logic has been used with behavioural RT measurements. Given that the dependent measures were biological in nature, it was concluded that an 'objective', biological measure of intelligence was observed. Later studies have indicated that the IQ-evoked potential relationship is highly dependent on the age, sex and race of the subject, the modality and intensity of the stimulus and the evoked potential component under question. There is always the possibility that non-cerebral sources might have contributed to the results. Recall that it is always preferable to assume the negative – unless proven otherwise, the waveform is probably of a non-cerebral origin, due to some artifact. Children of low intelligence might not have followed instructions to refrain from movement, from blinking, and so forth. Simultaneous recordings from artifact monitors were not provided. Moreover, Ertl does not offer any evidence that low IQ children's visual gaze was actually fixated on the stimulus. The evoked potential data might have been more convincing had replicate waveforms been provided. Given the present knowledge of the endogenous influences on these waveforms (particularly the influence of selective attention), the possibility that non-sensory factors such as the subject's level of attention might account for the findings cannot be ruled out. By this, it is not implied that there should be no relationship between intelligence and attention. It may well be that intelligent children are able to sustain attention for longer periods than less intelligent children. Few would, however, claim that the two should be equated. It is certain that the child's level of attention may vary, yet his level of intelligence remains constant.

More recent studies have employed different types of physiological measurement: its amplitude, asymmetry or variability[15–17]. Robinson[18] has used complex visual steady-state responses at different frequencies of stimulation. Although a number of the physiological assumptions he makes are highly questionable, at least one of his measures, which he labels 'V', does show a small (about 0.35), but significant correlation with some of the subscales of the Wechsler Adult Intelligent Scale. It is claimed that the differences that arise in even these limited number of subscales is due to the mediation of the diffuse thalamocortical system. Even here, however, Robinson's physiological model may well be too simple to be useful, being based on the now outdated proposals of admitted giants, Pavlov and, later, Magoun.

Hendrikson and her colleagues, in a series of studies[19, 20], have proposed a complex theory of the functioning of the nervous system as it relates to intelligence. Their claim that information is coded in complex neuronal pulse codes is very much in keeping with classical neurophysiology. Their explanation of how these pulses relate to intelligence deviates so far from what is known in neurophysiology as to place it in the realm of speculation if not fantasy. Intelligent information processing is characterized by the stability of neuronal pulse trains. They are 'noise-free'. The averaged evoked potential in a very intelligent subject would be quite complex with multiple deflections related to stable pulse-train coding of stimulus information. By contrast, single trial evoked potentials in a less intelligent individual would be less complex (less stable). The average of these noise-induced variable evoked potentials would thus reduce the number and amplitude of the deflections. The averaged evoked potential would thus be 'smoother'. There are various means of measuring the 'complexity' of a waveform. Hendrikson and Hendrikson have opted for what they term a 'string' measure: beginning with peak 1, the distance between it and peak 2 is computed, then the distance between 2 and 3, then 3 and 4 and so forth until the end of the sweep. The sum of the total of these distances shows a correlation of approximately 0.5 with IQ. A correction for attenuation increases the correlation to about 0.8, which more or less equals the reliability of most standard IQ tests and, not to be overlooked, also equals the shared variance between variance in IQ and genetic makeup. (It should however be pointed out that such corrections for attentuation have been seriously questioned[21].) Apart from the fact that the model does not appear to be based on any accepted neurophysiological theory or data, there are also a number of methodological problems that serve to question the validity of possible interpretations. As in many other studies purporting to show a relationship between evoked potentials and IQ, the authors fail to provide convincing evidence that their evoked potentials are indeed cerebral in origin. It is mentioned that the raw EEG was visually scanned for possible sources of artifact. As noted in the Chapter 6, artifact is often hardly visible in the EEG. The objective, presumably computer-based criteria for rejection of a trial are not clear in these studies. Slight changes in muscle or jaw tension could cause the averaged waveform to become quite 'complex' with many peaks and valleys. Perhaps highly intelligent individuals are more restless, fidgety and bored because of monotonous experiments. Hendrikson does not provide sample waveforms from her *own* data in any of her publications. Instead, she draws upon data from only 20 of the many hundreds of subjects that were originally run by Ertl. Artifact monitors are not illustrated. Again, as in many of these sorts of studies, it is never really clear what the subject is doing. They are told to sit still and avoid movement while a series of visual or auditory stimuli are presented. Again, it is possible that highly intelligent persons are more attentive than those that are less intelligent and these differences in the level of attention cause the variation in the evoked potential waveform.

To conclude, there appears to be little solid evidence that evoked potentials are able to provide a measure of intelligence. Futhermore, even if there were evidence that evoked potentials were related to intelligence, simply because the dependent measure is biological in nature does not imply that it is genetically determined. There is little support for the notion that late components of the evoked potential are genetically determined. As well, the physiological differences that exists amongst subjects that vary in intelligence arise at a time when non-sensory influences can affect the evoked potential waveform. The possibility that non-cerebral artifact can account for the findings looms very large. It must be concluded that a great deal more research employing much more sophisticated methodology is required before even a preliminary answer to the issue can be made.

## EXTRAVERSION

There have been relatively few studies of RT related to groups varying in degree of extraversion. Two points of view on the matter might be postulated. Eysenck's original theory[22] was largely centred on sensory input. Introverts were thought to be characterized by an overly active reticular formation – they are thus more sensitive to external input than their opposites, the extraverts. One might also postulate that this being the case, information should therefore be processed more rapidly. If RT is a measure of stimulus evaluation time, then it should occur faster for introverts than for extraverts. On the other hand, extraverts are thought to be more impulsive than introverts. Thus, in the choice RT paradigm, they may emphasize speed more than accuracy. Their mean RTs might therefore be faster than introverts', yet their error rate will be higher. As a result, because RT is a measure of both the timing of stimulus evaluation and response bias processes, predictions of differences due to extraversion are difficult, if not impossible, to make. Over the past decade, John Brebner[23, 24] (see also Chapter 2) has carried out a series of studies and arrived at essentially this point of view:

'. . . if instead of assuming central excitation to derive only from stimulation and inhibition as a consequence of either the absence of stimulation or of high response rates, it is accepted that the central mechanisms are capable of being in one of two different states, excitation or inhibition, and that either can be induced by the demands of stimulus analysis (S-excitation or S-inhibition) or response organization (R-excitation or R-inhibition) acting upon the person' (Brebner and Cooper[25], p. 265).

Introverts tend to generate 'excitation' from stimulation yet are 'inhibited' from active responding (at least in perceptual or cognitive tasks). Extraverts show the reverse. Thus, introverts are 'geared to inspect' – they are slow, but accurate – whereas extraverts are 'geared to respond' – they are fast, but less accurate. In a test of his model, Brebner provides data from different experiments to support his claim. In vigilance-type tasks, when stimuli are presented at very slow rates (every 18 s), over time the extraverts' performance, in terms of RT and missed signals, deteriorates. This was thought to be due to S-inhibition. On the other hand, in more typical simple RT tasks (when stimuli are presented at a faster rate), very different results were observed. In one well-designed study, subjects were presented with a warning stimulus (WS) and told to respond as soon as possible to the digit '1' that followed it. In different conditions, 'catch' trials were presented on 10, 40 or 70% of the trials. In these trials, no actual stimulus was presented following WS. Extraverts were found to alter their response strategy over the course of the experiment. As the number of catch trials increased, their RTs slowed, but the number of errors decreased. Moreover, anticipatory responses (defined as those in which RTs were less than 80 ms) were readily apparent in extraverts, the number decreasing as the number of catch trials increased. Introverts maintained stable performance across conditions. They did not have any anticipatory responses in any of the conditions.

In an as yet unpublished study, our laboratory has carried out an event-related potential study designed, amongst other reasons, to test Brebner's theory. Bob Stelmack, who happens to occupy an office next door, had earlier noted that the N1–P2 waveform was larger in introverts than in extraverts, but only for low 500 Hz tone pips[26]. Similar differences were reported in the somatosensory modality within the same latency range by Shagass and Schwartz[27]. The Stelmack et al. study is exemplary in that it controlled for possible sources of artifact. Moreover, aware that N1 differences could arise by varying levels of attention, the authors asked the subjects to count the number of stimuli. Unfortunately, across conditions the number of stimuli was always the same. Hence, it was possible for a subject to maintain an apparently accurate count but to remain inattentive all the while.

We decided to take a closer look at the mesogenous nature of N1–P2 and to use P3 as a possible index of Brebner's theory (in liaison with RT). Introverts and extraverts were presented with a train of regularly occurring 500 Hz tone pips (the stimuli for which Stelmack et al. reported significant differences[26]). On 20% of the trials, at random, the 500 Hz tone pip was changed to a 'target'. In one condition, the target was 'easy' to detect, its frequency being 2000 Hz. In another condition it was 'difficult' to detect, its frequency being 525 Hz. On certain conditions, for half the subjects the task was to keep a running mental count of these targets. The count was subsequently verified. To prevent subjects from using the knowledge of counts in previous conditions, the number of stimuli presented in each condition was varied. The other half of the subjects were asked to button press upon detection of the target. In other conditions, subjects were asked to ignore all stimuli by reading a book. Our suspicion was that earlier differences between the groups may have been due to variation in the level of selective attention. Thus, in this study we systematically manipulated the degree of attention paid to the auditory stimuli (in one condition, subjects were actively engaged in a target detection task – their hit rate served as an index of their attentiveness – while in another condition, the subjects ignored the auditory stimuli by reading a book). We also examined the effects of varying stimulus parameters since N1–P2 is determined, in part, by sensory factors. In one condition, stimuli were loud (90 dB SPL), while in another, soft (60 dB SPL).

The evoked potentials following the standard and target stimuli were recorded from midline frontal, central and parietal electrodes. Care was taken to reject trials in which excessive eye movement artifact was recorded.

The results are presented in Figures 7.2, 3 and 4. When the subjects were actively engaged in the target detection task (and recall, we could prove it by

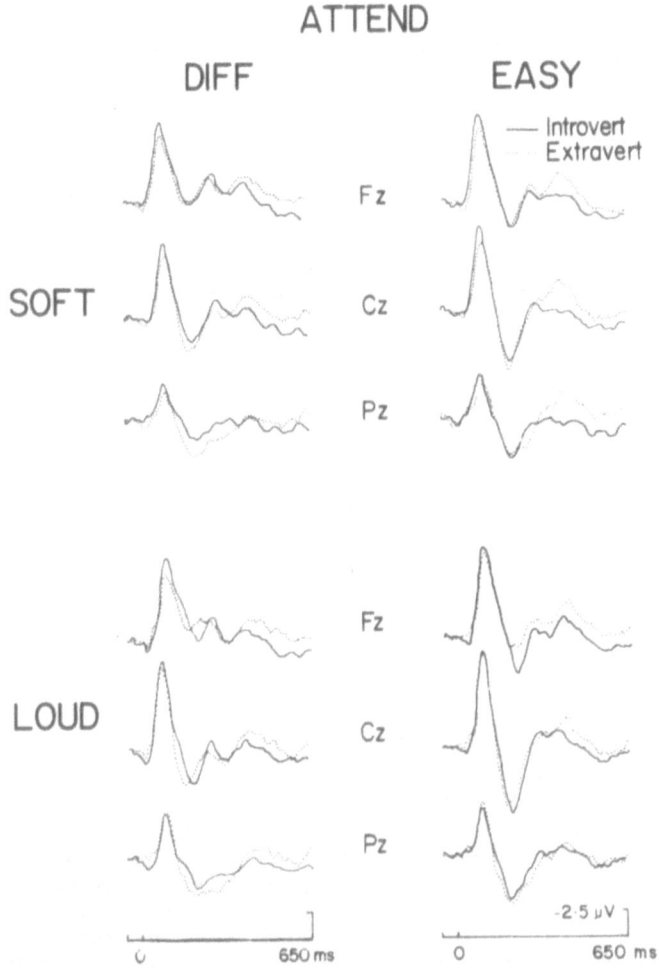

Figure 7.2  The effects of selective attention on the mesogenous evoked potentials in groups varying in extraversion. During 'ATTEND' conditions, subjects were actively engaged in a signal detection rate in which they were asked to detect a rare target presented amongst a train of more frequently presented 500 Hz standards. Target probability was 0.20. In one condition, targets were difficult to detect, while in another, they were easy to detect. In different conditions, the stimuli were presented at either a low ('SOFT') or high ('LOUD') intensity. The waveforms presented are the group grand averaged evoked potentials following the standard stimulus. Note that components (N1–P2) do not discriminate between the groups

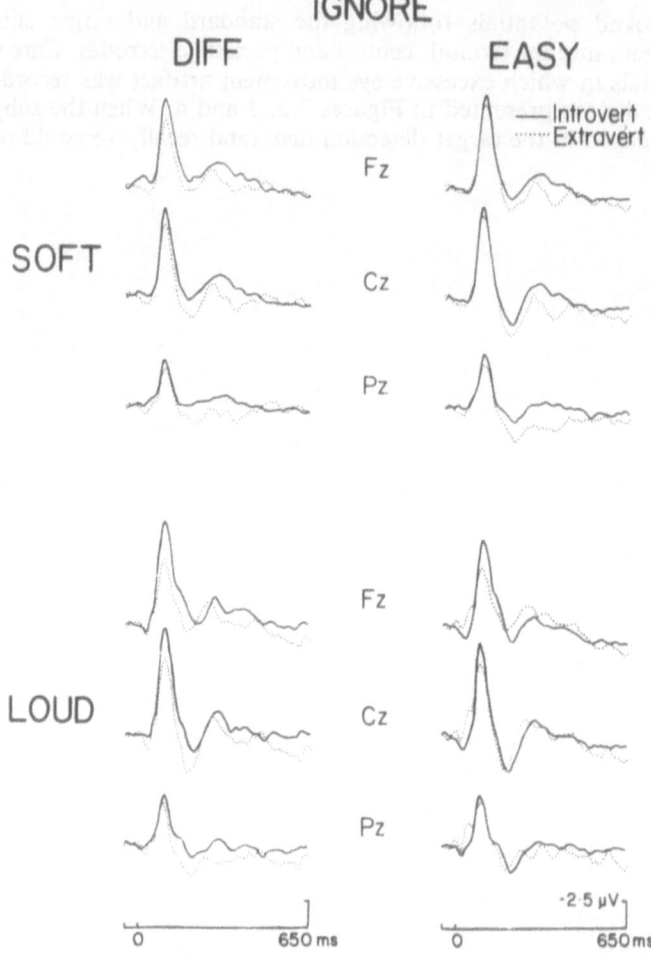

*Figure 7.3 As in Figure 7.2, but when subjects were asked to ignore the stimuli by reading a book. Although N1–P2 did not differ between the groups when subjects were selectively attending to the auditory stimuli, when they were attending elsewhere (reading a book), differences begin to emerge. This is especially the case when the standard stimuli were loud. Introverts appeared to be unable to ignore the stimuli. The group differences (greater negativity in the introverted group) last over several hundred ms. Such a baseline shift has been termed 'processing negativity' or 'Nd'. Extraverts therefore manifest greater processing negativity (difference between attend and ignore conditions). They are thus better able to ignore irrelevant information*

behavioural verification), there were no N1 or P2 between group differences following the standard 500 Hz stimulus, regardless of stimulus intensity (Figure 7.2). Hence, when the level of the subject's attention is tightly controlled, we were unable to find differences in components that had previously been used to support the claim that introverts are biologically more sensitive than extraverts.

On the other hand, when subjects were asked to ignore the stimuli, N1 was significantly smaller in the extraverts. In actual fact, introverts showed what seemed to be a long-lasting 'processing negativity' (Figure 7.3). Beginning before N1 and lasting for several hundred ms, there appears to be a negative baseline shift in the introvert's waveform. Thus, the actual N1 peak is of higher amplitude and the P2 peak of lower amplitude (i.e. it is more negative). That differences only arose when subjects were inattentive was somewhat unexpected. We suspect that the introverts were unable to ignore the stimuli, even if they were asked to do so. Further experimentation will be required before this can be demonstrated to be the case.

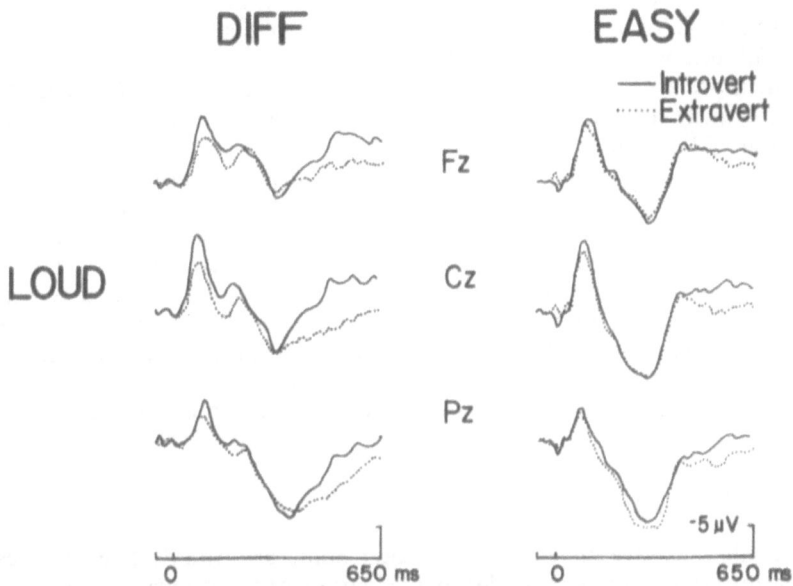

*Figure 7.4   As in Figure 7.3 except the waveforms presented are the grand averages following the target stimulus. Note the appearance of the late positive wave, P3. Under all conditions (although only the event-related potential to the LOUD target is illustrated) and at all scalp locations, the responses are almost identical in both groups. If P3 represents the termination of stimulus evaluation processing, then it appears to be identical in both introverts and extraverts. RT, however, was significantly longer in the extraverts*

The evoked potentials following the target stimulus are presented in Figure 7.4. Although half the subjects were asked to count the targets, while the other half responded by button pressing, as it turned out, the waveforms were essentially identical (we feared that button pressing might act as a contamination, perhaps for one group more than another). The data illustrated in Figure 7.4 were therefore collapsed across these conditions. Of particular interest to this discussion, the extraverted RT was slower than that of the introverts.

From what was said above, it might be concluded that, contrary to Brebner's expectations, introverts displayed R-excitation and extraverts R-inhibition. If so, the hit and false alarm rates should have discriminated between the groups. In actual fact, the hit rate for both groups was virtually perfect and the false alarm rate almost zero. Clearly, both groups emphasized accuracy. Recall from the discussion in Chapter 6 that very small differences in the false alarm rate can be associated with substantial differences in speed of responding[28]. RT differences between the groups are impossible to interpret – they could be due to real differences in stimulus evaluation time (in which case, there may be some evidence to support the notion that introverts are biologically more 'sensitive' or are characterized by S-excitation) or perhaps due to a response bias (the extraverts might simply have been bored by the whole task and 'took their time' to button press, or more formally stated, they were characterized by S-inhibition). Subjects were asked to button press upon detection of the targets and these were presented quite infrequently (on average, every 7.5 s). This is therefore effectively a vigilance task and as Brebner has already noted, in these conditions RTs are long in extraverts.

P3 however, remained unaltered in spite of variation in the intensity of the stimuli. This confirms that P3, a cognitive evoked potential, is independent of stimulus characteristics. Regardless of target intensity, neither the latency nor the amplitude of P3 was able to discriminate between the two groups. This being the case, stimulus evaluation times for the two groups may be assumed to be identical, even though mean RT is different. The speed of information processing (assuming stimulus evaluation time) for both introverts and extraverts is the same. RT differences probably therefore reflect variation in response bias. Reliance on mean RT data alone would perhaps lead to a false conclusion.


## CLOSED HEAD INJURY

Individuals who have suffered severe head trauma or 'injury', often as a result of a motor vehicle accident, are left with a variety of temporary and permanent disabilities. Amongst the most frequently cited are problems of attention (distractibility, inability to remain vigilant) and slowed decision-making. As long ago as 1944, Ruesch[29] noted that reaction times of head-injured patients were much slower than those of matched controls. These findings have since been replicated many times. It is now known that simple RT is not nearly as affected as choice RT (i.e. the slowing is probably not due to concomitant motor difficulties). Recently, van Zomeren[30] carefully controlled for possible motor deficits by providing measures of both DT and MT. The time to move from a homebase to the correct response key in a choice decision task did not differ between patients and controls. This suggests that neither primary motor deficits nor slowness in 'finding' the appropriate key (a response bias) could account for the slowing of RT. However, van Zomeren did suggest that the slowing could be due to another form of response bias – the now familiar emphasis on accuracy at a cost of speed. It is quite possible that the head-injured are far less certain of their decisions than controls. As such, they may require considerably more evidence before initiating their behavioural response.

Over the past 2 years, we have run several experiments[31] aimed, in part, at a clarification of this issue. The head-injured patients we have studied have had from 1 to 2.5 years of recovery prior to testing. A number of variants of the oddball task have been run: the effects of stimulus intensity, rate of stimulus presentation, probability of target presentation, modality of target presentation and duration of the condition. The results are very consistent and are highly reliable. Figure 7.5 is an example of the results obtained from several different conditions in one of these studies.

In the uppermost portion of the figure, an auditory 'oddball' task is illustrated. Standard stimuli were presented on 90% of the trials and targets on 10%. The subject's task in this and other conditions was to count the targets. P3 was smaller and later in the patients. To verify that the potential we recorded in both the patients and a control was a true 'P3', we ran a variety of other conditions that are known to affect P3. In each of these conditions, we also verified scalp distribution (although this is not illustrated in Figure 7.5). When we recorded a P3, it was almost always largest in parietal-central areas of the scalp, a classic and essential part of its definition. When we increased target probability (making it less informative), its amplitude became attenuated. When we changed modalities from the auditory to the visual (the subject's task being to detect the rare presentation of a green LED compared to the more frequent presentation of a red LED), P3 maintained its auditory scalp distribution and morphology. When the auditory target was omitted (i.e. the subject was asked to detect the omission of a stimulus occurring in a train of regularly presented standards), although no N1–P2 was apparent in the emitted waveform (since a physical stimulus is required for its appearance), P3 was nevertheless visible. It was thus evoked by the cognitive event of decision-making and not the presence of a physical stimulus. Finally, when the subject was asked to read a book and thus ignore the auditory stimuli, only a minimal P3 was apparent (since it is evoked by the actual detection of the target and not its mere presentation).

In spite of the particular condition, when P3 was present (in all except the 'ignore' task), it was always attenuated and delayed from 50 to 75 ms in patients compared to controls. This suggests that there is a true delay in stimulus evaluation time in these patients. Behaviourally, the hit rate, as determined by verification of the subject's count, was very high, being about 0.98 for both groups depending on the actual condition.

Convinced that there was a very real delay in stimulus evaluation processes in this group, we decided to return to the issue of the delayed reaction time. In subsequent experiments we have concurrently recorded both physiological and RT measures. These studies have found that across a variety of conditions, the patient RT is indeed prolonged – typically by as much as 150 ms. RT usually occurs before the peak of P3 in controls and after P3 in patients. This suggests that controls respond on the basis of minimal evidence in these relatively simple tasks. Much as van Zomeren predicted, the strategy adopted by the head-injured is quite different. They require much more evidence before responding. The net effect of the differential response bias may well be that mean RT exaggerates the cognitive deficit underlying head-injury.

159

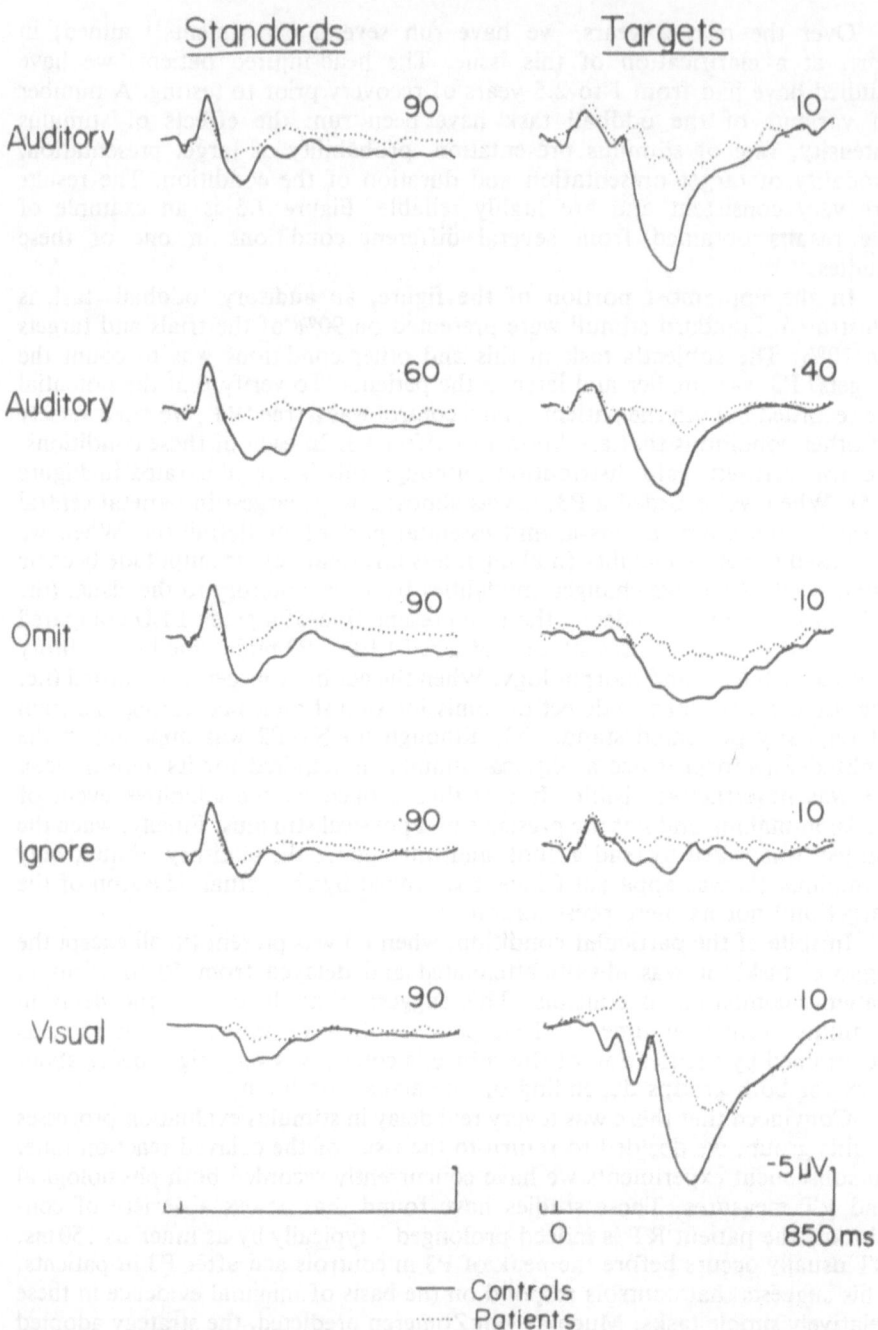

*Figure 7.5 Standard and target grand averages for head-injured outpatients and matched controls. In a wide variety of conditions, P3 is attenuated and prolonged in the head-injured. Stimulus evaluation processing may thus be delayed in this group*

## HYPERACTIVITY

A large volume of data now exists indicating that RTs of hyperactive children are significantly slower than matched controls. Stimulant drugs appear to improve vigilance in these children and to enhance RT[32, 33]. On the other hand, these drugs appear to have little effect on RTs of normal peers. Unfortunately, this field has also been plagued by inadequate analysis of RT, relying mainly on mean or median measures of central tendency. Lip service has been paid to greater variability in the hyperactive group, but little systematic analysis of a trial-by-trial breakdown of the cause of this variability has been attempted. Once again, we are left with a fairly substantial volume of data which shows fairly consistent trends but due to inadequate analysis makes interpretation of these findings quite difficult. Why is RT slower? Why do stimulants speed the response?

The American Psychiatric Association now classifies the hyperkinetic syndrome as an attentional deficit disorder. RT is slowed because the children are inattentive. In a fine example of circularity, one of the proofs used to demonstrate that hyperactives manifest attentional deficits is that they have slowed RTs. As has already been explained, the behavioural measure, RT, while it may be affected by a failure to adequately attend to the task at hand, cannot in itself be used as a measure of attention. A very fast RT probably does mean the subject was attentive. A slowed RT is much more difficult to interpret. The subjects might indeed have been inattentive. They might also have been very cautious even though they might have been highly attentive. Or, given the acknowledged wide variability in the RT distribution, extreme scores may have simply skewed the distribution. It appears that we again have another body of literature plagued by an inability to separate stimulus evaluate and response bias processes.

Two prominent laboratories in the United States have employed event-related potentials to help resolve the issue. Halliday and colleagues[34] in San Francisco and Klorman and his co-workers[35] in Rochester, New York have both noted that in oddball paradigms, the target P3 is attenuated in hyperactives while RT is slowed. RT, however, tends to be later than P3 latency. The effects of methylphenidate on the behavioural physiological relationship are extremely interesting. Callaway[36] has indicated that while RT latency decreases, P3 latency is unaltered. Similarly, RT in the Klorman *et al.* study decreased from 60 to 92 ms, depending on drug dosage whereas the P3 change was less than 4 ms[35]. It would therefore appear that methylphenidate functions to alter the response production stage of information processing and has very little effect on stimulus evaluation. These data are also supported by Frowein[37] who varied both stimulus and response complexity. The details of the study need not be of concern in this discussion. What is important is that he measured both the time between stimulus presentation and the initiation of a response – initiation of a response from 'home' towards the response key (decision time) and the time between leaving the home key and striking the response key (movement time). Stimulants were found to affect the response execution stage of information processing without affecting the earlier processes.

161

## AGEING

Salthouse and Somberg[38] have suggested that ageing causes a general slowing of human information processing by means of an increase in 'cycle time'. Furthermore, it is believed that this increase is independent of the type of information being processed. A series of physiological studies now suggest that this is not the case.

Pfefferbaum et al.[39] have indicated that in simple tasks, the latency of P3 is significantly later in the elderly compared to the young. The behavioural RT, however, does not differ, at least in the auditory modality. An increase in RT was noted for the elderly when visual stimuli were employed. Picton et al.[40] have replicated the P3 findings using an auditory, visual and somatosensory oddball task. Within the auditory modality, the latency of P3 to a detected target increased at a rate of 1.36 ms per year. Contrary to Pfefferbaum et al., no RT differences were found regardless of stimulus modality. The differing results might be explained by variant methodologies. Although both studies employed an oddball task, in the Pfefferbaum et al. study, two targets were presented, the subject having to respond to one and refrain from responding to the other while in the Picton et al. study, only a single target was presented. In the visual oddball task, Pfefferbaum et al. asked subjects to make the standard/target discrimination on the basis of shape whereas Picton et al. employed a colour discrimination. Again, seemingly minor procedural changes may in fact radically alter the cognitive demands of a task. The RT–P3 latency relationship differences in the young and elderly point to varying cognitive strategies. In the auditory tasks, for the younger subjects, P3 generally occurred about 20–30 ms before RT whereas for the older subjects, it occurred some 50–75 ms later. The elderly therefore appear to respond following less than complete stimulus evaluation (assuming of course that P3 latency serves as a metric of stimulus evaluation time). There should be a cost to such a strategy – namely, an increase in errors. This is precisely what Ford et al.[41] observed in an oddball task in which subjects had to respond one way to a 1000 Hz tone pip and another way to a 1500 Hz stimulus, the probability of each being 0.50.

Oddball tasks assume, implicitly or explicitly, that the subjects are continually 'updating' their expectancy for one event or another based on the preceding sequences of events. We have already seen that even the mentally retarded appear to carry on a sequence-by-sequence memory of past events in order to alter cognitive strategy to optimize speed of responding. Rabbitt and Vyas[42] suggest that the elderly are poor statistical predictors of events because they are unable to base their expectancies on 'long samples simply because, unlike the young, they cannot remember long sequences of past events' (p.918). In the Ford et al. study, P3 and RT were concurrently recorded during long sequences. Recall that P3 amplitude is highly dependent on the probability of occurrence of an event such that a highly improbable event elicits a large P3. Repetitions of an event lead to small amplitude P3s (in the behavioural context, they lead to fast RTs). The discontinuation of an expected stimulus elicits a large P3 (and a slowed RT). Ford and her colleagues have indicated that contrary to Rabbitt and Vyas's prediction, the effects of local sequential probability are quite similar in the elderly and the young. For both groups, P3 was larger and RT

162

longer for discontinuations than continuations. If anything, the elderly showed a larger P3 following a discontinuation of the repeated sequence than did the younger subjects. This may mean that the elderly expect repetitions to a greater extent than do the young. This could thus explain the failure to find age differences in RT in the oddball paradigm. Furthermore, as mentioned above, the expectation for a repetition would also explain the elderly's greater tendency toward error.

In complex memory retrieval tasks, the disassociation between RT and P3 latency takes on a new twist in the elderly. Pfefferbaum *et al.*[43] and Ford *et al.*[44] have both employed the Sternberg task, in which the response to a probe stimulus indicates whether the probe was a member of a previously presented memory set. The consistent finding in the Sternberg paradigm is that RT is an increasing, linear function of the number of items in the memory set size. Concurrent recordings of P3 indicate a larger effect of memory load on RT than P3 latency[45]. This effect seems to be exaggerated in the elderly. Increasing memory size increased the RT for both groups, but had a greater effect on the elderly. Although P3 increased in latency with increasing memory sizes for the young, this was not the case for the elderly. Furthermore, although making a negative response increased RTs in both groups, only the young subjects showed a parallel P3 latency change. Thus, in these complex tasks, P3 latency in the elderly is not as sensitive to response type or set size as it is in the young. This is precisely the opposite trend to what was found with the simple oddball task.

The conclusion based on very different cognitive tasks is that the usual RT–P3 relationship typically seen in young subjects, reflecting the parallel processing of separate processes, may become decoupled in the elderly. One process appears to generate RT and the other P3. These processes seem to be differentially affected by age and the cognitive demands of the task.


## CONCLUSIONS

The two chapters falling under the general rubric 'Mental Chronometry' have attempted to summarize a vast array of literature. Obviously, space does not permit more than a brief overview of most of the areas that have been discussed. No doubt, many readers will ask why study X or study Y was not included. The intent was to present 'typical' or 'sample' studies, not necessarily the best, hopefully, not the worst.

We also realize that we risk damnation from both the behavioural and physiological camps. In our emphasis on the less well-known physiological methods, one may be left with the impression that we are claiming that behavioural studies in and by themselves are somehow inferior or inadequate. Modern experimental and cognitive psychology have developed some highly sophisticated techniques for the analysis and the understanding of reaction time. The identification of the stages of information processing remains a very 'hot' issue. Certainly, it is true that a number of behavioural techniques can adequately handle the 'stimulus evaluation–response bias' question. To do so, however, requires very complex and time-consuming methodology. Providing physiological measures such as P3 can provide us with the same information (in itself, a highly controversial claim), then the considerable economy of time certainly justifies their use.

Recent developments in cognitive psychophysiology can no longer be ignored. We have admittedly stressed the P3–RT relationship. It is readily apparent that the physiological measure complements the behavioural, providing more information than would otherwise be available. However, just as we may be accused of simplifying the behavioural field, the same can also be said of the physiological. A number of recent studies have indicated that the concept of a single, solitary P3 or N1 or N2 can no longer be accepted. Just as there are probably many parallel processes generating 'N1' (N1a, N1b, N1c, Nd), so also there are overlapping processes at the time of P3. Furthermore, the very averaging process employed in most evoked potential studies may serve to distort late, cognitive waveforms. The theory of signal averaging holds that the component in consideration is constant in amplitude and in latency. It is highly doubtful that cognitive processes that generate waveforms such as P3 are always constant in time. It should be noted, however, that several techniques have been developed to deal with this very question.

Even if P3 is a measure of stimulus evaluation time, this tells us very little about the stages of information processing that lead to its generation. Several steps must surely precede the 'final' output that generates P3. In a similar vein, although we have assumed a 'serial' stage model of information processing, even the data we have presented can be interpreted to favour a 'parallel' model or some sort of hybrid of the two. For example, it was earlier stated that in a serial approach, the processing of one stage must be completed before a later one can begin. It has been suggested that RT represents the sum of the time taken for both stimulus evaluation and response production, whereas P3 latency reflects only the former. Very often, however, RT occurs before P3. In these cases, response production begins and may terminate *before* stimulus evaluation processes have been completed. If we stay with our same stage analysis, the conclusion must surely be that some form of parallel processing is taking place.

The intent of this chapter was to review methodological issues underlying mental chronometry as related to individual differences. It is fairly evident from the literature that in very many cases, the analysis of RT data presently being carried out cannot in any way be conclusive. Few modern experimental psychologists would place much credence in average (or mean) RT between group differences. Such differences can arise in so many ways as to make interpretation essentially impossible. Until researchers interested in the study of individual differences begin to adopt a level of analysis on par with recent behavioural and/or physiological advances, little in the way of progress can be expected.

## ACKNOWLEDGEMENTS

A variety of colleagues have assisted in the writing of these chapters. Many of my students, past and present, have been involved in various phases of different experiments. They include Lin Arcand, Libbie Bartoli, Ian Bell, Diana

Deacon-Elliott, Sylvie Houle, Diane Keeling, Dominique Lorrain, Cathy Malizia, Roxane Marois, Nancy Saunders, Braxton Suffield and Sharon Todd. Terry Picton has provided me with invaluable advice on evoked potential research. Bob Stelmack and I have had many discussions centred around the study of individual differences. Guy Proulx continues to be an inspiration for many of the studies of head injuries. Technical support was provided by Herman van den Bergen and Bob Spratt. Madan Makasare has written most of the lab's software.

Financial support was provided by the Natural Sciences and Engineering Research Council (NSERC) of Canada and the Faculty of Social Sciences of the University of Ottawa.

## References

1. Sternberg, R. J. (1984). Toward a triarchic theory of human intelligence. *Behav. Brain Sci.*, **7**, 269–315
2. Jensen, A. R. (1984). Mental speed and levels of analysis. Commentary to Sternberg, R. J. Toward a triarchic theory of human intelligence. *Behav. Brain Sci.*, **7**, 295–6
3. Smith, G. A. and Stanley, G. (1983). Clocking *g*: relating intelligence and measures of timed performance. *Intelligence*, **7**, 353–68
4. Galton, F. (1883). *Inquiries into Human Faculty and its Development*. 2nd. Edn. (New York: Dutton)
5. Jensen, A. R. and Munro, E. (1979). Reaction time, movement time, and intelligence. *Intelligence*, **3**, 121–6
6. Jensen, A. R. (1982). Reaction time and psychometric *g*. In Eysenck, H. J. (ed.) *A Model of Intelligence*. pp. 93–132. (New York: Springer-Verlag)
7. Vernon, P. A. (1983). Speed of information processing and general intelligence. *Intelligence*, **7**, 53–70
8. Carlson, J. S. and Jensen, C. M. (1982). Reaction time, movement time and intelligence: a replication and extension. *Intelligence*, **6**, 265–74
9. Carlson, J. S., Jensen, C. M. and Widaman, K. E. (1983). Reaction time, intelligence and attention. *Intelligence*, **7**, 329–44
10. Baumeister, A. A. and Kellas, G. (1968). Reaction time and mental retardation. In Ellis, N. R. (ed.) *International Review of Research in Mental Retardation*. Vol. 3, pp. 163–93. (New York: Academic)
11. Nettlebeck, T. and Kirby, N. H. (1983). Measures of timed performance and intelligence. *Intelligence*, **7**, 39–52
12. Nettlebeck, T. and Brewer, N. (1981). Studies of mild mental retardation and timed performance. In Ellis, N. R. (ed.) *International Review of Research in Mental Retardation*. **10**, pp. 61–106. (New York: Academic)
13. Brewer, N. and Smith, G. A. (1984). How normal and retarded individuals monitor and regulate speed and accuracy of responding in serial choice tasks. *J. Exp. Psychol.: Gen.*, **113**, 71–93
14. Ertl, J. and Schafer, E. W. P. (1969). Brain response correlates of psychometric intelligence. *Nature*, **223**, 421–2
15. Callaway, E. (1975). *Brain Electric Potentials and Individual Psychological Differences*. (New York: Grune and Stratton)
16. Shagass, C., Roemer, R. A., Straumanis, J. J. and Josiassen, R. C. (1981). Intelligence as a factor in evoked potential studies of psychopathology. I. Comparison of high and low IQ subjects. *Biol. Psychiatry*, **16**, 1007–30
17. Rhodes, L. E., Dustman, R. E. and Beck, E. C. (1969). The visual evoked response: a comparison of bright and dull children. *Electroenceph. Clin. Neurophysiol.*, **27**, 364–72

18. Robinson, D. L. (1982). Properties of the diffuse thalamocortical system, human intelligence and differentiated vs. integrated modes of learning. *Pers. Individ. Diff.*, **3**, 393–405

19. Hendrickson, A. E. and Hendrickson, D. A. (1975). An auditory illusion predicted by a theory of brain function. *Percept. Motor Skills*, **41**, 279–89

20. Hendrikson, D. E. and Hendrikson, A. E. (1980). The biological basis of individual differences in intelligence. *Pers. Ind. Diff.*, **1**, 3–33

21. Winne, P. H. and Belfry, M. J. (1982). Interpretive problems when correcting for attenuation. *J. Educ. Measure.*, **19**, 125–34

22. Eysenck, H. J. (1967). *The Biological Basis of Personality*. (Springfield: Thomas)

23. Brebner, J. (1980). Reaction time in personality theory. In Welford, A. T. (ed.) *Reaction Times*. (London: Academic)

24. Brebner, J. (1983). A model of extraversion. *Austr. J. Psychol.*, **35**, 349–59

25. Brebner, J. and Cooper, C. (1974). The effect of low rate of regular signals upon the reaction times of introverts and extraverts. *J. Res. Pers.*, **8**, 306–11

26. Stelmack, R. M., Achorn, E. and Michaud, A. (1977). Extraversion and individual differences in auditory evoked response. *Psychophysiology*, **14**, 368–74

27. Shagass, C. and Schwartz, M. (1965). Age, personality and somatosensory evoked responses. *Science*, **148**, 1359–61

28. Pachella, R. G. (1974). The interpretation of reaction time in information processing research. In Kantowitz, B. (ed.) *Human Information Processing: Tutorials in Performance and Cognition*. pp. 41–82. (Hillsdale, NJ: Erlbaum)

29. Ruesch, J. (1944). Dark adaptation, negative after images, tachistoscopic examinations and reaction time in head injuries. *J. Neurosurg.*, **1**, 243–51

30. van Zomeren, A. H. (1981). *Reaction Time and Attention after Closed Head Injury*. (Lisse: Swets and Zeitlinger B.V.)

31. Campbell, K. B., Houle, S., Lorrain, D., Deacon-Elliott, D. and Proulx, G. B. (1985). Event-related potentials as an index of recovery from severe head-injury. *Electroenceph. Clin. Neurophysiol.* (special suppl.), in press

32. Weiss, B. and Laties, V. G. (1962). Enhancement of human performance by caffeine and the amphetamines. *Pharmacol. Rev.*, **14**, 1–36

33. Conners, C. K. and Werry, J. S. (1979). Pharmacotherapy, In Quay, H. C. and Werry, J. S. (eds.) *Psychopathological Disorders of Children.*, pp. 333–86. (New York: Wiley)

34. Halliday, R., Callaway, E. and Naylor, H. (1983). Visual evoked potential changes induced by methylphenidate in hyperactive children: dose/response effects. *Electroenceph. Clin. Neurophysiol.*, **55**, 258–67

35. Klorman, R., Saltzman, L. F., Bauer, L. O., Coons, H. W., Borgstedt, A. D. and Halpern, W. I. (1983). Effects of two doses of methylphenidate on cross-situational and border-line hyperactive children's evoked potentials. *Electroenceph. Clin. Neurophysiol.*, **56**, 169–85

36. Callaway, E. (1983). The pharmacology of human information processing. *Psychophysiology*, **20**, 359–70

37. Frowein, H. W. (1981). Selective effects of barbiturate and amphetamine on information processing and response execution. *Acta Psychol.*, **47**, 105–15

38. Salthouse, T. A. and Somberg, B. L. (1982). Isolating the age deficit in speeded performance. *J. Gerontol.*, **37**, 59–63

39. Pfefferbaum, A., Ford, J. M., Wenegrat, B. G., Roth, W. T. and Kopell, B. S. (1984). Clinical applications of the P3 component of event-related potentials. I. Normal aging. *Electroenceph. Clin. Neurophysiol.*, **59**, 85–103

40. Picton, T. W., Stuss, D. T., Champagne, S. C. and Nelson, R. F. (1984). The effects of age on human event-related potentials. *Psychophysiology*, **21**, 312–25

41. Ford, J. M., Duncan-Johnson, C. C., Pfefferbuam, A. and Kopell, B. S. (1982). Expectancy for events in old-age: stimulus sequence effects on P300 and reaction time. *J. Gerontol.*, **37**, 696–704

42. Rabbitt, P. M. A. and Vyas, S. (1980). Selective anticipation for events in old age. *J. Gerontol.*, **35**, 913–19

43. Pfefferbaum, A., Ford, J. M., Roth, W. T. and Kopell, B. S. (1980). Age differences in P3-reaction time associations. *Electroenceph. Clin. Neurophysiol.*, **49**, 266–76

44. Ford, J. M., Pfefferbaum, A., Tinklenberg, J. R. and Kopell, B. S. (1982). Effects of perceptual and cognitive difficulty on P3 and RT in young and old adults. *Electroenceph. Clin. Neurophysiol.*, **54**, 311–21
45. Adam, N. and Collins, G. I. (1978). Late components of the visual evoked potential to search in short-term memory. *Electroenceph. Clin. Neurophysiol.*, **44**, 147–56

# 8
# Neurophysiology of emotions and some general brain mechanisms

## *Natalia P. Bechtereva and Diliara K. Kambarova*

The use of long-term electrode implantation for diagnostic and therapeutic means has opened up new vistas for studying intracerebral dynamics of physiological processes[1-4]. Clinical studies require modern techniques for specifying the location of pathological foci, the functional states of particular brain areas, the structures associated with emotional expression as well as for decoding complex neurodynamics of mental activity. For this purpose, a technique has been developed and tested, which monitors brain physiological rearrangements at rest, in the process of performing diverse functional tests, and during spontaneous fluctuations of mood. The technique also analyses physiological and behavioural effects of electrostimulation and polarization (employed in therapeutic sessions)[1, 5-7].

Analysis of emotional brain organization demands an adequate subset of methods in which point electrical stimulation is complemented by recordings of slow physiological processes and their shifts (within the millivolt range) for a variety of normal and pathological responses during many tasks. By investigating neuronal impulse activity, a technique is available which detects subtle dynamics of the cortex as well as subcortical regulation related to the type and stage of mental activity, and provides a basis for developing a neural model of human thinking[1, 8-10]. This contrasts with previous studies on brain structural-functional bases of cognitive processes[1, 11].

*Electrical stimulation (ES)* analysed together with recordings of *infraslow physiological processes (ISPP)*[12-14] provide an effective methodological basis for determining cerebral regulation of emotional behaviour. There are of course obvious ethical limitations imposed on electrostimulative techniques. Great care must be taken to obviate the effects that externally-induced stimulation, particularly synchronous *multistimulative* procedures could have on routine brain functions (by means of an effect on its modulating formations). Nevertheless, careful recording of ISPP possesses distinct advantages in tracing the dynamics of neurophysiological concomitants of emotional behaviour.

Emotions can be determined by a variety of exogenous and endogenous factors, which in turn involve quite different processes. Consideration of cerebral neurodynamics ought to provide insight into the intimate interrelationship between emotions and such phenomena as motor processes, an area of significance for a more thorough understanding of healthy and pathological expressive states. The present study generalizes ISPP investigations during emotional states/responses in epileptic patients providing unique data on those neural processes reflecting the interdependence of emotional and speech-motor processes.

## METHOD

Fifteen epileptic patients, with and without significant disturbances at the emotional level, were investigated during the course of their treatment using long-term implanted intracerebral electrodes. Emotional behaviour was studied by recording ISPP in different brain regions (limbic structures, thalamic nuclei, different cortex areas of temporal and frontal lobes) during spontaneous and evoked changes of emotional state[14, 15]. The total number of ISPP recordings in 150 brain sites amounted to 54 000 (most of which had been conducted by G. G. Ivanov).

Six gold electrodes were gathered into single bundles, insulated by neutral plastic up to their tips and implanted into the brain target-structures, the active surface of the electrode ranging from 0.05 to 0.2 mm$^2$. Electrode implantation was performed using the computerized stereotactic approach, a method developed by A. D. Anitchkov and Y. S. Polonsky (Patent N4228799, Oct. 21, 1980)[16, 17]. The reference electrode, cylindrical in form with an active surface of 150–200 mm$^2$ – was implanted either into the frontal skull bone, or, in some cases, subcutaneously under the aponeurosis in the same area.

A couple of simultaneous recordings of fluctuations in infraslow physiological processes were conducted daily in many structures throughout the entire phase of treatment/therapy (3–5 months). The ISPP involve numerous physiological phenomena possibly of various genesis, characterized by different amplitude, period and fluctuation regularity. Their amplitude may be as high as, or in excess of, 100 mV.

The investigation was based primarily on data associated with changes of a relatively stable component of the ISPP (the so-called *permanent potential*, a consistent millivolt range potential difference). The recordings were made between each of the intracerebral electrodes and the reference electrode. A special eight-channel DC-amplifier with an input impedance of 150 MΩ was used as a measuring device together with the digital microvoltmeter B-7-22. It should be emphasised that the potential difference measures are summated values acquired over a period of approximately six seconds. Since the process of averaging involved a relatively long period of time, the distortion by high frequency range events ought to be minimal. The signals are of quite different frequency spectra as well as temporal characteristics to those associated with EEG studies. The registration techniques involve filtering low frequencies – the frequency band of the amplifiers range from 0 to 0.05 Hz and the frequency slope in beyond the cut-off 6 dB/octave. The linear filtering in the amplifier cannot create slow potentials – it only filters slow components that are *actually* present in the complex signal.

In characterizing emotional behaviour, a distinction was drawn between emotional *condition* and *state*. Emotional condition refers to the relatively enduring, inert changes which, when manifested, persist for hours or even days, influencing the patient's emotional behaviour and responsivity. Emotional states refer to *transient* feelings.

It is necessary to reiterate the medico-ethical aspects of such studies. The implementations of the procedures outlined are only considered indispensable when they involve selective expedience of usage for any particular patient, with sound justification of its efficacy as well as demonstration of minimal side-effects. The data accumulated during ES-techniques should be restricted to diagnosis and therapy, 'experimentation' being inadmissible.

For local electrical stimulation of the brain we used an ESC-I electric stimulator. Biphasic rectangular impulse stimulation was made through insulating blocks[18,19]. A series of short, weak electrical pulses (1 ms, 0.15–15 V, frequency of 1–60 Hz) were provided over sessions of 5–10 s duration.


## RESULTS AND DISCUSSION

The recording of ISPP during various emotional states offers quantitative estimates of the *intensity* of brain correlates of emotions as well as the character of these changes, their *duration* and *spatial* distribution. Thus ISPP enables one to describe changes in the brain in terms of millivolts, and their duration in seconds or more often, minutes or hours (Figure 8.1).

Figure 8.1 shows the dynamics of the relatively stable ISPP components in the frontal lobe area, uncus gyri hippocampi and the right amygdala for an emotionally stable patient during an emotional episode elicited by unexpected pleasant or unpleasant information. When emotions of joy were experienced, ISPP dynamics were usually characterized by considerable (from 20 to 40 mV), transient (5–10 min) deviations of ISPP in one area of the structure under investigation. During the negative emotion (in this case fear prior to an oncoming operation), ISPP intensity (in one area investigated) grew slower (15–20 min) and was accompanied by reciprocal (decrease in the ISPP intensity) ISPP dynamics in the adjacent area.

Figure 8.2 reveals the ISPP shift associated with an emotional reaction of paroxysmal violent fear lasting approximately 3 min. After the reaction had subsided, the patient characterized her condition as the 'premonition of violent fear'. She had, however, remained conscious throughout and was able to adequately assess her experience. The ISPP level was found to change in only three areas of the right amygdala. In the remaining three areas of this formation as well as several other structures (left amygdala and hippocampus, both uncuses, and symmetrical cortex area in the temporal lobe poles) the ISPP remained stable.

Of particular interest were the initial changes in the physiological index a minute before the emotional response was exhibited, during which fluctuations

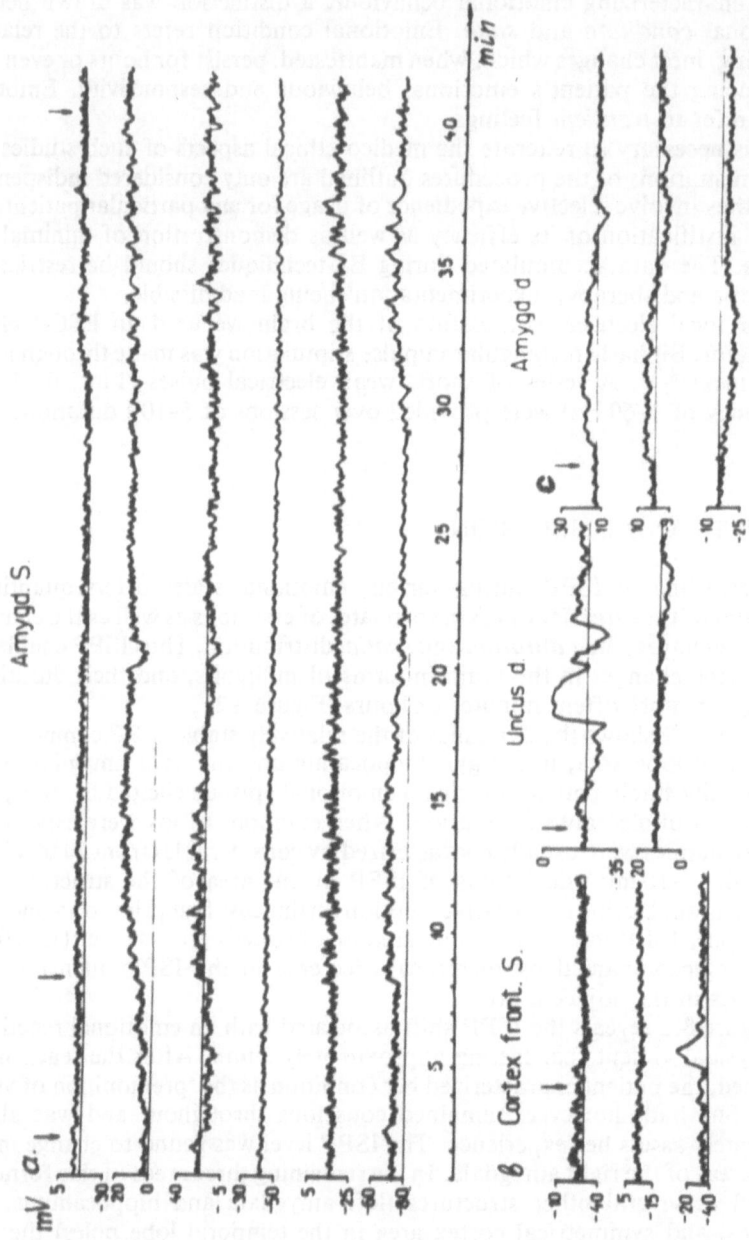

in ISPP were registered within a limited number of structures and reciprocal ISPP dynamics monitored in adjacent brain areas spaced at a distance of 2–3 mm.

The behavioural fear response coincided with three types of ISPP dynamics – anticipation of fear was accompanied by ISPP increase (more than 15 mV) in the third electrode area and its simultaneous decrease (by 5 mV) in the second. In the area of the first electrode it remained unchanged. This reaction lasted about 20 s and was followed by a sharp potential decrease in the third electrode area (more than 35 mV) together with a rapid increase in adjacent areas (by about 30 and 20 mV respectively in the areas of the second and third electrode). Then 30–90 s later a tendency to regain resting ISPP levels developed in all three areas of the right amygdala. The initial resting values were restored when the premonition of fear vanished.

Figure 8.2 reveals that emotional response is correlated with ISPP shifts recorded within the three areas of the right amygdala. There are clearly methodological limitations, such as the maximum number of electrodes which can safely be embedded in any one patient. Consequently, the infraslow physiological events developing in other anatomical brain structures cannot always be recorded. The data do prove, however, the possibility of spatially circumscribed brain area ISPP shifts which correlate with emotional response. Despite the limitations mentioned, there is every reason to suppose that an emotional reaction is likely to develop when, in their maintenance, a limited number of brain areas are involved. This implies that emotional responses are structurally timed within the brain and not every emotional reaction, no matter how intensive, is maintained by generalized changes in the brain (or evokes them). Such limited changes, recorded in the brain during emotional reactions emerging from a relatively normal emotional condition, have to be considered in cerebral mechanisms of emotional maintenance. Furthermore, it should be emphasized that the area of the brain involved in emotional organization, as well as the magnitude

---

*Figure 8.1    Dynamics of ISPP values for the patient with evident emotional disturbances (a), and patient with relatively preserved emotional sphere (b). (a) ISPP level variation (mV) in six areas of amygdala s. Arrows mark the moments of conversation with the patient (from left to right); neutral question is asked and not answered by the patient, the mimics express indignation; patient is asked to calm herself (second arrow) and she says angrily that now she has some 'unpleasant reminiscences'. Being asked, 'what are you thinking about?' (third arrow), she says she thinks about her father whom she hates. Diffuse changes of ISPP are of particular interest (an exception being the area under electrode 4). 45 min after the first conversation with the patient, ISPP are still not at the initial level.*

*(b) Arrows represent administration of emotional test. Patient smiles, and immediately after the presentation in the limited number of areas within cortex of the left hemisphere, and uncus of the right hemisphere intensive oscillations of level are seen, but for 1.5–15 min (for the cortex and uncus areas correspondingly) ISPP level returns back to initial value.*

*(c) The case of test connected with negative emotions is presented. ISPP level changes only in three areas (increase in two and decrease in one area). Return to initial values 10 min after presentation*

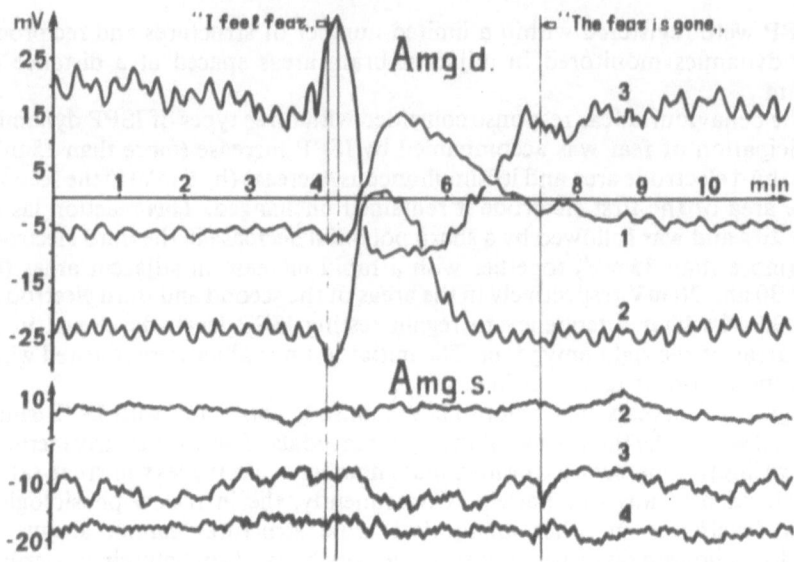

*Figure 8.2   Dynamics of ISPP values during the development of fear affect. Highest initial ISPP level was observed near electrode 3, in this particular area ISPP increase is seen to develop 15 s prior to clinical manifestations of paroxysm. Note reciprocal was significantly increased*

of the local ISPP changes, depends not only on intensity of emotions, but on their content and duration.

Figure 8.3 presents the ISPP dynamics during the expression of emotion in a patient who suffered from psychosensory (emotional-mnestic) paroxysms and mood disorders. Investigations were carried out after a one week remission when the patient's behaviour had been judged as adequate by medical/psychological specialists. ISPP dynamics were also analysed when the patient's condition suddenly began deteriorating. During this period the patient's condition was characterized by changeable moods with negativistic periods.

The ISPP changes in this particular case were induced by recollecting unpleasant experiences in the past. Such a diagnosis serves to elucidate the structural functional basis of emotional disorders.

The comparison of ISPP dynamics typical of the paroxysm affect (Figure 8.2) during violent emotions demonstrated that persistent negative emotional states differed from the transient fear affect not only in terms of the involvement of a considerable number of formations, particularly areas of the right amygdala, but also by the character of the ISPP changes. The areas not involved in the formation of the paroxysm affect in the right amygdala participated in the organization of the emotional state. Only the area of the third electrode was involved in the formation of negative emotions in both cases. However, the changes were markedly different. During enduring fluctuations of depressive moods, ISPP in both amygdalas gradually increased reaching the climax 10–14 min after the onset of the reaction (by 20 mV and 5 mV respectively in the area of the third and fifth electrodes). The same tendency had been observed in the left amygdala – ISPP increased by 20 mV in the second electrode area and by 10 mV in the fourth electrode area at about the same time. During this period the patient's eyes were filled with tears coupled with behavioural signs

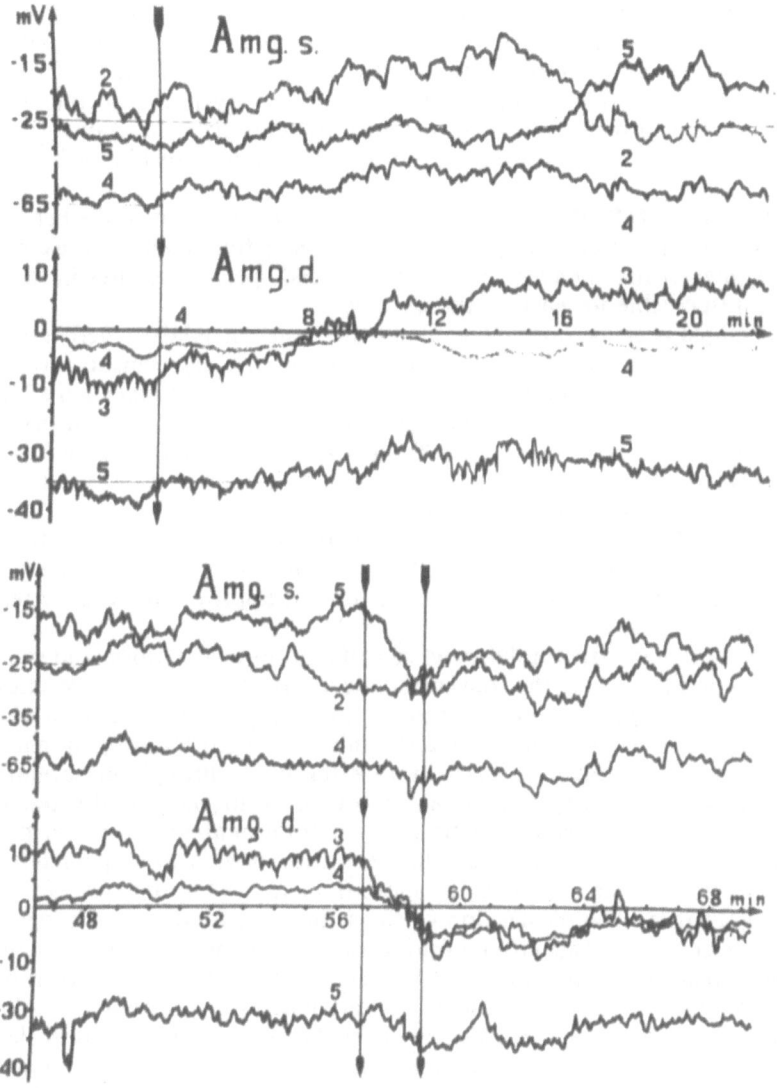

*Figure 8.3 Dynamics of ISPP during intensely experienced feelings associated with remembering unpleasant events in the past. One arrow shows the beginning of the test – the patient recalls the quarrel with her mother, two arrows indicate the period of psychotherapy which resulted in the patient becoming completely calm (return to initial state). For detailed description of investigation see text*

of a violent emotional experience. In the right amygdala the main tendencies in the ISPP dynamics remained the same though the *intensity* of emotion was found to change. In the left amygdala, however, reciprocal changes in the ISPP were recorded within the same period between the fifth electrode and the second and fourth electrode areas. In the area of the fifth electrode the potential increased rapidly (by 20 mV) whereas in two others it decreased (by 25 and 5 mV respectively). The same cycle of ISPP changes was then recorded and 49 min after the onset of the emotiogenic test (the patient was crying), ISPP dynamics reproducing the first pattern re-emerged. The psychotherapeutic talk the investigator had with the patient reassured her entirely, and against this background all the areas of both amygdalas tended to rapidly regain the initial ISPP level.

The study of ISPP dynamics combined with the analysis of the behavioural expressive states (fear paroxysm and a lasting negative change in the emotional state), suggest the involvement of common and specific features in the mechanism responsible for each of these states.

The area near the third electrode of the right amygdala (where a dramatic increase had been registered during the evolution of fear) seems to play the part of a *pathogenic factor* in the onset mechanism of this reaction (Figure 8.2). The resting level of ISPP in the same area is probably important in organizing negative emotional states (Figure 8.3). Furthermore, reference ought to be made to considerable ISPP fluctuations in the left amygdala as well as to reciprocal potential changes due to expressive emotional reactions.

From this it may be concluded that both these states result from a single source (the *hyperactivity focus in the right amygdala*) but the localization of linkages and the mechanism responsible for the appropriate brain systems are different.

The notion of structural dependence of emotional condition and state does not completely exclude the conventional concept that emotional reactions are maintained and accompanied by generalized changes in the brain. In instances of changes in the initial emotional state, shifts in the ISPP during the emotional reactions are generally recorded more extensively throughout several brain structures (Figure 8.4). Figure 8.4 shows that in the initially unchanged emotional state, the spontaneous positive emotional reaction (the patient's mood was stable, she remembered her favourite song) is accompanied by ISPP changes (their value decreasing by more than 15 mV) in only one area of the right amygdala. The recollection of the same song by this patient against an unstable emotional background (mood fluctuations with a high anxiety level) is accompanied by initial ISPP changes in the same brain area. Apart from these ISPP changes related to the patient's condition, the ISPP shifts are also detected in other brain areas. The reaction involves the area around the third electrode of the right amygdala, two areas in the left amygdala and the left hippocampus. The patient's 'report' is of special interest here. The report, which implies *speech motor activity* in the compensated emotional state, causes no significant changes in ISPP. On the contrary, the patient's report, comparable in content to the first one (since the patient spoke again about the tune and the words of her favourite song) was accompanied by dramatic ISPP dynamics throughout the course of the patient's worsening condition. There are two features that

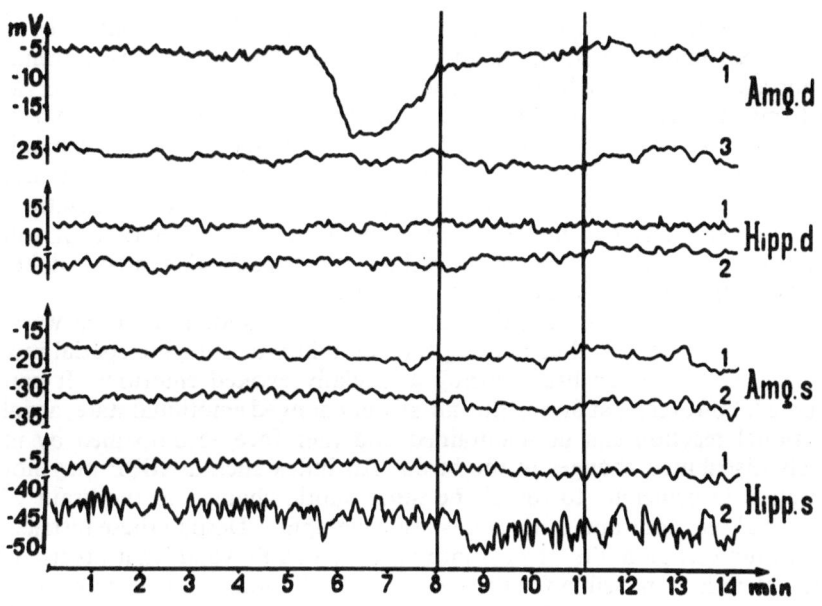

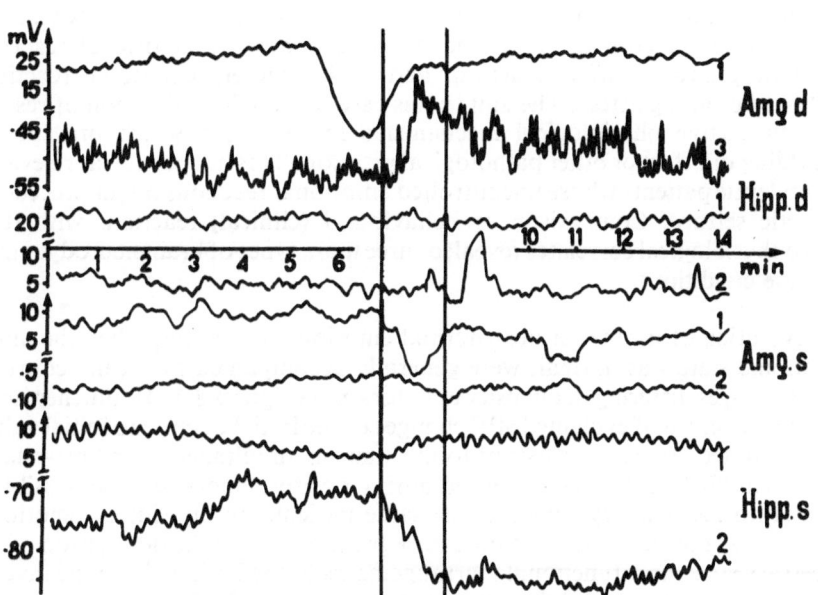

Figure 8.4  ISPP dynamics during a spontaneous recollection of a tune, lyrics of a favourite song during compensated emotional state (above) and a pathological emotional state (negativism, tears) (below). Two vertical lines represent the patient's report

characterize the ISPP dynamics in the latter case – the involvement of most brain areas under investigation in the response and the opposite trend (as compared to that preceding the 'report') of ISPP changes. This observation confirms the idea that in instances of pathologically changed emotional state, not only does the brain area involved in the emotional organization expand but the selectivity of involvement of some of its formations in maintenance of activity of a different modality may disappear. In the above investigation the shifts of ISPP differ in intensity, duration, trend and onset time. It will be demonstrated, however, that generally the pattern of shifts is similar in different areas during more marked changes in emotion.

For medical and ethical considerations strong emotional reactions were not evoked in the patients, thus limiting the possibility of studying spatial mosaic changes in the human brain during artificially evoked emotions. It can be assumed, however, that during the initially unchanged emotional state, a violent emotional reaction can be maintained and therefore accompanied by more widely distributed changes in the brain. An index such as ISPP may not be expected, in principle, to reveal the more subtle changes in the brain when emotional reactions and other states are developing. Despite these restrictions and within certain limits, the assumption is probably valid, that precisely the initial state is responsible for the degree of limitation, or, *vice versa*, for the generalization of ISPP shifts in the brain correlating with the emotion which is comparable by its character and intensity.

Data on neurophysiological mechanisms associated with preserving emotional states/responses provide an analysis of cerebral neurodynamics correlating with both the initiation of an uncontrolled emotional response developing into an affect reaction, and during violent emotional reactions without becoming affect. The aim in this case was the identification of restrictive, protective physiological mechanisms in the brain which prevent the unfolding of affect or other pathological reaction. This has particular relevance for epileptic patients whose uncontrolled emotional reactions might precede an epilectic seizure. Comparison of behavioural (clinical) reactions with their neurophysiological correlates revealed three main types of brain neurodynamics in these conditions.

(1) Evolution of normal or near-normal emotional responses, when the initial emotional state was normal, were generally accompanied by locally confined ISPP changes differing in intensity and duration (Figures 8.1, 4). Furthermore, typically a return of evolving ISPP changes to the initial or close to initial values was exhibited. It was commonly found that no simultaneous or time-related reciprocal ISPP shifts were recorded during positive emotions. The possibility of monitoring neurodynamics in the same patients during similar emotional reactions against a stable emotional background enabled the description of the necessary structural-functional rearrangements in the brain (within the investigated structures), ascertaining those major areas involved in such a reaction.

(2) The development of an emotional response against an unfavourable emotional background revealed, as was mentioned above, the spreading of simultaneous or *time-related* ISPP changes within the structures under

study. When we investigated the neurodynamics evolving against an adverse emotional background, the changes were manifested through reciprocal ISPP shifts evolving in the main area or some distance from it (Figures 8.2, 3, 4). These data are evidence of reciprocal physiological changes in the brain in these conditions. However, elucidation of the physiological importance of these reciprocal trends only became possible when we succeeded in recording and comparing the ISPP dynamics during intensive spontaneous emotions which occasionally ended abruptly after having been intense, whilst in other cases they became increasingly complex (Figure 8.2). Observations of ISPP over many days enabled the recording of dynamics in varied conditions. Special techniques used for daily analysis of the dynamics revealed physiological conditions which were likely to foster expression of pathological emotions of different intensity, or, contrarily, those preventing their formation.

Figure 8.5 presents the dynamics of daily average ISPP values. It illustrates an analysis of ISPP dynamics in the *mediobasal temporal* structures of both hemispheres conducted in such a manner that an independent estimate of mean ISPP value could be made for those brain areas which displayed a tendency for increasing or reducing ISPP value.

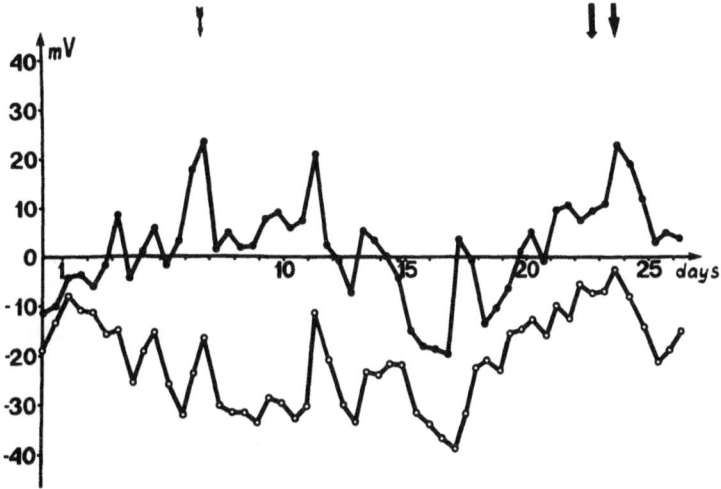

*Figure 8.5  Dynamics of mean ISPP values in amygdala, hippocampus and uncus g. hippocampus. Black circles denote the mean ISPP values over the areas with stable tendency towards the increase of ISSP value during the periods preceding the paroxysmal state; white circles denote the same for areas with tendency towards decrease of ISPP value. The trend towards a growth of the differences between ISPP mean values due to an increase in some areas and a decrease in others is related to the period of remission (days 6–11). Long-term trends in the form of an increase of ISPP mean values for both groups of brain areas is the symptom of approaching critical state. The development of single paroxysms, fear affects and dysphoria with frequent psychosensory paroxysms and psychomotoric is marked with arrows*

A critical condition (*disphoria*, frequent paroxysms of affect disorders, as many as ten per day) evolved only when both groups of cerebral areas exhibited similar ISPP trends tending to increase (Figure 8.5: 19th, 23rd day). Conversely, the emotional state returned to normal with reciprocal potential dynamics (Figure 8.5: 6th, 11th day). Of particular relevance for the patient was the index of the long-term tendencies in the ISPP dynamics. There was a general tendency for increasing differences between the mean ISPP values. This occurred when the index increased in one area of the brain whilst decreasing in another, coinciding with the period of improvement in the patient's condition (Figure 8.5: from 3rd to 17th day).

Further investigations of this phenomenon confirmed the assumption that pathological emotional states/responses do not evolve when the reciprocal ISPP shifts appear commensurable by intensity.

Clinical physiological analysis of all these data, particularly reciprocal ISPP shifts during a violent reaction, which does not develop into affect or seizure, suggested that negative ISPP trends were limiting, protective mechanisms of the

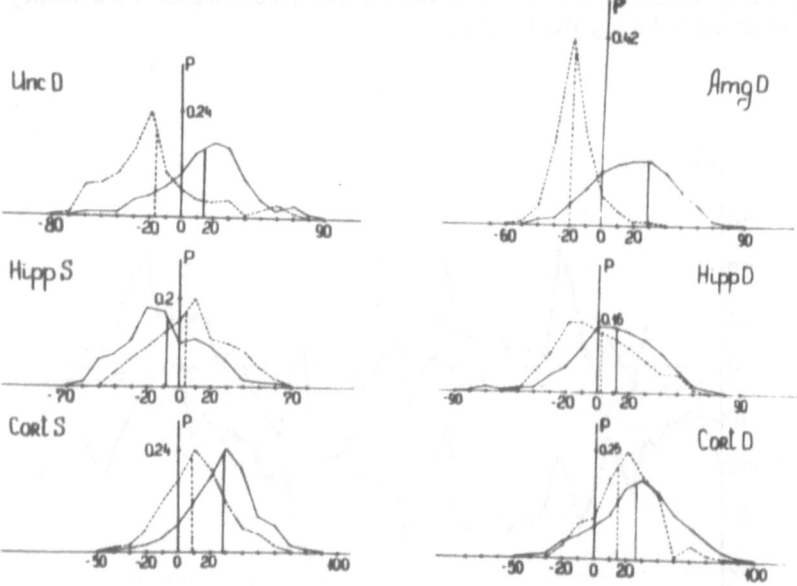

*Figure 8.6   Histogram of ISPP values distribution corresponding to pathological shifts of emotional state of dysphoric type (solid line) and after local electric therapeutic actions causing stable remission (dashed line). On the ordinate axis, frequency of ISPP value occurrences within the given range; on the abscissa axis, ISPP values in mV. Data are presented of summary ISPP values analysis in six areas of uncus g.hippocampus (Unc), hippocampus (Hipp), temporal cortex (Cort), amygdala (Amyg.) of the right (D) and left (S) hemispheres. Vertical lines correspond to mean ISPP values. The number of measurements (n) prior to and after electric actions are correspondingly: in unc.d. – 256 and 287; in hipp.s. – 287 and 132; in cort.s. – 839 and 366; in amyg.d – 841 and 413; in hipp.d. – 849 and 379; in cort.d. – 449 and 182. Correction of emotional disturbances causes significant (p < 0.01) decrease in ISPP values in all structures except hipp.s., where the ISPP level changes near electrodes 1 and 2*

brain. This conclusion has been replicated in instances when patients with emotional disorders were treated by local electrostimulation. During the ES therapy, when pathological emotional states were found to weaken, eventually disappearing entirely, the shifts of the summary ISPP index tended to become negative (Figure 8.6). In future it may be possible to intensify these cerebral protective mechanisms for therapeutic purposes in much the same way as delta-like electrical evoked inhibitory effect is presently being implemented in clinical practice[7].

(3) Neurodynamics of the third type were recorded when the emotional reaction developed into affect, or when a violent emotional reaction preceded an epileptic seizure. This was accompanied by more or less widespread but remarkably similar trends in ISPP changes. Recording ISPP during a transient

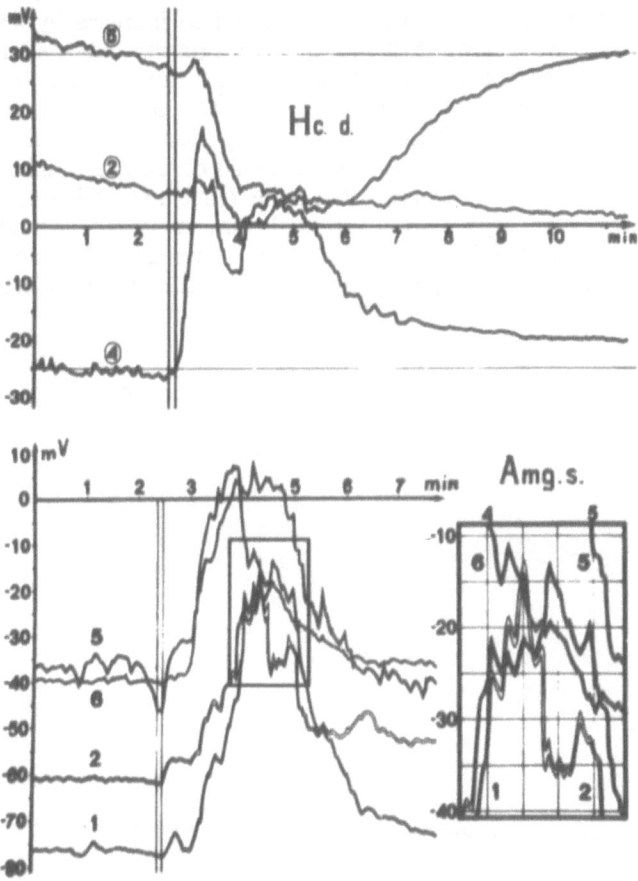

*Figure 8.7   Dynamics of ISPP in amygdala s. (epileptogenic area) and hippocampus d. during the development of impetuous laugh followed by psychomotor seizure. Numerals above the curves correspond to the electrode numbers. Period of partial consciousness and automatic movements is presented separately within the rectangular frame.*

psychomotor seizure demonstrated that the return of the ISPP level to its original value simultaneously with the cessation of the seizure was preceded by reciprocal ISPP shifts.

Figures 8.7, 8 show the ISPP characteristics in the left amygdala (the focus of pathological hyperactivation – epileptogenic focus), in the right hippocampus and in the polar area of the left temporal lobe during the evolution of a psychomotor seizure preceded by the affect of uncontrolled laughter.

The first sign of laughter coincided temporally with minor fluctuations in ISPP level for the area of the fifth electrode of the left amygdala, gradual decrease of ISPP in two areas of the right hippocampus and a different degree of ISPP level decrease in three pole areas of the temporal cortex. The psychomotor seizure developed at the height of violent laughter. The onset of the seizure coincided with a rapid increase of ISPP magnitude in all areas of the left amygdala, in one area of the right hippocampus and in two cortex areas of the temporal lobe. The ISPP value was found to increase by 45–55 mV in different amygdala areas, by 45 mV in the hippocampus and by 40 mV, 42 mV, and 46 mV in the cortex (in the first, second and third electrode areas). The increase in ISPP level concurred with transient loss of consciousness. During the third minute of the seizure (the second period) reciprocal trends were monitored in the ISPP level. A thorough analysis of ISPP dynamics within this period revealed that in some amygdala areas (first and fifth electrode areas) ISPP level remained high for more than 1 min, in others (second and sixth electrode areas) it dropped drastically, then increased a little, thereafter decreasing. Since ISPP changes in the area of each of the six electrodes were

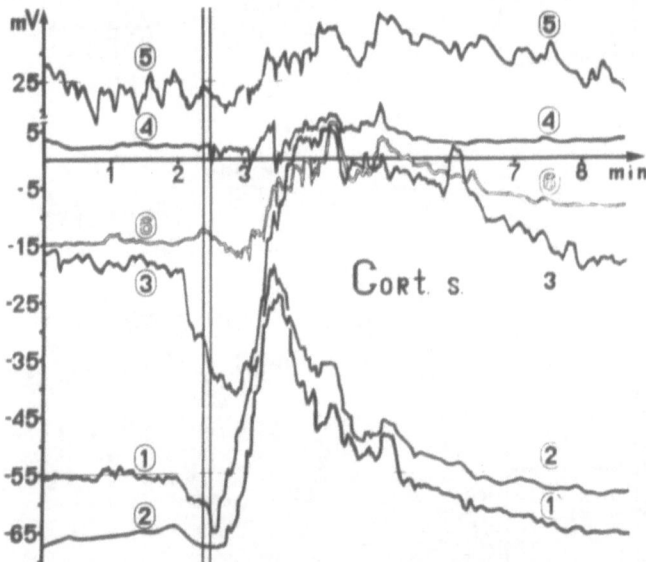

*Figure 8.8   ISPP dynamics in six areas of the left temporal lobe cortex (cort. s.) during a psychomotor seizure. For designations see previous figure*

unsynchronized, reciprocal relations (according to the ISPP data) evolved between some amygdala areas during each time interval. A dramatic decrement in ISPP level in the hippocampal areas and two of the cortex areas coincided with the total increase of ISPP level in all amygdala areas.

During the heterochronous decrease of ISPP values in the amygdala the basal level in all areas of the hippocampus fluctuated within the range of low positive values (5–8 mV). The levelling of the potential occurred due to the ISPP level increase by 30 mV in the fourth electrode area and an equivalent decrease in the fifth electrode area. In the cortex, however, co-instantaneous with the rapid drop in the ISPP level to its original value in the first and second electrode area, the potential level in the third and sixth electrode areas remained at a high level compared to initial values. The behaviour during this period was characterized by automatic movements and 'confused' consciousness. The end of the seizure and the total recovery of consciousness was accompanied by restabilization towards initial ISPP level in all the explored brain areas. These findings combined with ISPP dynamics presented in Figure 8.2, give supplementary information on the *spatial-temporal* and *structural-functional* organization of paroxysmal pathological states differing by the degree of generalized pathological disorders in the brain. The differences in nature between the paroxysmally evolving affect and psychomotor seizure are detected in slow physiological processes. The principal feature characterizing the ISPP dynamics during the psychomotor seizure is the *total* potential increase in all the left amygdala areas (*epileptogenic structure*). At this stage, when the pathological system is being consolidated, the ISPP changes are diffusive, their level tending to increase. During this period ISPP dynamics display no intra-structural reciprocal trends but the seizure is not generalized. It may be accounted for by the fact that it is the functional state in the formations in different structures of *ipsi-* and *contralateral hemisphere* (some areas in the right hippocampus and in the area of cortex pole in the left temporal lobe) rather than individual areas in the amygdala that restrict the expansion of pathological excitation in the brain. Heterochronous changes in ISPP dynamics for different structures serve, in such instances, as a factor preventing a generalized pathological paroxysm. Reciprocal ISPP dynamics, arising after originally similar changes of the index, predetermine the increase of functional heterogeneity inside one or different brain formations. Heterochronous and reciprocal changes in the areas of pathological hyperexcitation decrease the intensity of the impulse train in this area thereby weakening its control over other brain structures. These observations indicate that the reciprocal ISPP changes during the pathological reactions appear to represent protective cerebral systems whose operations extend beyond the limitation of emotional reactions alone. Hence when ISPP trends are characterized by an increase in intensity and especially when coupled with a reduction in asymmetry between the hemispheres it is indicative of evolving pathological reactions and of profound pathological changes in the brain.

Diagnostic and therapeutic usage of implanted electrodes suggest that medio-basal limbic formations are frequently the structures responsible for triggering the chain of pathological reactions culminating in an epileptic seizure. Experiments on animals, in addition to clinical studies involving electrostimulation in

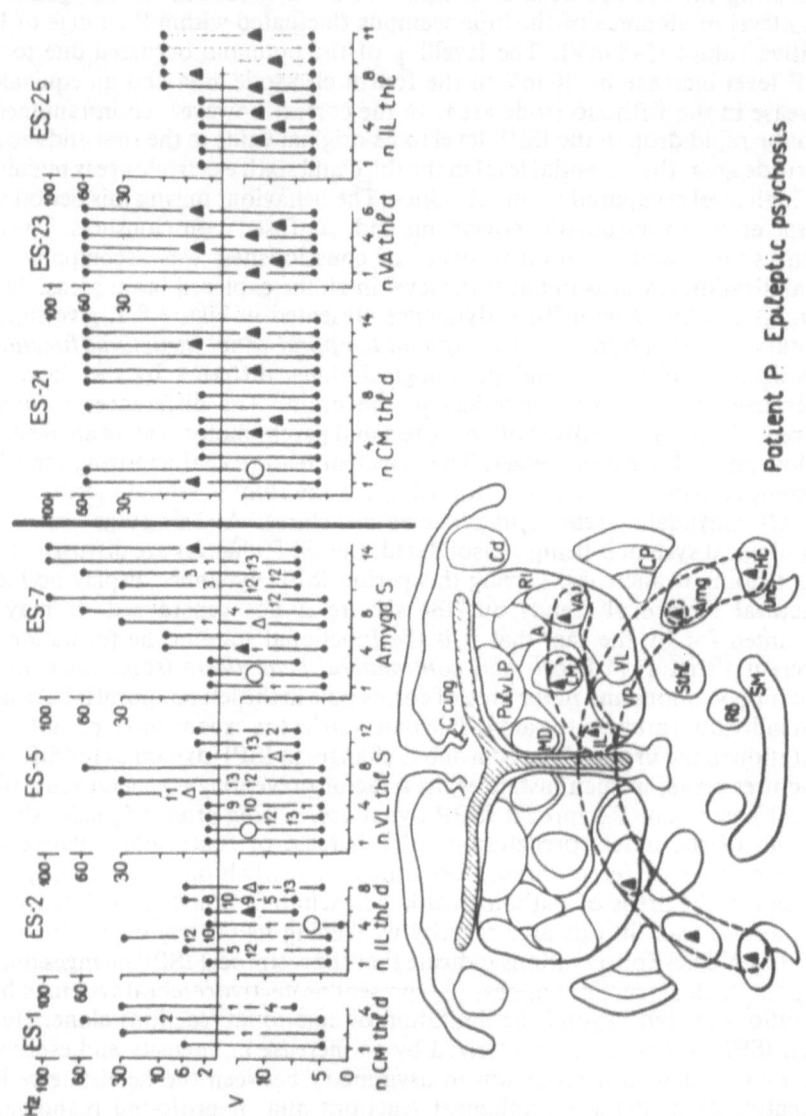

Patient P. Epileptic psychosis

humans, demonstrate *polyfunctionality* of these brain formations. This property forms the foundation for brain plasticity. Electrical stimulation permits monitoring of a wide range of reactions including motor, sensory, perceptual-motor, vegetative and visceral symptoms. Repeated stimulation of secondary emotiogenic zones resulted in a diminution (inhibition) of effects previously observed, such that reproducibility was mainly confined to emotional responses (Figure 8.9.) Thus, for instance, at the beginning of diagnostic electrical stimulation of different cerebral structures in an epileptic patient with psychic disorders this caused her to have reproducible responses in terms of motor, sensory, vegetative, psychosensory and epileptic phenomena. During repeated ES the range of evoked reactions grew narrower with only a limited number of stable clinical effects. During the first ES of thalamic and some temporal limbic structures, the patient manifested variations in activation level in the direction of improved mood, cheerfulness, and higher efficiency coupled with sensory-motor changes. Later, practically all previously evoked ES changes in the patient's condition vanished under the influence of repetitive therapeutic electrical stimulation with the exception of the activation syndrome based on positive emotions. From this and other evidence it appears that during the natural development of epilepsy with frequent seizures of temporal origin, some emotional features of limbic structures may also be prevalent.

The development of epileptic seizures, when epileptic areas are localized in limbic brain structures in accordance with the nature of the seizure, results from the pathological excitation propagating within these structures or within large brain territories. Whereas such pathological excitation accounts for the appearance of seizures, it it the recurrent activation of *temporal limbic* structures that leads to the expression of *emotional disorders*, typically of epilepsy.

---

*Figure 8.9   Changes of brain properties under the influence of local electrical stimulation (ES). Upper part: affects caused by ES of some brain areas. Numerals, triangles and white circles – reactions and states of different modality. Ordinate axis: above – frequency; below – amplitude of bipolar stimulating impulse (duration 1 ms, applied for 5–6 s). Parameters of stimulating impulses in each case are marked with black dots. Above the graphs – ordinal number of ES. Lower part – schematic map of a cross-section of the brain with black triangles showing areas where ES caused activation syndrome with positive emotions. During the first ES, positive emotions arose together with other reactions in single current application in a limited number of brain areas (intralaminar nucleus of the thalamus, amygdala s.). Later on, the increase in the number of brain areas was observed responding upon ES with development of positive emotional states and reactions. Activation syndrome manifested as positive emotions was provoked by ES of practically all brain areas in which electrodes were implanted for diagnosis and therapy. n. CM thl – centrum median of the thalamus; n. IL thl and VL thl – intralaminal and ventrolateral nuclei of the thalamus of the right (d) and left (s) hemispheres. (1) Involuntary reminiscences; (2) Itching of the face; (3) Hyperaesthesia; (4) Non-local pain; (5) Hyperhydrosis; (6) Psychosensory seizure; (7) Pain in temporal area; (8) Double image seen by the eyes; (9) Asymmetry of the face; (10) Feeling of hunger; (11) Senestrophotia; (12) Bad mood; (13) Feeling of uncertainty. White triangle – aura; circle – psychomotor seizure; dark triangle – improvement of mood, feeling of cheerfulness*

Numerous observations made by relatives of epileptic patients suggest that emotional disorders are frequently characterized by 'explosive' behaviour rather than epileptic disorders[20]. This makes the relationship between epileptic and motor seizures, and emotional disorders in epileptic patients quite comprehensible and simple, although, as far as the mechanisms are concerned, it does not fit the clinical concept of emotional disorders during epilepsy as a secondary phenomenon. This approach to the investigation of some mechanisms of pathological emotions and epilepsy provides a better insight into the study of correlations of emotional and other brain functions, especially different variations of motor behaviour. This special analysis has been based on studying interrelationships between emotional and speech-motor processes.

The investigation of human emotional activity and thinking as well as their neurophysiological maintenance was conducted using constant, periodic and sporadic verbal communication with the patient. Thus several emotional reactions were elicited by the investigator speaking with a patient. They developed during the speech contact, either unfolding or ceasing entirely dependent on the investigator's aim in directing the content of the conversation. Figure 8.10 shows ISPP dynamics in a patient in an euphoric state. When the investigator addressed the patient with the words, 'you look happy today', the patient responsed with the emotion of uncontrolled laughter. The increase of ISPP level was registered in the fifth and sixth amygdala areas prior to the onset of behavioural signs of laughter. ISPP value was at a maximum during the peak of behavioural response. The intensity of physiological reactions appeared to be greater during initial ISPP changes. At this moment, the investigator had asked the patient about the health of her sick child with the intention of eliminating the fit of laughter. The patient stopped laughing and began discussing her child's health. During this period, ISPP dynamics differed from the original in terms of trends and characteristic fluctuations. ISPP variations similar to those observed at the beginning of the emotiogenic test were registered immediately after the patient's talk about her child's health had been interrupted and she was questioned about her reasons for laughing. ISPP level was found to increase in three right amygdala areas preceding the uncontrolled behavioural reaction of laughter. When the expressive emotional component was at maximum, the ISPP level stabilized. When the ISPP level tended to decrease, more intense fluctuations were recorded during a second attempt to interrupt the patient's reaction of laughter. In this case, the patient succeeded in suppressing the emotion but the level of the emotional tension remained high as evidenced by occasional outbursts of constrained laughter. The delayed reaction registered as a decrease in level and a specific pattern of ISPP dynamics correlated with the patient's efforts to attenuate the intensity of the emotion.

In the above example, the main factors influencing emotional intensity were the *semantic content* of the investigator's speech addressed to the patient, and his *intonation* which conveyed considerable semantic connotation. Almost every such investigation of evoked emotional state included the patient's verbal response activating the system responsible for speech-motor functions.

The study of neurophysiological mechanisms of thinking[9] has shown that the components of a complex speech-motor system can hardly be considered separately in terms of neuronal mechanisms of speech production. This indicates that cerebral processes implicated in the unfolding of emotions both during spontaneous and evoked speech can be assumed to result from the interaction of phenomena maintaining emotional and speech-motor activity. We observed the neurophysiological result of interaction of all these components many times whilst recording ISPP. There are two types of observation that are of special interest here:

(1)  ISPP dynamics in the course of rapidly evolving pathological emotions accompanied by delirious speech with some interval in the ISPP dynamics.

(2)  ISPP dynamics which developed after the investigator had persuaded the patient to cease talking about an unpleasant topic.

A progressive increment in ISPP intensity was recorded during rapidly evolving uncontrolled pathological emotional states in a patient suffering from *epileptic psychosis*, which is illustrated in Figure 8.11. During one session (45 min), the stable component of ISPP increased from 5 to 40 mV. The patient's delirious speech was monitored against this background within a range of 5 to 25 mV. Not a single sentence uttered by the patient could be considered as normal speech, yet every episode of the patient's speech activity evoked a marked phasic decrease in ISPP level. When ISPP reached 35–40 mV, speech production ceased entirely. This observation when compared with the second type is of importance for understanding its physiological mechanism.

As ISPP had been recorded many hours daily for a period of weeks, and even months, various spontaneous and evoked emotions could be observed. Furthermore, it has been demonstrated that emotional conditions correlating with ISPP shifts differ in terms of intensity, duration and propagation in the brain. In fact, such differences may permit detection of spontaneous reactions and states which could then be related to the patient's verbal report of his state of health. Emotional states were also monitored prior to speech utterances. The postinvestigation and ISPP records reveal, however, that not every unpleasant conversation the patient had with the investigator was necessarily followed by development of an emotional reaction. For example in one session, the patient suddenly began talking about a topic very painful for him (concerning his relationship with girls and the difficulties his illness caused him when confronting them socially). Then the investigator suggested that they discontinue discussing it. There were no ISPP shifts registered during the conversation. The situation altered, however, immediately afterwards; considerable variations in ISPP level arose in many areas (in both uncuses gyri hippocampus, left hippocampus) as shown in Figure 8.12. There was a drastic, transient decrease in ISPP followed by a sharp increase that was recorded simultaneously in six areas of the left uncus giri hippocampus. As has been mentioned, these ISPP shifts are correlated with a violent emotional reaction. In epileptic patients, should the shifts intensify, an epileptic seizure might develop. There were no clinical signs of a seizure recorded in this case. It is of interest, however, that responses to questions that the investigator had asked the patient, after the ISPP had regained its resting level, revealed amnesia to events preceding ISPP shifts. ISPP shifts give every reason to suppose that the interruption of speech-motor activity at the request of the investigator was immediately followed by a

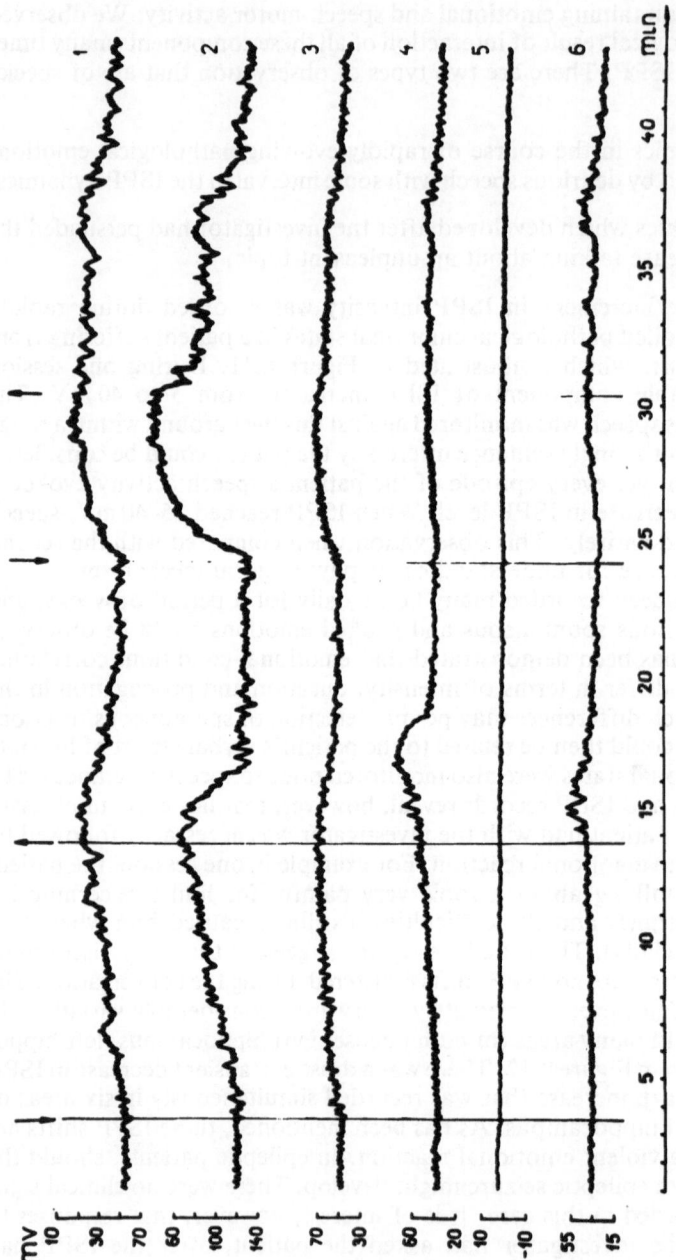

*Figure 8.10  Changes of ISPP level in six areas of amyg.s. (numbers of electrodes are given at the right of each trace) during spontaneous development of impetuous laugh in the state of euphoria (first arrow); after the attempt to interrupt the laugh by reminding about the sick child of the patient (second arrow). In response to the question, 'Why did you laugh' (third arrow) the impetuous laugh starts again, and a new attempt is made to stop it (fourth arrow)*

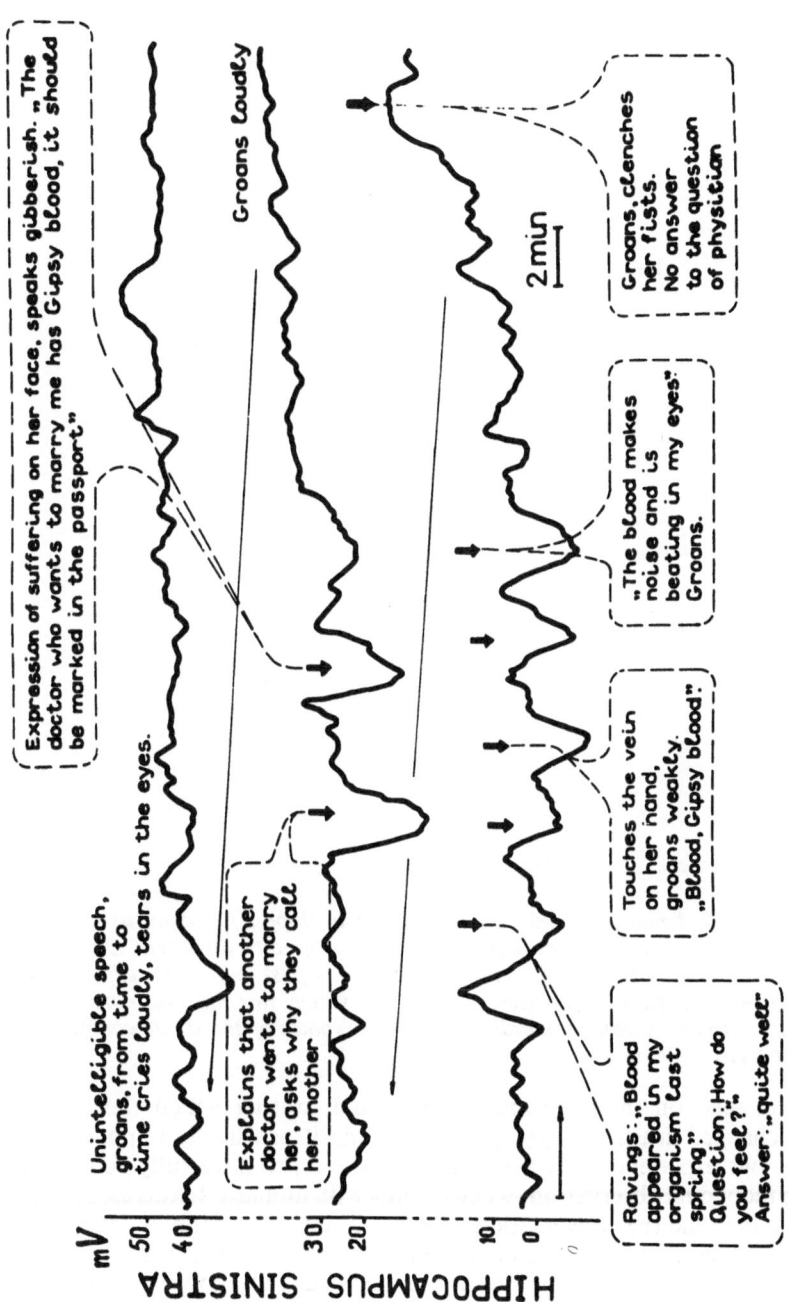

*Figure 8.11  ISPP dynamics in the left hippocampus in a patient with epileptic psychosis during the deterioration of psychopathological disorders. Lower curve – the beginning of the investigation, upper curve – the end. The arrows show the speech-motor activity. ISPP value – ordinate axis; time (min) – abscissa axis*

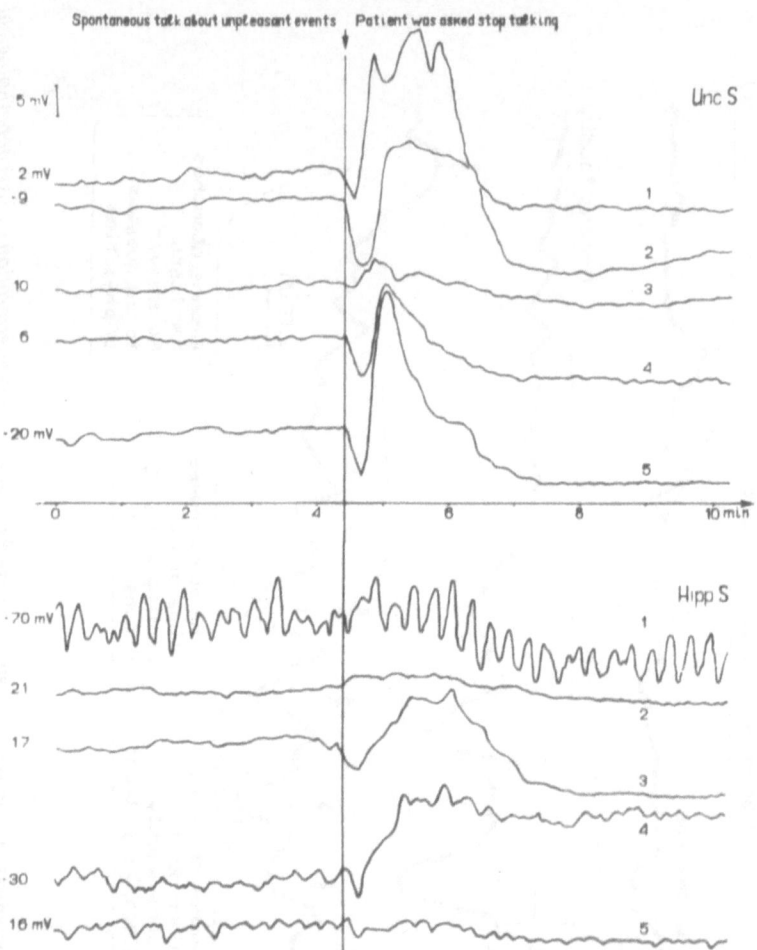

*Figure 8.12   ISPP dynamics in the left hippocampus (hipp.s.) and uncus g.hippo-campus (unc.s.) in a patient with pronounced emotional-mnestic disorders. On the left – ISPP dynamics during the patient's report concerning past unpleasant experiences. On the right – the period of manifested emotions which was not accompanied by speech-motor activity. Arabic numerals on the left – values of the stable component; on the right – electrode numbers*

pathological reaction, most probably emotional, during which the brain's condition changed drastically (the patient finding it practically impossible to retain previous experiences). It is difficult, however, to have fully controlled studies for individual observations when dealing with humans. In this case, it can be assumed that had the conversation relating to unpleasant topics continued, it might have gradually elicited an emotional response. Previous observations of spontaneous and evoked emotional reactions suggest, however, that it is improbable that such an induced pathological response would be as intensive and violent as during the unanticipated interruption of the conversation.

190

Thus if a comparison is made of the two above-mentioned observations, no matter how different they might at first appear, it can be assumed that, in addition to different variants of correlations between emotions and speech-motor processes, relationships may exist in which speech-motor activity contributes to phasic ISPP shifts characteristic of a more favourable condition. Conversely, its 'forced' interruption contributes to ISPP rearrangements characteristic of the pathological (emotional?) state.

## SUMMARY

The study of emotions using infraslow physiological processes offers a quantitative description of rearrangements in the brain under diverse conditions. It was possible to record, from those brain areas in which electrodes were implanted, the sequence and degree of involvement of various structures in the cerebral maintenance of emotional processes. By analysing the neurophysiological correlates of behavioural responses, it was possible to demonstrate the existence of hitherto unknown cerebral protective mechanisms which manifested themselves as ISPP shifts of a negative polarity in adjacent and remote brain areas, compared to those in which positive shifts developed, maintaining the given reaction. A more complete understanding of emotional behaviour is offered by studying neurophysiological indices of various emotional responses developing against a diverse background of emotional states. These investigations provide a foundation for further study of brain maintenance of emotional states and reactions, as well as yielding information concerning the brain processes involved in maintaining other aspects of human activity. The possibility of recording slow physiological processes, both from intracerebral electrodes and from the scalp (which is widely used), makes the method more promising. The latter approach is not expected, however, to offer information associated with more complex intracerebral neurodynamics; nor do we know whether this will become a reality in the future. Hence data obtained from recording ISPP by means of implanted electrodes remain unique despite all limitations already discussed. A most important problem requiring more detailed study is directed at methodological issues of neurodynamics during the interaction of different forms of activity, more specifically, the ISPP dynamics during the interaction of emotional and motor processes. Some preliminary data on this problem have been treated in this contribution based on recording cerebral neurophysiological concomitants of emotional and speech-motor activity. From these data we have been led to believe that a controled organization of motor activities may contribute to the mobilization of protective mechanisms of the brain.

### References

1. Bechtereva, N. P. (1978). *The Neurophysiological Aspects of Human Mental Activity*. 2nd Edn. (New York: Oxford University Press)

2. Bechtereva, N. P., Gratchev, K. V., Orlova, A. N. and Jatzuk, S. L. (1963). Ispolzovanie mnozshestvennykh elektrodov, vzshivlennykh v podkorkovye obrazovanija golovnogo mozga tcheloveka, dlja letchenija giperkinezov. *Zsh. Nevropatol. i Psykhiatr.*, **1**, 3–8
3. Bechtereva, N. P., Bondartchuk, A. N., Smirnov, V. M. and Trokhatchev, A. I. (1967). *Fiziologija i patofiziologija glubokikh struktur golovnogo mozga.* Moskow, Leningrad. (Translated into German and published, Berlin: Volk und Gesundheit, 1969)
4. Bechtereva, N. P., Bondartchuk, A. N., Smirnov, V. M., Melutcheva, L. A. and Shandurina, A. N. (1975). Method of electrostimulation of the deep brain structures in treatment of some chronic diseases. *Confinia Neurologica*, **37**, 136–40
5. Bechtereva, N. P. (1966). *Nekotorye printizipialnye voprosy izutchenija neirofiziologitchestikh oszov psikhitcheskikh javlenii v norme i patologii.* pp. 18–21. (Moscow, Leningrad: Nauka)
6. Bechtereva, N. P. (1971). *Neirofiziologitcheskie aspekty psikhitcheskoi dejatelnosti tcheloveka.* (Leningrad: Meditzina). (Translated into English and published, New York: Oxford University Press, 1978, see ref. 1)
7. Bechtereva, N. P. (1980). *Zdorovyi i bolnoi mozg tcheloveka.* (Leningrad: Nauka)
8. Bechtereva, N. P., Bundzen, P. V., Matveev, Yu. K. and Kaplunovskii, A. S. (1971). Funktzionalnaja reorganizatzija aktivnosti neironnykh populjatzii mozga tcheloveka pri kratkovremennoi pamjati. *Fiziol. zshurn SSSR*, **57**, 1745–61
9. Gogolitsin, Yu. L. and Kropotov, Yu. D. (1983). *Issledovanie tchastoty razpjadov neironov mozga tcheloveka.* (Leningrad: Nauka)
10. Bechtereva, N. P., Gogolitzin, Yu. L., Kropotov, Yu. D. and Medvedev, S. V. (1985). *Neirofisiologitcheskie mekhanismy myshlenija.* (Leningrad: Nauka)
11. Bechtereva, N. P. (1967). Nekotorye vosmozshnosti isseledovanija glubokikh otdelov mozga tcheloveka. In *Problemy klitcheskoi i experimentalnoi fiziologii golovnogo mozga.* pp. 7–13. (Leningrad: Meditzina)
12. Bechtereva, N. P., Kambarova, D. K. and Ivanov, G. G. (1972). Mozgovaja organizatzija emotzionalnykh reaktzii i sostojanii. *Fizio. tcheloveka (Human Physiology – USA)*, **8**, 691–706
13. Bechtereva, N. P. (1983). Neurophysiology of intellectual and emotional processes in man. *Int. J. Psychophysiol.*, , **1**, 7–12
14. Bechtereva, N. P., Kambarova, D. K. and Ivanov, G. G. (1984). Investigation and treatment of emotional disorders. In *Theoretical Problems of Modern Psychiatry.* pp. 143–56. (Basel: Sandoz Ltd.)
15. Kambarova, D. K. (1981). Vozmozshnosti neirophysiologii v isutchenii i letchenii psikhitcheskikh narushenii pri epilepsii. *Fiziol. tcheloveka (Human Physiology – USA)*, **7**, 143–56
16. Anitchkov, A. D. (1977). Stereotaxitcheskii apparat dlja vvedenija dolgosrotchnykh mnozshestvennykh vnutrimozgovykh elektrodov. *Fiziol. tcheloveka (Human Physiology – USA)*, **3**, 372–5
17. Polonsky, Yu. Z. (1977). O vozmozshnostjakh optimizatzii stereotaxitcheskoi metodiki s ispolzovaniem EVM. *Fiziol. tcheloveka (Human Physiology – USA)*, **4**, 376–8
18. Danko, S. G. and Kaminskii, Yu. L. (1978). Portativnyie pribory dlja elektritcheskikh stimuljatzii mozga. *Fiziol. tcheloveka (Human Physiology – USA)*, **4**, 169–72
19. Danko, S. G. and Kaminskii, Yu. L. (1982). *Sistema technitcheskikh sredstv neirofiziologitcheskikh issledovanii tcheloveka.* (Leningrad: Nauka)
20. Savtchenko, Yu. N. (1968). *Funktzionanalno-morfologitcheskaja kharakteristika epilepsii i skhodnykh sostojanii.* Avtoref dokt. diss. Omsk-Leningrad

# 9
# Personality and motor activity: a psychophysiological perspective

## Robert M. Stelmack

The view that differences in personality are influenced by constitutional, genetically determined predispositions is one which is gathering increasing support from a variety of sources[1,2]. This notion is endorsed by evidence from biometric analyses of personality inventories which have examined the heritability of personality traits[3], from biochemical assays which link differences in personality to differences in neurohormonal and catecholamine activity[4] and from psychophysiological measures which ascribe differences in personality to differences in physiological arousal systems[5]. With regard to psychophysiological studies of personality, the research has largely focused on individual differences in the effects of sensory stimulation on autonomic and cortical activity. Psychophysiological investigation of individual differences in the expression of motor behaviour has not been so intensively pursued, and research in this area is quite fragmented. However, the emergence of impulsiveness as a fundamental personality factor[6,7] that is relevant to the conceptually similar dimensions of extraversion, Type A behaviour and sensation-seeking behaviour, has fostered a growing recognition of the importance of individual differences in motor performance for the understanding of personality. An analysis of individual differences in the expression of motor activity, by means of psychophysiological techniques, may serve to focus the neurological bases of differences along those personality dimensions.

In this chapter, a brief overview is presented that outlines the context in which psychophysiological research on personality has been pursued. A perspective from which research on the psychophysiology of individual differences in motor expression may be considered is also noted. The review considers two psychophysiological techniques that are sensitive to variation in motor activity and that have been related to personality differences – specifically, the contingent negative variation, which describes a waveform derived from the recording of electrocortical activity, and, secondly, cardiac activity. The functional significance of these measurement techniques with regard to motor activity is outlined for the purpose of establishing the interpretative limits of the techniques. The results of studies that have applied these psychophysiological measures to personality research and some of the methodological and theoretical issues that emerge from this work are discussed.

## INDIVIDUAL DIFFERENCES IN RESPONSE TO SENSORY STIMULATION

The most widely researched personality domain to which psychophysiological methods have been applied is Eysenck's theory of extraversion. For ease of exposition, this brief discussion is limited to that subject in this section. To begin, it should be noted that the enhanced sensitivity to stimulation of introverts has been observed in several sensory modalities using a variety of psychophysical methods. Lower sensory thresholds or greater sensitivity for introverts have been demonstrated for auditory[8], visual[9] and somatosensory[10] modalities and with painful stimulation[11]. This evidence of enhanced sensitivity for introverts supports the hypothesis that introverts are characterized by stronger excitatory potential[12] or lower thresholds of reticulocortical arousal[13].

In a previous report[14], we argued that a large literature treating the psychophysiology of extraversion could also be understood in terms of differences in sensory sensitivity to stimulation and that these differences may be referred to the level of the sensory nerve. The argument was based on the following considerations. First, studies comparing introverts and extraverts on electroencephalographic indices of cortical arousal offer little support for differences in endogenous or resting level of cortical arousal, i.e. under 'non-stimulus' conditions. In studies which report higher levels of cortical arousal for introverts, the effects seem to be determined by stimulus conditions or task demands. Secondly, there is a good deal of evidence that introverts display enhanced or more frequent electrodermal responses, a measure of autonomic activity, to stimuli of moderate intensity or arousal potential. Similarly, introverts display enhanced cortical evoked responses to auditory stimuli of moderate intensity. In general, the electrodermal and evoked potential effects concur with the view that introverts are characterized by lower thresholds of reticulo-cortical arousal than extraverts. Recently, however, we have found that extraverts display longer latency of auditory brainstem evoked responses than introverts. These cortical evoked potential components emanate from the level of the auditory nerve and cochlear nucleus and they are independent of the reticular system. The findings are consistent with the lower sensitivity of extraverts evident in psychophysical tasks and with their lower responsiveness on electrodermal and evoked potential measures. Since auditory brainstem evoked responses are largely unaffected by differences in attention, sleep and arousal, the findings may require the elaboration of the neurophysiological bases of extraversion to accommodate differences in neural transmission that are present in peripheral nervous system processes. At the very least, the results of these psychophysiological inquiries suggest clear differences between introverts and extraverts in their response to sensory stimulation that are quite consistent with their heightened sensitivity to stimulation observed in psychophysical tasks.

While the electrodermal and evoked potential measures can be linked to individual differences in sensory sensitivity and extraversion in a straightforward way, a similar association cannot be readily observed between psychophysiological measures and individual differences in motor activity and extraversion. Introverts and extraverts have been found to differ in the expression of motor behaviour in social and athletic activities (cf. Chapters 13 and 14) and in a variety of experimental paradigms (cf. Chapter 2). In general, it appears that introverts perform with more effective control than extraverts in tasks which require refined motor control, such as pursuit-rotor tracking tasks[15, 16] and they make fewer false-positive errors in reaction time tasks[17]. In free response situations, on the other hand, extraverts have been found to respond faster and more often than introverts and to have more involuntary rest pauses in a tapping task[18].

In early work, rest pauses on motor tasks were conceived as measures of inhibitory potential which Eysenck[12] had proposed as a determinant of extraversion. As the analysis of the reminiscence phenomenon has shown (Chapter 4), these motor measures of inhibitory activity have proved to be far more complicated than initially supposed. Brebner[19] has also attempted to reconcile some of the complex effects observed in reaction time tasks by distinguishing between response excitation and inhibition and between stimulus excitation and inhibition. The psychophysiological analysis of individual differences in motor activity, which has been a relatively neglected topic of investigation, could provide useful information both in regard to differences in motor behaviour between introverts and extraverts and in regard to the neurological bases of extraversion. In approaching this problem, two psychophysiological techniques, the contingent negative variation and cardiac activity, provide measures which are functionally related to motor activity and for which some evidence of consistent variation with personality differences has been observed.

## PERSONALITY AND THE CONTINGENT NEGATIVE VARIATION

In a reaction time task, where the subject is given a warning signal ($S_1$) followed by an imperative stimulus ($S_2$) that signals the subject to initiate a motor response, an increase in negative potential is observed from scalp electrodes prior to the imperative signal. This waveform was first described by Walter, Cooper, Aldridge, McCallum and Winter[20], who gave the name 'contingent negative variation' (CNV) to the effect. This term emphasized the associative stimulus features of the paradigm for the facilitation of motor activation. Enhanced CNV amplitude, for example, has often been associated with quicker reaction times. At the present time, there is some consensus that when the $S_1$–$S_2$ interval is greater than 3 or 4 s, two distinct components are observed[21]. The first component, which appears within 1 s after $S_1$, is referred to as the orienting or O-wave, since it is similar in some respects to the orienting response described by Sokolov[22]. That is, it is sensitive to variation in physical stimulus parameters, novelty and stimulus significance[23]. A second component, featuring an increasing negative potential, develops prior to $S_2$. This component is commonly referred to as the expectancy or E-wave. The biphasic nature of the CNV is illustrated in Figure 9.1.

There is a strong case for the view that the E-wave reflects preparation for a motor response[24]. The E-wave is consistently present when a motor response to $S_2$ is required and it is considerably diminished or absent when a motor response is not required[25]. CNV is also enhanced when increased muscular effort or fast

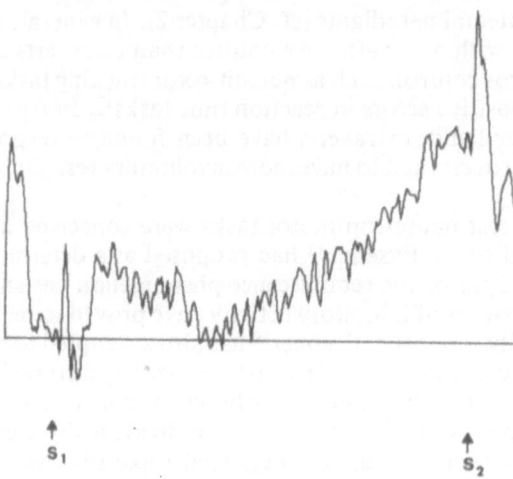

$S_1$ $S_2$

*Figure 9.1   Contingent negative variation for one subject with a 4 s interval between the warning signal ($S_1$) and the imperative signal to respond ($S_2$)[23] (reprinted with kind permission from N. E. Lovelace and A. J. Sandford, 1974, **1**, 303–14, Biological Psychology, Elsevier Science Publishers B.V.)*

*reaction times are requested*[26]. In general, the CNV is sensitive to the motor task demands and conditions which have been shown to influence reaction time performance. Differences in CNV amplitudes have also been related to differences along a number of personality dimensions. The question remains, however, what, if anything, can individual differences in CNV tell us about individual differences in the expression of motor behaviour and personality?

## ANXIETY AND THE CNV

Anxiety was recognized as a contributing factor to individual differences in CNV in the very earliest research reports. Walter[27], for example, observed that the CNV developed slowly and irregularly in anxious patients. Despite the sampling and diagnostic problems which are frequently encountered with clinical populations, the reduced CNV amplitude of anxious psychiatric patients has been reported quite consistently[28, 29]. When questionnaire measures of trait anxiety have been employed with non-psychiatric subjects, no differences in CNV are evident in non-stressful experimental conditions[30–32]. However, significant relationships between trait anxiety and CNV amplitude have been observed in experiments which have manipulated stress or arousal levels through task demands or stimulus conditions.

Knott and Irwin[32] described an experiment which examined the effects of stress on the CNV amplitude for groups defined as high and low anxiety on the basis of extreme scores on the Bendig[33] social introversion–extraversion and emotional stability scales. In the high stress condition, the $S_2$ was a flash of light and the $S_1$ was an electric shock previously judged 'uncomfortable' by the subject. High anxious subjects displayed reduced CNV amplitude relative to their performance in a low stress condition, where $S_2$ was also a light flash, and relative to the low anxious subjects. The authors accounted for this reduction of CNV amplitude in terms of a ceiling effect in which a 'long-term, slow potential shift occurs in the high anxiety group with the creation of stress which persists over the entire time that high intensity shock is expected'. That is, a maximum degree of negativity develops, which limits the extent to which the negative potential can increase.

Similar findings have been reported by Low and Swift[34] who manipulated difficulty levels in an auditory discrimation task. High and low anxiety groups were defined on the basis of extreme scores on the IPAT anxiety scales. In this study, the subject's task was to discriminate the frequency of $S_2$ from the frequency of $S_1$. For all subjects, CNV amplitude diminished with increasing task difficulty. High anxious subjects displayed smaller CNV amplitudes than low anxious subjects for the more difficult discrimination tasks. Thus, the reduced CNV observed in moderately stressful conditions for subjects classified as high anxious, by means of trait measures, concords with the reduced CNV observed in high anxious clinical subjects.

The suggestion that the CNV reduction in high anxious subjects is due to a ceiling effect does not address the principal question of what determines the sustained negative shift. Increased muscular force applied in response to $S_2$ has the effect of enhancing CNV magnitude[35,36], rather than diminishing it. However, Papakostopoulos and Jones[37] have shown that CNV amplitude is reduced when muscular effort is maintained or varied with the $S_1$–$S_2$ interval. Thus, it is quite plausible that motor preparation is disrupted in high anxious subjects by sustained or variable muscle tension. Indeed, muscular overactivation is widely regarded as an important characteristic of chronic anxiety.

A broader interpretation of reduced CNV amplitude in high anxious subjects has been advocated by Tecce[38] in terms of a distraction–arousal hypothesis. When subjects are distracted by the necessity to perform mental tasks, such as a memory task[39] or mental arithmetic during the $S_1$–$S_2$ interval[40], arousal, as indexed by increased heart rate levels and blink rates[41], is increased and CNV amplitude is reduced. From this evidence, it may be argued that high anxious subjects are more susceptible to distraction by stimuli or ideation that are not relevant to the task. Consequently, CNV amplitude is reduced in those subjects. Moreover, there is some debate concerning the extent to which CNV development is dependent on motor components in view of evidence of a dissociation of CNV amplitude and peripheral electromyographic activity which has been reported in distraction paradigms[24,42].

Virtually all of the studies investigating individual differences in CNV amplitude between high and low anxious subjects have employed $S_1$–$S_2$ intervals of 2 s or less. Thus, a clear distinction between the early O-wave and late E-wave components of the CNV was not possible. Recently, Glanzmann and Froehlich[43] have reported a study which compared high and low anxious subjects in a CNV paradigm with a 4 s ISI. In their report, subjects were assigned to either an ego threat condition, where they were advised that their intelligence was being assessed, a pain-threat condition, where non-contingent electric shocks were announced but not applied, or a control condition. Within each condition subjects were instructed to either respond (Go) with a button press or not respond

(NoGo), depending on whether $S_1$ was a high or low frequency tone. No clear differences between high and low anxious groups emerged. Although this study was inconclusive, the design of the experiment has a good deal of merit, which should be noted. In addition to the separation of E- and O-waves afforded by the long $S_1$, the Go/NoGo instructions within the same series enable some assessment of ceiling effects. A sustained negative potential would result in lowered CNV amplitude in both Go and NoGo sets. In fact, in the ego threat condition there was no difference in CNV amplitude between Go and NoGo trials for the high anxious subjects. Secondly, the pain and ego threat conditions enable some assessment of current hypotheses concerning the nature of anxiety. The pain condition, for example, is relevant to Gray's model of anxiety where it is proposed that high anxious subjects are characterized by a heightened sensitivity to punishment or threats of punishment[44]. The ego threat condition is also relevant to the hypothesis that high anxious subjects are particularly sensitive to situations of perceived threat to self-esteem[45]. There are a number of variations in this design which would be worthwhile to pursue in the context of these theories of anxiety. Of particular interest would be examination of the distraction–arousal hypothesis where a mental task is required during the $S_1$–$S_2$ interval. It would also be worthwhile to consider the application of a negative valence stimulus or threat of punishment at the imperative stimulus, as in the studies with anxious patients, to explore hypotheses concerning anxiety and individual differences in susceptibility to threat of punishment.

Overall, the evidence suggests that high anxious subjects in psychiatric settings tend to display smaller CNV amplitudes than low anxious patients. Similarly, non-psychiatric subjects classified as high anxious on the basis of trait anxiety questionnaires tend to display smaller CNV amplitude than low anxious subjects when stressful task demands are introduced in the $S_1$–$S_2$ interval, although these effects are not consistently observed. For the most part, the structure of the CNV, in terms of O-wave and E-wave components, has not been extensively examined and thus the sensory and motor contributions to the CNV effects for groups that differ in degree of anxiety have not been assessed.

## EXTRAVERSION AND THE EFFECTS OF DRUGS ON CNV

Research on the effects of drugs on CNV is remarkable for demonstrating paradoxical effects and striking individual differences[46]. Analysis of those effects, however, provides a promising approach for examining the biological bases of individual differences in personality. The Eysenck personality typology has been particularly useful in focusing paradoxical individual differences in a number of CNV studies[47]. Moreover, since both extraversion and neuroticism are independent dimensions that correlate with measures of anxiety, the contribution of extraversion and neuroticism in the effects of anxiety on the CNV can be considered.

The greater CNV amplitude of extraverts than introverts in non-stressful conditions has been reported by a number of investigators[48-51]. Null effects have been reported in other cases where the typology has been employed[52,53].

In those studies which report positive findings, the effects are adduced in support of the arousal hypothesis with the lower CNV of introverts taken as evidence of their higher levels of arousal[13]. None of the studies has reported a significant relationship between neuroticism and CNV amplitude. Thus, it may be that the CNV differences between high and low anxious subjects that have been discussed may be attributable to differences that are associated with introversion–extraversion rather than neuroticism. Of those studies which report positive findings for non-stress conditions, only Plooij-Van Gorsel and Janssen employed interstimulus intervals which allowed the O-wave and E-wave of the CNV to be distinguished[51]. The enhanced response of extraverts was evident for both components, though the effects were more prominent for the E-wave. On the other hand, those studies which report significant effects between high and low anxious subjects have introduced manipulations which were designed to increase stress levels.

Since Eysenck's theory of extraversion holds that introverts are characterized by higher levels of reticulocortical arousal[13], some investigators have argued that introverts and extraverts should respond differently to the effects of central nervous system stimulant and depressant drugs and that these effects can be expressed in differences in the CNV waveform. Individual differences in the effects of high and low doses of chlordiazepoxide, a cortical inhibitory drug, and of caffeine, a cortical excitatory drug, on CNV amplitude were examined for independent groups of introverts and extraverts under noise and no-noise conditions by Janssen, Mattie, Plooij-Van Gorsel and Werre[54]. Introverts in the noise condition displayed smaller CNV amplitudes than introverts in the no-noise condition but no differences between introverts and extraverts were observed in any drug condition.

In an early report, Ashton, Millman, Telford and Thompson[52] noted that nicotine intake during cigarette smoking had differential effects on CNV magnitude for subjects classified as introverts or extraverts on the Eysenck Personality Inventory[55]. Extraverted smokers had a slower rate of nicotine intake, and displayed increased CNV amplitudes from pre-smoking levels than introverts who had a faster rate of nicotine intake and who displayed decreased CNV amplitude. In this case, however, it was not clear whether the effects were due to rate of nicotine intake or to differences in personality. In a more recent study, cannabis, which, like nicotine, is known to have both stimulant and depressant effects on various measures of central nervous system activity, was also found to have different effects on CNV amplitude for introverts and extraverts[56]. In this experiment, CNV increased, relative to predrug levels, after a low cannabis dose for introverted subjects and for subjects with high neuroticism scores. Extraverts and low neuroticism scorers displayed a decrease in CNV amplitude with the low dosage. Thus, for introverts and high neuroticism scorers, the low dosage acts as a stimulant while it acts as a depressant for extraverts and low neuroticism subjects. The opposite effects were observed with high doses of cannabis. That is, with high doses, introverted and high neuroticism scorers showed a decrease in CNV magnitude while the extraverts and low neuroticism scorers showed an increase in CNV magnitude. Within the $S_1$–$S_2$ presentations, the interstimulus interval was randomly varied between 2, 3 and 4 s. This should have the effect of attenuating CNV magnitude since an expectancy set will be less likely to develop. In fact, CNV magnitude was greater at the longer $S_1$–$S_2$

interval. Despite this confounding of interstimulus interval, however, the effects are quite remarkable and potentially important. Such dramatic reversals are a rare phenomenon in personality research and it would be very informative if the neural generators of the CNV which are activated by cannabis could be specified.

In a recent series of experiments, O'Connor observed differences in CNV amplitude between introverts and extraverts which confirm the effects of nicotine noted by Ashton *et al.*[52, 53, 57]. In his first experiment, extreme groups of introvert and extravert subjects performed choice and simple reaction time tasks with either a short 1.25 s $S_1$–$S_2$ interval or a longer 4 s interval. For introverts, CNV amplitude tended to decrease in amplitude from sham to real smoking while for extraverts amplitude increased during smoking. Examination of the slow cortical wave components indicated that for the extraverts the O-wave decreased and the E-wave increased during smoking while for the introverts the E-wave decreased. These effects are illustrated in Figure 9.2. In a subsequent study, the prominent effect indicated that the E-wave amplitude decreased during smoking for introverts and increased for extraverts[57]. Overall, this well-controlled series of experiments confirms the previously observed paradoxical effects of nicotine on the CNV amplitude of introverts and extraverts.

Since introverts and extraverts differ in their response to nicotine, consideration of the neurophysiological effects of nicotine should be helpful in focusing the neurophysiological bases of individual differences in extraversion. An excellent summary of the neurochemical action of nicotine has recently been published by Edwards and Warburton in a paper which attempts to delineate the usefulness of electrocortical measurement techniques for the study of smoking

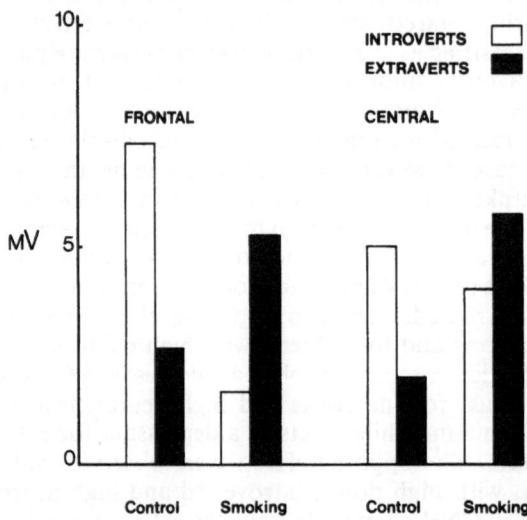

*Figure 9.2   Mean amplitude of the E-wave of the contingent negative variation for introverts and extraverts during sham and smoking conditions*[53] *(reprinted with kind permission from K. O'Connor, 1982, 3, 271–85, Personality and Individual Differences, Pergamon Press Ltd.)*

behaviour[58]. They point out that, 'the major finding from animal studies using smoking doses is that nicotine acts on nicotinic, cholinergic receptors in the mesencephalic reticular formation and activates the ascending cholinergic pathway to the cortex. This pathway releases acetylcholine and controls electrocortical activity.' At smoking doses, nicotine appears to mimic acetylcholine and induces the same neural changes that are produced by the natural activation of cholinergic synapses. Although extrapolating from animal studies to human behaviour must be done with considerable caution, the notion that introverts and extraverts may differ with respect to acetylcholine release is one which fits quite well with the sensory facilitation and motor inhibition that may characterize extraversion.

It should be noted that not all of the studies which investigated the relationship between CNV and personality reported reaction times. Moreover, the negative association of CNV magnitude with reaction time was not observed in those studies which did report them[32, 50–52, 56]. Thus, although there is general agreement that the development of CNV reflects preparation for a motor response and that quicker reaction times are associated with enhanced E-waves[59], there is little evidence of a direct relationship between CNV magnitude and reaction time for subjects who differ in degree of anxiety or extraversion. Nevertheless, consistent individual differences in CNV magnitude have been observed which can be attributed to differences in personality and the technique may be usefully applied to explore those differences.

## PERSONALITY AND CARDIAC ACTIVITY

The recording of cardiac activity gained prominence some 30 years ago as an effective means of investigating arousal and activation states[60]. Cardiac measures were employed, for example, to study anxiety; increased heart rate and blood pressure were often observed as symptoms of chronic anxiety. The efficacy of heart rate as an index of arousal was challenged by demonstrations that tonic cardiac activity did not invariably increase with increased motivational conditions, but in fact, decreased in some situations. A novel stimulus change of moderate intensity, for example, was seen to consistently elicit heart rate deceleration. Decreasing heart rate was also observed in anticipation of aversive stimuli in classical conditioning paradigms. The bidirectional nature of cardiac activity is illustrated in the forewarned reaction time task in which a warning signal is followed in a few seconds by a stimulus to which the subject is instructed to respond with a motor action. A biphasic cardiac response is frequently observed in which there is an initial heart rate acceleration followed by a deceleration prior to the signal to respond. As illustrated in Figure 9.3, the biphasic heart rate acceleration–deceleration that precedes the signal to respond is paralleled by an increase in electromyographic recordings from the chin and in respiratory frequency.[61].

The functional significance of heart rate deceleration has been the subject of considerable debate. The argument has centred on the role of heart rate deceleration in sensory facilitation and/or somatomotor activity. Obrist and his

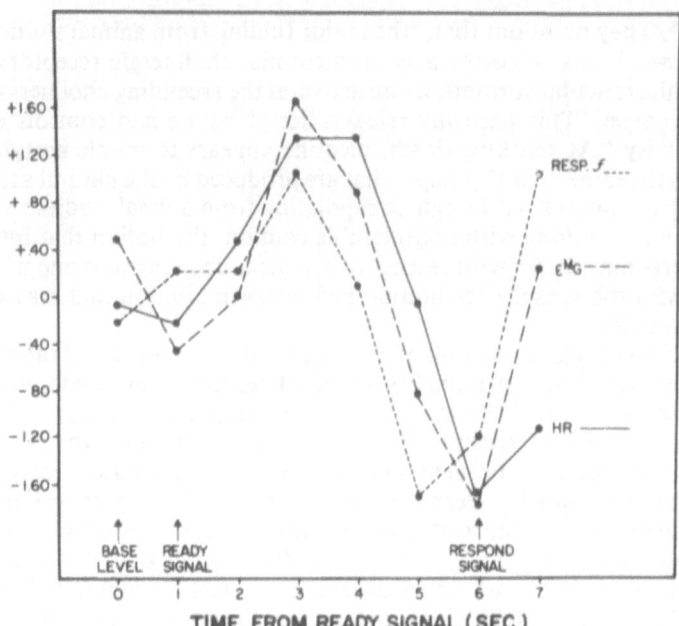

*Figure 9.3 Changes in heart rate, chin electro-myograph and respiratory frequency during a forewarned reaction time task[61] (reprinted with kind permission from P. A. Obrist, R. A. Webb and J. R. Sutterer, 1969, 5, 696–723. Psychophysiological Research)*

co-workers have emphasized the covariation between heart rate and somato-motor activity in a number of behavioural paradigms such as simple reaction time[62]. In their view, cardiac deceleration accompanies a reduction in somatic activity that is not relevant to the execution of the task signalled by the warning stimulus. On the other hand, Lacey and Lacey argue that cardiac deceleration is a component in a feedback loop which increases cortical arousal and serves to facilitate both sensory and motor action[63].

There is greater consensus concerning the functional significance of heart rate acceleration. In the most direct example, heart rate is seen to increase during physical exercise and to provide the increased cardiac output that is required by the increased metabolic demands. In early work, heart rate acceleration was regarded as a good index of psychological activation[60]. More recent interest has focused on the defensive or protective function of heart rate acceleration[64]. In this regard, heart rate acceleration is consistently elicited by high intensity stimulation and may be seen to serve a motor readiness function. Heart rate acceleration is also seen to prevail in circumstances where an individual has the opportunity to control aversive events[62].

Overall, there appears to be an abundance of evidence showing that heart rate is directly coupled to increases and decreases in muscle activity even in situations which require minimal task demands such as reaction time or classical aversive conditioning[65–67]. The relationship between cardiac activity and motor performance, however, is not clear. A monotonic relationship between response

202

latency in a simple reaction time task and the heart rate deceleration which precedes the response has been frequently reported[68, 69] but the relationship has not been consistently endorsed[70, 71]. Similarly, the amplitude of heart rate acceleration does not relate to reaction time performance unequivocally.

In general, the task parameters and cardiac components that mediate sensorimotor performance interact in a complex manner that remains to be delineated. Progress in this direction has been made by investigating reaction time responses which occur at different points in the cardiac cycle. Variation in performance as well as in cardiac responses may depend on the point in the cardiac cycle at which warning stimuli and responses occur. In an elegant series of experiments, for example, Somsen, van der Molen, Jennings and Orlebeke systematically varied cardiac cycle time and response time[72]. This work indicated 'that initiation rather than completion of the reaction time responses seems to control the inhibitory vagal input to the heart that is responsible for anticipatory deceleration'. Although the association of motor behaviour with specific cardiac events continues to develop, the present state of knowledge is sufficient to encourage the application of cardiovascular measurement to the question of individual differences in the expression of motor behaviour and personality.

## CARDIOVASCULAR ACTIVITY AND TYPE A BEHAVIOUR

The concept of Type A behaviour emerged from clinical observations that aggressive, ambitious, competitive individuals were prone to develop coronary heart disease[73]. These clinical impressions were endorsed by a large scale prospective study which classified individuals as either Type A or Type B on the basis of a structured interview[74]. Despite some inconsistencies, there appears to be a good deal of evidence that Type A behaviour is linked to heart disease. To put the matter in perspective, however, it should be noted that only a small portion of individuals who are classified as Type A develop coronary heart disease. Although the incidence of coronary heart disease amongst individuals classified as Type A may be almost twice as great as those classified as Type B, the Western Collaborative Group Study which surveyed 3000 employed men for 8.5 years indicated that some 74% of those classified as Type A remained disease-free during the study period[74]. Given the prospect that Type A behaviour indicates a predisposition to develop coronary heart disease, there has been a good deal of interest in determining the physiological mechanisms which distinguish Type A behaviour. Of particular interest are the cardiovascular adjustments of Type A and Type B individuals to stressful task demands. This research has attempted to determine whether Type A individuals would display the elevated blood pressure and exaggerated cardiac response that are regarded as precursors to coronary heart disease.

In general, it has been found that Type A individuals do in fact display exaggerated cardiac activity but only under some conditions. There is rather little evidence of differences between Type A and Type B in either heart rate or blood pressure under neutral or resting conditions. No consistent effects have emerged when the stressor has been a mental task[75, 76]. Similarly, no differences are evident when stressors such as the cold pressor (holding one's hand in near freezing water) have been applied[77, 78]. However, increases in blood pressure have been observed for Type A individuals under conditions of harassment and reward. For example, in a recent project, Glass and his colleagues examined the cardiovascular responses of Type A individuals in a competitive situation[79]. In this study, subjects competed in an electronic game with a tennis-type format in which the ball was manipulated by a hand controlled electronic paddle. A monetary reward was also offered as an incentive for good performance. In the first experiment, half of the subjects were exposed to insulting harassment by a confederate who posed as an opponent to the subject. In the harassment condition, the Type A subjects displayed greater increases in systolic blood pressure, heart rate and plasma epinephrine than Type B subjects. In a second experiment, reward was manipulated, with half of the subjects being offered the monetary incentive and the other half simply engaging in the competition. Type A individuals displayed greater systolic and diastolic blood pressure elevation than Type B individuals in the incentive condition. Thus, in this case, incentive alone was sufficient to differentiate the two groups with blood pressure measures. Similar cardiovascular effects of incentives for Type A and Type B individuals have been reported both with a motor requirement in the task[80] and without an explicit motor response requirement[81-83]. Although this review is by no means comprehensive, it is clear that there is a good deal of evidence which indicates that individuals classified as Type A display exaggerated cardiac reactivity in competitive, provoking situations and when incentives are introduced.

It should also be noted that the effects seem to be somewhat more robust when individuals are classified using the structured interview technique rather than a questionnaire measure, specifically, the Jenkins Activity Survey (JAS)[84]. Perhaps this is not surprising since the interview method specifically introduces elements of provocation and challenge that are somewhat similar to those introduced in the experimental procedures. Analysis of the structure of the JAS has revealed three main factors (hard-driving competitiveness; job involvement; speed and impatience) which are moderately intercorrelated. The extent to which one or all of these factors are predictive of coronary heart disease or cardiac responsivity has not been established. The classification scheme seems not to have been extensively examined in the context of contemporary personality theory; thus, it is not at all clear *why* Type A personality individuals are coronary prone. There is some evidence which indicates that Type A behaviour is positively related to scores on the Extraversion and Neuroticism dimensions of Eysenck's typology[85, 86]. Given the apparent importance of incentives in differentiating Type A and Type B with cardiac measures, it is also noteworthy that differences in susceptibility to reward have been proposed by Gray as a basis for individual differences in degree of impulsivity, that is high extraversion and high neuroticism in Eysenck's typology[87].

# HEART RATE, REWARD AND PERSONALITY

Fowles and his students have developed a reliable paradigm to investigate the effects of monetary incentives on heart rate[88]. They have employed a continuous motor task, a button press adjacent to one of five signal lights, to demonstrate that heart rate increases with increases in monetary incentive. The paradigm was inspired, in part, by Gray's model of personality which proposed that reward seeking and active avoidance behaviour are determined by an appetitive motivational system and that this system may exercise a causal influence on individual differences in impulsiveness[89]. Fowles has developed the argument that heart rate may serve as an index of activity of the appetitive motivational system[90]. The successful demonstration of an increasing monotonic relationship between incentives and heart rate endorses this view and provides the basis for linking individual differences in cardiac activity to personality theory. From this perspective, the enhanced heart rate for Type A individuals in incentive conditions observed by Perkins leads to the conclusion that differences in the sensitivity of the appetitive motivational system to incentives may be responsible for differences in heart rate reactivity between Type A and Type B individuals[80]. As Perkins points out, this interpretation differs from prevailing cognitive interpretations which focus on the attempt of Type A individuals to control competitive, challenging situations. More importantly, however, the liaison between heart rate activity and Gray's theory which Fowles has drawn provides a comprehensive framework that facilitates the application of heart rate measures in accounting for differences in personality.

In developing his paradigm, Fowles has followed Malmo and Belanger by emphasizing incentive effects on heart rate that are apparently not attributable to somatic activity[90, 91]. As previously noted, there are strong links between cardiac and somatic activity and it is no mean feat to disassociate this coupling. In Fowles' experiments, heart rate is recorded during a continuous motor task. Nevertheless, the heart rate effects are attributed to incentives rather than somatic activity since no relationship between rate of responding and heart rate was observed across the incentive conditions. This null argument regarding response rate, that is affirming the null hypothesis, is not a compelling one. Although increased heart rate is not reflected in increased rate of responding, somatic influences may be expressed in increased muscle tension or pressure that also influence heart rate. Nevertheless, the evidence parallels the Malmo and Belanger[91] demonstrations which showed that in animal experiments responding was not necessary to elicit an increase in heart rate. These arguments underscore the importance of incentive cues in inducing the heart rate effects. On the other hand, it is difficult to reconcile susceptibility to incentives and this feature of heart rate function as determinants of individual differences in motor activity between introverts and extraverts that were outlined earlier in this paper. Reward was not a condition which distinguished those demonstrations.

## SENSATION-SEEKING AND CARDIAC RESPONSE

Cardiac measures have also been employed to investigate the biological bases of the sensation-seeking trait[2]. Individuals who obtain high scores on this trait are motivated to seek sensation through participation in exciting activities, drug taking and through social stimulation. High sensation-seekers generally tend to be more active and more involved in contact sports[4], and physical movement than low sensation-seekers[92]. However, there does not appear to be any work that has considered differences in motor performance tasks. Rather, interest has focused on those stimulus conditions which promote interest and attention.

Zuckerman has argued that high sensation-seekers are disposed to seek variation in stimulation in order to maintain an optimal level of arousal[2]. In this context, it was proposed that high sensation-seekers would be more responsive to novel stimulation than low sensation-seekers and thus, high sensation-seekers would be expected to display enhanced orienting responses. With respect to the cardiac component of the orienting response, it was predicted that high sensation-seekers would exhibit larger amplitude decelerative cardiac responses than low sensation-seekers. Overall, this prediction has been confirmed in four independent studies. The interpretation of the effects, however, remains open to some questions.

There has been a good deal of similarity in the procedures applied and of the findings obtained between investigators who have examined differences in cardiac response between high and low sensation-seekers[93-96]. In these studies, high sensation-seekers, or more specifically those high on the disinhibition subscale, displayed a decelerative response to brief auditory tones. This effect is illustrated in Figure 9.4.

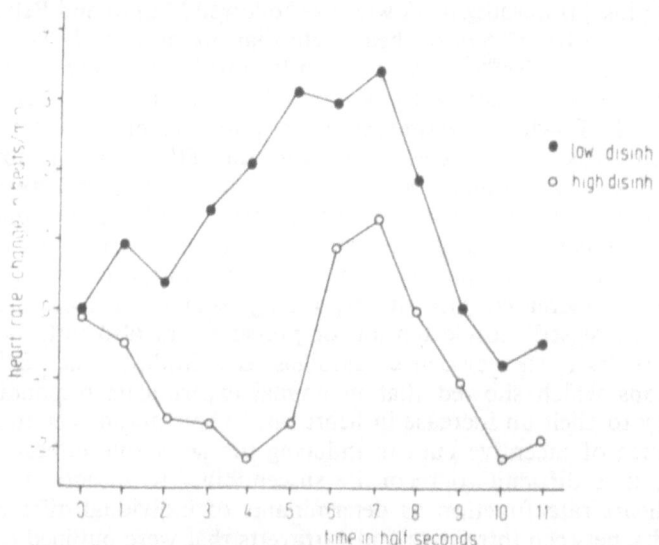

*Figure 9.4   Heart rate response to 80 dB, 1000 Hz, tones for subjects classified as high and low disinhibitors on the Sensation Seeking Scale[93] (reprinted with kind permission from J. F. Orlebeke and J.A. Feij, 1979, Laurence Erlbaum Associates, Inc.)*

The effects were obtained with moderate intensity (50–80 dB) auditory stimuli (1000 Hz) that were presented in a simple repetitive habituation series. Both the accelerative and decelerative cardiac responses decrease in amplitude and return to the prestimulus heart rate level after the first few stimulations. The decelerative response of high sensation-seekers can be regarded as an orienting response, which is a non-specific response to novel stimulus change. Zuckerman suggests that 'the differences may reflect the biological propensity to elicit interest and "seeking" in high sensation-seekers, and lack of interest and avoidance of novel stimuli – in the low sensation-seekers'[4].

The orienting response has been shown to play an important role in the facilitation of stimulus reception, attention and in the elaboration of conditioned responses[22]. From this perspective, it would be expected that high sensation-seekers would display greater sensitivity on psychophysical tasks and enhanced performance in conditioning and vigilance tasks. What little evidence there is available on this point suggests that the *opposite* is the case. That is, high sensation-seekers have been shown to be less sensitive on psychophysical tasks than low sensation-seekers[97] and to be more tolerant of intense stimulation[98]. In general, the cardiac 'orienting response' evident for high sensation-seekers in these demonstrations is not consistent with their behaviour on measures of sensory sensitivity or conditioning in a manner that concords with enhanced orienting responses[99].

The accelerative response to auditory stimulation of low sensation-seekers does not meet the criteria or conditions suggested for distinguishing orienting responses from defensive or startle responses[64]. Defensive responses tend to be elicited by high intensity tones and they are thought to be resistant to habituation. With the low sensation-seekers, however, the accelerative responses are elicited by moderate intensity tones and they habituate quickly. Startle responses, on the other hand, are characterized by cardiac accelerations that habituate quickly and they are elicited by abrupt auditory stimuli, such as clicks that have fast rise times. Only two of the studies cited[94, 96] report rise time and they are relatively slow (30–50 ms). Ridgeway and Hare argue that the heart acceleration probably reflects a blending of both startle and defensive components[94]. In a similar vein, one could argue that the accelerative responses are intensity effects, with low sensation-seekers responding as if the stimuli were more intense. This is suggested by the fact that with increasing intensity, there is a shift from heart rate deceleration to acceleration[100]. This shift may simply occur earlier for the low sensation-seekers.

The interpretation of these effects has important implications for the understanding of sensation-seeking behaviour. What is at issue is whether the adventurous, risk-taking activities of high sensation-seekers are determined by a 'need for novelty', a view which interprets the greater decelerative cardiac response of high sensation-seekers as an orienting response, or whether sensation-seeking behaviour is predisposed by lower sensitivity to stimulation, particularly intense stimulation, a view which interprets the decelerative responses of high disinhibition subjects in terms of a higher threshold in the transition to an accelerative response to increased stimulus intensity. It is also important to note that in the most recent exposition of his model, Zuckerman has given more emphasis to the rewarding effects of novel stimulation[4]. Although there does not seem to be any evidence of differences in cardiac response between high and low sensation-seekers in incentive conditions, the fact that Type A individuals tend to have high scores on the sensation-seeking scales suggests that such a relationship might be found. Such effects would be consistent with the higher levels of general activity in which sensation-seekers are disposed to engage and they would implicate response-mediated or motor mechanisms in the biological bases of sensation-seeking.

In a previous paper, we suggested that the psychophysiology of personality, specifically the extraversion dimension, would be parsimoniously viewed in terms of sensory and motor effects[14]. In particular, we developed the argument that differences between introverts and extraverts in the response to sensory stimulation and in the expression of motor activity may be referred to differences at the level of the sensory and motor nerve. In some respects, this approach articulates the general concept of arousal by drawing attention to the functional significance of the specific psychophysiological measures employed. In this context, it is tempting to extend this view by addressing cardiac activity in terms of distinctions that are similar to those proposed by Brebner in addressing contradictory differences between introverts and extraverts in reaction time tasks[19]. From this perspective, differences between high and low sensation-seekers in heart rate deceleration to moderate intensity stimulation would be viewed as stimulus-mediated motor inhibition, whereas the heart rate acceleration to more intense stimulation would be viewed as stimulus-mediated motor excitation. The increased heart rate activity of Type A individuals which persists throughout incentive task paradigms and which is thought to characterize extraverted impulsive individuals[44], can be conceived as response-mediated motor excitation (or at least somatomotor activity) while decreased heart rate which may develop during the course of an unpleasant, repetitive or boring activity could be viewed as response-mediated motor inhibition. Applying such distinctions to individual differences in cardiac activity may be helpful in clarifying the biological bases of extraversion, Type A behaviour and sensation-seeking.

## SUMMARY

Psychophysiological methods provide a useful, non-invasive means to explore the biological bases of individual differences in sensitivity to stimulation and in the expression of motor behaviour. With respect to the extraversion dimension, introverts have been shown to be more sensitive to stimulation in several sense modalities. Electrodermal measures of autonomic activity and measures of electrocortical activity indicate that introverts display an enhanced response to stimulation of moderate intensity or arousal potential. There is also evidence that the enhanced sensitivity of introverts may be referred to the level of the auditory nerve; such effects cannot be easily ascribed to individual differences in reticulocortical arousal mechanisms. There is also a good deal of evidence that introverts and extraverts differ in the expression of motor activity, with extraverts tending to show less control in tasks which require motor containment.

The biological bases of differences in motor activity between introverts and extraverts have not been extensively investigated.

The contingent negative variation (CNV) is an electrocortical measure which is widely regarded as an expression of preparation for a motor response. High anxious psychiatric subjects tend to display smaller CNV amplitudes than low anxious patients. When stressful task demands are applied, non-psychiatric high anxious subjects classified by personality inventories also tend to display smaller CNV amplitudes. Some investigators also report lower CNV amplitudes for introverts in non-stressful conditions. Nicotine has been found to have differential effects on CNV amplitude for introverts and extraverts, enhancing CNV amplitude in extraverts and decreasing CNV in introverts. In general, there is little direct evidence linking differences in CNV amplitude between introverts and extraverts to differences in motor performance between these groups. Further, there have been few attempts to distinguish the sensory and motor contributions to the development of the CNV in research which has investigated personality differences.

There is an abundance of evidence showing that heart rate is directly coupled to increases and decreases in muscle activity. Measures of cardiac activity provide an appropriate means of investigating personality and differences in the expression of motor behaviour. Type A behaviour, extraversion and sensation-seeking are personality measures which share common descriptive characteristics. Incentive and reward also feature prominently as determinants of individual differences along those dimensions. Type A individuals display exaggerated cardiac reactivity in competitive situations and when incentives are introduced. High sensation-seekers display decelerative cardiac responses and low sensation-seekers display accelerative cardiac responses to moderately intense stimulation. These effects may be clarified by viewing them in terms of stimulus and response-mediated motor excitation and inhibition.

## References

1. Eysenck, H. J. (ed.) (1981). *A Model for Personality*. (Heidelberg: Springer-Verlag)
2. Zuckerman, M. (1979). *Sensation Seeking: Beyond the Optimum Level of Arousal*. (Hillsdale, NJ: Erlbaum)
3. Fulker, D. W. (1981). The genetic and environmental architecture of psychoticism, extraversion and neuroticism. In Eysenck, H. J. (ed.) *A Model for Personality*. pp. 88–122. (Heidelberg: Springer-Verlag)
4. Zuckerman, M. (1984). Sensation-seeking: a comparative approach to a human trait. *Behav. Brain. Sci.*, 7, 413–71
5. Stelmack, R. M. (1981). The psychophysiology of extraversion and neuroticism. In Eysenck, H. J. (ed.) *A Model for Personality*. pp. 38–64. (Heidelberg: Springer-Verlag)
6. Barratt, E. S. (1983). The biological basis of impulsiveness: the significance of timing and rhythm disorders. *Pers. Individ. Diff.*, 4, 387–91
7. Eysenck, S. B. G. and Eysenck, H. J. (1977). The place of impulsiveness in a dimensional system of personality description. *Br. J. Soc. Clin. Psychol.*, 16, 57–68
8. Stelmack, R. M. and Campbell, K. B. (1974). Extraversion and auditory sensitivity to high and low frequency. *Percept. Mot. Skills*, 38, 875–9
9. Siddle, D. A. T., Morrish, R. B., White, K. D. and Mangan, G. L. (1969). Relation of visual sensitivity to extraversion. *J. Exp. Res. Pers.*, 3, 264–7

10. Dunstone, J. J., Dzendolet, G. and Henckeruth, O. (1964). Effect of some personality variables on electrical vestibular stimulation. *Percept. Mot. Skills*, **18**, 689–95
11. Haslam, D. R. (1967). Individual differences in pain threshold and level of arousal. *Br. J. Psychol.*, **58**, 139–42
12. Eysenck, H. J. (1957). *The Dynamics of Anxiety and Hysteria*. (London: Routledge and Kegan Paul)
13. Eysenck, H. J. (1967). *The Biological Basis of Personality*. (Springfield, Ill.: Thomas)
14. Stelmack, R. M. and Plouffe, L. (1983). Introversion–extraversion: the Bell–Magendie law revisited. *Pers. Individ. Diff.*, **4**, 421–7
15. Frith, C. D. (1971). Strategies in rotary pursuit tracking. *Br. J. Psychol.*, **62**, 187–97
16. Horn, P. D. (1975). Evidence for the generality of reminiscence as a function of extraversion and neuroticism. *J. Psychol.*, **90**, 41–4
17. Brebner, J. and Flavell, R. (1978). The effect of catch-trials on speed and accuracy among introverts and extraverts in a simple RT task. *Br. J. Psychol.*, **69**, 9–15
18. Eysenck, H. J. (1964). Involuntary rest pauses in tapping as a function of drive and personality. *Percept. Mot. Skills*, **18**, 173–4
19. Brebner, J. (1983). A model of extraversion. *Aust. J. Psychol.*, **35**, 349–59
20. Walter, W. G., Cooper, R., Aldridge, V., McCallum, W. C. and Winter, A. L. (1964). Contingent negative variation: an electric sign of sensorimotor association and expectancy in the human brain. *Nature (London)*, **203**, 380–4
21. Connor, W. H. and Lang, P. J. (1969). Cortical slow-wave and cardiac rate responses in stimulus orientation and reaction time conditions. *J. Exp. Psychol.*, **82**, 310–20
22. Sokolov, E. N. (1963). *Perception and the Conditioned Reflex*. (New York: Macmillan)
23. Loveless, N. E. and Sandford, A. J. (1974). Slow potential correlates of preparatory set. *Biol. Psychol.*, **1**, 303–14
24. Rohrbaugh, J. W. and Gaillard, A. W. K. (1983). Sensory and motor aspects of the contingent negative variation. In Gaillard, A. W. K. and Ritter, W. (eds.) *Tutorials in Event Related Potential Research: Endogenous Components*. pp. 269–310. (Amsterdam: North Holland)
25. Loveless, N. E. (1975). The effect of warning signal interval on signal detection and event-related slow potentials of the brain. *Percept. Psychophys.*, **17**, 565–70
26. Rebert, C. S. and Tecce, J. J. (1973). A summary of CNV and reaction time. In McCallum, W. C. and Knott, J. R. (eds.) Event-related slow potentials of the brain: their relations to behavior. *Electroencephalogr. Clin. Neurophysiol.*, **33** Suppl., pp. 173–8
27. Walter, W. G. (1965). Effects on anterior brain responses of an expected association between stimuli. *J. Psychosom. Res.*, **9**, 45–9
28. McCallum, W. C. and Walter, W. G. (1968). The effects of attention and distraction on the contingent negative variation in normal and neurotic subjects. *Electroencephalogr. Clin. Neurophysiol.*, **25**, 319–29
29. Small, J. C. and Small, I. F. (1971). Contingent negative variation (CNV) correlations with psychiatric diagnosis. *Arch. Gen. Psychiatry*, **25**, 550–4
30. Low, M. D., Coats, A. C., Rettig, G. M. and McSherry, J. W. (1967). Anxiety, attentiveness-alertness: a phenomenological study of the CNV. *Neuropsychologia*, **5**, 379–84
31. Knott, J. R. and Irwin, D. A. (1967). Anxiety, stress and the contingent negative variation. *Electroencephalogr. Clin. Neurophysiol.*, **22**, 188
32. Knott, J. R. and Irwin, D. A. (1973). Anxiety, stress and the contingent negative variation. *Arch. Gen. Psychiatry*, **29**, 538–41
33. Bendig, A. W. (1962). The Pittsburg scales of social extroversion–introversion and emotionality. *J. Psychol.*, **53**, 199–209
34. Low, M. D. and Swift, S. J. (1971). The contingent negative variation and the 'resting' D.C. potential of the human brain: effects of situational anxiety. *Neuropsychologia*, **9**, 203–8
35. Low, M. D. and McSherry, J. W. (1968). Further observations of psychological factors involved in CNV genesis. *Electroencephalogr. Clin. Neurophysiol.*, **25**, 203–7
36. Rebert, C. S., McAdam, D. W., Knott, J. R. and Irwin, D. A. (1967). Slow potential change in human brain related to level of motivation. *J. Comp. Physiol. Psychol.*, **63**, 20–3
37. Papakostopoulos, D. and Jones, J. G. (1980). The impact of different levels of muscular force on the contingent negative variation (CNV). In Kornhuber, H. H. and Deeke, L. (eds.) Motivation, motor and sensory processes of the brain: electrical potentials, behaviour and clinical use. *Prog. Brain Res.*, **54**, 195–202

38. Tecce, J. J. (1971). Contingent negative variation and individual differences: a new approach in brain research. *Arch. Gen. Psychiatry*, **24**, 1–16

39. Tecce, J. J. and Scheff, N. M. (1969). Attention reduction and suppressed direct-current potentials in the human brain. *Science*, **164**, 331–3

40. Tecce, J. J. and Hamilton, B. T. (1973). CNV reduction by sustained cognitive activity (distraction). *Electroencephalogr. Clin. Neurophysiol.*, Suppl. **33**, 229–37

41. Tecce, J. J., Savignano-Bowman, J. and Meinbresse, D. (1976). Contingent negative variation and the distraction–arousal hypothesis. *Electroencephalogr. Clin. Neurophysiol.*, **41**, 277–86

42. Tecce, J. J., Cattanach, L., Boehner-Davis, M. B. and Clifford, T. S. (1984). CNV and myogenic functions. II. Divided attention produces a double dissociation of CNV and EMG. In Karrer, R., Cohen, J. and Tueting, P. (eds.) Brain and information: Event-related potentials. *Ann. N.Y. Acad. Sci.*, **425**, 289–94

43. Glanzmann, P. and Froehlich, W. D. (1984). Anxiety, stress and contingent variation reconsidered. In Karrer, R., Cohen, J. and Tueting, P. (eds.) Brain and information: event related potentials. *Ann. N.Y. Acad. Sci.*, **425**, 578–84

44. Gray, J. A. (1981). A critique of Eysenck's theory of personality. In Eysenck, H. J. (ed.) *A Model for Personality*. pp. 246–76. (Heidelberg: Springer-Verlag)

45. Speilberger, C. D. (1972). Anxiety as an emotional state. In Speilberger, C. D. (ed.) *Anxiety: Current Trends in Theory and Research*. Vol. 2, pp. 481–93. (New York: Academic Press)

46. Tecce, J. J., Savignano-Bowman, J. and Cole, J. O. (1978). Drug effects on contingent negative variation and eyeblinks: the distraction–arousal hypothesis. In Lipton, M. A., DiMascio, A. and Killam, K. F. (eds.) *Psychopharmacology: A Generation of Progress*. pp. 745–58. (New York: Raven)

47. Eysenck, H. J. and Eysenck, S. B. G. (1975). *Manual for the Eysenck Personality Questionnaire*. (San Diego: Hodder and Stoughton)

48. Werre, P. F., Favery, H. A. and Janssen, R. H. C. (1973). Contingent negative variation and personality. *Electroencephalogr. Clin. Neurophysiol.*, **34**, 739

49. Lolas, F. and Andracca, I. (1977). Neuroticism, extraversion and slow brain potentials. *Neuropsychobiology*, **3**, 12–22

50. Dincheva, E. G. and Piperova-Dalbokova, D. L. (1982). Differences in contingent negative variation (CNV) related to extraversion–introversion. *Pers. Individ. Diff.*, **3**, 447–51

51. Plooij-Van Gorsel and Janssen, R. H. C. (1978). Contingent negative variation (CNV) and extraversion in a psychiatric population. In Barber, C. (ed.) *Evoked Potentials. Proceedings of an International Evoked Potentials Symposium*, University of Nottingham. (Lancaster: MTP Press)

52. Ashton, H., Millman, J. E., Telford, R. and Thompson, J. W. (1974). The effect of caffeine, nitrazepam and cigarette smoking on the contingent negative variation in man. *Electroencephalogr. Clin. Neurophysiol.*, **37**, 59–71

53. O'Connor, K. (1982). Individual differences in the effect of smoking on frontal-central distribution of the CNV: some observations on smokers' control of attentional behaviour. *Pers. Individ. Diff.*, **3**, 271–85

54. Janssen, R. H. C., Mattie, H., Plooij-Van Gorsel and Werre, P. F. (1978). The effects of a depressant and a stimulant drug on the contingent negative variation. *Biol. Psychol.*, **6**, 209–18

55. Eysenck, H. J. and Eysenck, S. B. G. (1964). *Manual for the Eysenck Personality Inventory*. (San Diego: Educational and Industrial Testing Service)

56. Ashton, H. J., Golding, J., Marsh, V. R., Millman, J. E. and Thompson, J. W. (1981). The seed and the soil: effect of dosage, personality and starting state on the response to $\Delta^9$ tetrahydrocannibinol in man. *Br. J. Clin. Pharmacol.*, **12**, 705–20

57. O'Connor, K. P. (1980). The CNV and individual differences in smoking behaviour. *Pers. Individ. Diff.*, **1**, 57–72

58. Edwards, J. A. and Warburton, D. M. (1983). Smoking, nicotine and electrocortical activity. *Pharmacol. Ther.*, **19**, 147–64

59. Harkins, S. W., Thompson, L. W., Moss, S. F. and Nowlin, J. B. (1976). Relationship between central and autonomic nervous system activity: correlates of psychomotor performance in elderly men. *Exp. Aging Res.*, **2**, 409–23

60. Malmo, R. B. (1959). Activation: a neuropsychological dimension. *Psychol. Rev.*, **66**, 367–86

61. Obrist, P. A., Webb, R. A. and Sutterer, J. R. (1969). Heart rate and somatic changes during aversive conditioning and a simple reaction time task. *Psychophysiology*, **5**, 696–723
62. Obrist, P. A. (1981). *Cardiovascular Psychophysiology*. (New York: Plenum Press)
63. Lacey, B. C. and Lacey, J. I. (1974). Studies of heart rate and other bodily processes in sensorimotor behavior. In Obrist, P. A., Black, A. H., Brener, J. and DiCara, L. V. (eds.) *Cardiovascular Psychophysiology: Current Issues in Response Mechanisms, Biofeedback and Methodology*. pp. 93–114. (Chicago: Aldine)
64. Graham, F. K. (1979). Distinguishing among orienting, defense and startle reflexes. In Kimmel, H. D., van Olst, E. H. and Orlebeke, J. F. (eds.) *The Orienting Reflex in Humans*. pp. 137–67. (Hillsdale, NJ: Erlbaum)
65. Obrist, P. A. (1976). The cardiovascular–behavioral interaction – as it appears today. *Psychophysiology*, **13**, 95–107
66. Simons, R. F., Ohman, A. and Lang, P. J. (1979). Anticipation and response set: cortical, cardiac and electrodermal correlates. *Psychophysiology*, **16**, 222–33
67. Cohen, M. J., Johnson, H. J. and McArthur, D. L. (1980). Interaction of a motor response, and reaction time and time estimation tasks, on heart rate and skin conductance. *Psychophysiology*, **17**, 377–84
68. Lacey, B. C. and Lacey, J. I. (1977). Change in heart period: a function of sensorimotor event timing within the cardiac cycle. *Physiol. Psychol.*, **5**, 383–93
69. Wynn, V. T. (1980). Reaction time as a function of the cardiac cycle. *Br. J. Psychol.*, **71**, 155–62
70. Carroll, D. and Anastasiades, P. (1978). The behavioural significance of heart rate: the Laceys' hypothesis. *Biol. Psychol.*, **7**, 249–75
71. Paller, K. and Shapiro, D. (1983). Systolic blood pressure and a simple reaction time task. *Psychophysiology*, **20**, 585–90
72. Somsen, R. J. M., van der Molen, M. W., Jennings, J. R. and Orblebeke, J. F. (1985). Response initiation not completion seems to alter cardiac cycle length. *Psychophysiology*, **22**, 319–25
73. Friedman, M. and Rosenman, R. H. (1959). Association of specific overt behavior pattern with blood and cardiovascular findings. *J. Am. Med. Assoc.*, **169**, 1085–96
74. Rosenman, R. H., Brand, R. J., Jenkins, C. D., Friedman, M., Straus, R. and Wurm, M. (1975). Coronary heart disease in the Western Collaborative Group Study: final follow-up experience of 8½ years. *J. Am. Med. Assoc.*, **233**, 872–7
75. Dembrowski, T. M., MacDougall, J. M., Shields, J. L., Petitto, J. and Lushene, R. (1978). Components of the coronary-prone behavior pattern and cardiovascular responses to psychomotor performance challenge. *J. Behav. Med.*, **1**, 159–76
76. Steptoe, A. (1981). *Psychological Factors in Cardiovascular Disorders*. (London: Academic Press)
77. Simpson, M. T., Olewine, D. A., Jenkins, C. D., Ramsay, F. H., Zyzanski, S. J., Thomas, G. and Hames, C. G. (1974). Exercise-induced catecholamine and platelet aggregation in the coronary-prone behavior pattern. *Psychosom. Med.*, **36**, 476–587
78. Lott, G. G. and Gatchel, R. J. (1978). A multiresponse analysis of learned heart rate control. *Psychophysiology*, **15**, 576–81
79. Glass, D. C., Krakoff, L. R., Contrada, R., Hilton, W. F., Kehoe, K., Mannucci, E. G., Collins, C., Snow, B. and Elting, E. (1980). Effect of harassment and competition upon cardiovascular and plasma catecholamine responses in Type A and Type B individuals. *Psychophysiology*, **17**, 453–63
80. Perkins, K. A. (1984). Heart rate change in Type A and Type B males as a function of response cost and task difficulty. *Psychophysiology*, **21**, 14–21
81. Manuck, S. B. and Garland, F. N. (1979). Coronary-prone behavior pattern, task incentive and cardiovascular response. *Psychophysiology*, **16**, 136–42
82. Blumenthal, J. A., Lane, J. D., William, R. B., McKee, D. C., Haney, T. and White, A. (1983). Effects of task incentive on cardiovascular response in Type A and Type B individuals. *Psychophysiology*, **20**, 63–70
83. Contrada, R. J., Wright, R. A. and Glass, D. C. (1984). Task difficulty, Type A behavior pattern, and cardiovascular response. *Psychophysiology*, **21**, 638–46
84. Jenkins, C. D., Rosenman, R. H. and Zyzanski, S. J. (1974). Prediction of clinical coronary heart disease by a test for the coronary-prone behavior pattern. *N. Engl. J. Med.*, **290**, 1271–5

85. Rim, Y. (1981). Pattern-A behaviour and its personality correlates in students of both sexes. *Sci. Paedagogica Exp.*, **18**, 98–102
86. Eysenck, H. and Fulker, D. (1983). The components of Type A behaviour and its genetic determinants. *Pers. Individ. Diff.*, **4**, 499–505
87. Gray, J. A. (1973). Causal theories of personality and how to test them. In Royce, J. R. (ed.) *Multivariate Analysis and Psychological Theory*. pp. 409–63. (London: Academic Press)
88. Fowles, D. C. (1983). Appetitive motivational influences on heart rate. *Pers. Individ. Diff.*, **4**, 393–401
89. Gray, J. A., Owen, S., Davis, N. and Tsaltas, E. (1983). Psychological and physiological relations between anxiety and impulsivity. In Zuckerman, M. (ed.) *Biological Bases of Sensation Seeking, Impulsivity and Anxiety*. (Hillsdale, NJ: Erlbaum)
90. Fowles, D. C. (1980). The three arousal model: implications of Gray's two factor learning theory for heart rate, electrodermal activity, and psychopathy. *Psychophysiology*, **17**, 87–104
91. Malmo, R. B. and Bélanger, D. (1967). Related physiological and behavioral changes: what are their determinants? *Sleep and Altered States of Consciousness*, **45**, 288–318
92. Hocking, J. and Robertson, M. (1969). The sensation seeking scale as a predictor of need for stimulation during sensory restriction. *J. Consult. Clin. Psychol.*, **33**, 367–9
93. Orlebeke, J. F. and Feij, J. A. (1979). The orienting reflex as a personality correlate. In Kimmel, H. D., Van Olst, E. H. and Orlebeke, J. F. (eds.) *The Orienting Reflex in Humans*. pp. 567–85. (Hillsdale, NJ: Erlbaum)
94. Ridgeway, A. and Hare, R. D. (1981). Sensation seeking and psychophysiological responses to auditory stimulation. *Psychophysiology*, **18**, 613–18
95. Robinson, T. N. and Zahn, T. P. (1983). Sensation seeking, state anxiety and cardiac and EDR orienting reactions. Paper presented to the *23rd meeting of the Society for Psychophysiological Research*, Asilomar, California
96. Como, P. G., Simons, R. F. and Zuckerman, M. (1984). Psychophysiological indices of sensation seeking as a function of stimulus intensity. Paper presented at meeting of the *Society for Psychophysiological Research*, Milwaukee
97. Davis, C., Cowles, M. and Kohn, P. (1983). Strength of the nervous system and augmenting-reducing: paradox lost. *Pers. Individ. Diff.*, **4**, 491–8
98. Haier, R. J., Robinson, D. L., Braden, W. and Williams, D. (1984). Evoked potential augmenting-reducing and personality differences. *Pers. Individ. Diff.*, **5**, 293–301
99. Stelmack, R. M. (1984). Sensation seeking, orientation and defense: empirical and theoretical reservations. A commentary on M. Zuckerman's sensation seeking: a comparative approach to a human trait. *Behav. Brain Sci.*, **7**, 450
100. Turpin, G. and Siddle, D. A. T. (1983). Effects of stimulus intensity on cardiovascular activity. *Psychophysiology*, **20**, 611–24

# 10

## The effects of aerobic exercise on mood

## *Patricia J. Castell and James A. Blumenthal*

---

INTRODUCTION

It has been estimated that more then 30 million Americans engage in running or jogging. Exercise adherents claim that participation in physical exercise elevates their mood and produces a sense of well-being. In the past 10 years, a series of clinical and laboratory studies have been performed to provide a more objective assessment for these claims. The purpose of this chapter is to review the recent research on the relationship between exercise and mood, in clinical and in normal populations.

DEFINITION OF TERMS

Exercise is one form of physical activity that is undertaken to improve or maintain physical fitness. *Physical fitness* can be thought of as a set of attributes that people have or achieve through exercise training. Certain qualities associated with physical fitness such as agility, power, speed and balance are important to athletic performance. Four other qualities of physical fitness – cardiorespiratory endurance, muscular strength/endurance, body composition, and flexibility – are regarded as important to health, as well as to movement ability. These components, referred to as *health-related physical fitness*, are important for prevention of disease and/or promotion of health[1]. One efficient means to achieve health-related fitness is through *aerobic exercise*, the rhythmic, repetitive movement of large muscle groups. Aerobic exercise is usually performed at an intensity level that does not exceed the ability of the lungs, heart, and blood vessels to bring oxygen to the exercising muscles. Because aerobic exercises maintain a balance between the uptake and expenditure of oxygen, they can be engaged in over a relatively long time period and are thought of as endurance activities. In contrast, exercise of higher intensity that requires more energy than can be derived from aerobic metabolism is referred to as *anaerobic exercise*. Because the intensity and energy requirements of anaerobic exercises are high, they can be performed for only short periods of time.

Energy, stored in the form of two high energy compounds, adenosine triphosphate (ATP) and creatine phosphate (CP), is released when either ATP or CP are broken down within the cell. Muscle contraction results when ATP is reduced to adenosine diphosphate (ADP) and inorganic phosphate. CP is reduced to creatine and inorganic phosphate, and provides the energy for resynthesis of ATP. Oxidation or *aerobic metabolism* provides the energy to resynthesize CP. In the presence of sufficient oxygen, metabolism can proceed through the aerobic stages of metabolism to the point where oxygen is combined with hydrogen ions to form water and carbon dioxide. When sufficient oxygen is not available, the hydrogen ions and hydrogen atoms accumulate and effectively block the aerobic cycle so that the body must rely on *anaerobic metabolism*. During exercise at high work loads, the body is incapable of providing sufficient oxygen to regenerate the necessary ATP and anaerobic metabolism leads to the formation and accumulation of lactic acid.

The main criterion of aerobic exercise is that it is continuous and steady. When exercise is conducted aerobically, the movement is non-stop for at least 12 min with up to 80% maximum heart rate[2]. Measurement of the physical exertion associated with various physical activities is possible using units of metabolic equivalents (METs). One MET is the resting oxygen uptake relative to the total body mass and is generally ascribed the value of 3.5 ml of oxygen per kilogram per minute. The total amount of caloric expenditure associated with any physical activity, including exercise, is determined by the amount of muscle mass producing bodily movements and the intensity, duration, and frequency of muscular contractions. The calories spent per hour in a given activity can be approximated by multiplying the MET intensity level by total body mass (in kg)[3].

The level of activity above the basal, resting rate produces a variety of physiological changes referred to as a *training effect*. Changes due to physical fitness training are specific to the type of physical activity engaged in, and also depend on the frequency, duration, and intensity of participation. In healthy adults, endurance training produces cardiovascular adaptations such as reduction in heart rate at submaximal workloads, increased heart and blood volume, and reduction in resting heart rate and blood pressure. A more efficient respiratory system also results from regular physical exertion as indicated by lowered respiratory rate at rest and during submaximal exercise. Body composition changes such as decreased weight and reduction of percentage body fat also have been associated with training.

To achieve a training effect regular participation in aerobic-type exercise at least three times a week for 20 minutes or more is required. Some physical exercises produce a training effect more efficiently than others. Exercises such as running, jogging, cross-country skiing, jumping rope, cycling, or swimming usually can be performed as steady, endurance activities. Exercises such as tennis, downhill skiing, and football are often performed in a 'stop-and-go' manner with sudden bursts of energy expenditure and, therefore, typically have a significant anaerobic component. Exercises, such as weight lifting, sprinting, isometrics, square dancing, are usually of too short a duration to qualify as aerobic exercise, while exercises such as golf are of too low intensity to qualify as aerobic exercise.

216

Anecdotal reports that aerobic exercise elevated the mood of participants may have initiated the use of exercise, particularly running, as an adjunct to the treatment of mood disorders. Aerobic exercise as a therapy for depression and anxiety has advantages over some of the more traditional therapies. Exercise is inexpensive and can be performed by most people with little training or skill. Participants must assume an active role in their treatment. Moreover, exercise provides additional physical health benefits such as improvements in cardio-respiratory function and in body composition. Finally, exercise can provide mental health benefits and promote a sense of self-confidence and well-being. Because depression and anxiety are common problems in the American population[4], these advantages may make exercise an appealing form of therapy and may provide a rationale for widespread use in various clinical settings.

The term *depression* is used to refer to a spectrum of phenomena that are distinguished by duration, severity of symptoms, and extent of psychological impairment. The less severe forms of depression, such as sadness, the 'blues' or normal grief reactions are experienced by many adults. However, as many as 15% of the US adult population suffer from serious depressive disorders in any given year[5].

*Anxiety* is characterized by high levels of sympathetic arousal and may be accompanied by somatic complaints such as heart palpitations, tiredness or headaches. Anxiety is a concern for health professionals because the negative effects of anxiety increase the need for health care[6], and may be associated with decreased work effectiveness[7] and lowered morale. Researchers often make a distinction between two types of anxiety. *State* anxiety is a transient condition defined by how a person feels at a particular moment, whereas *trait* anxiety is a more stable disposition defined by how a person usually feels[8].

The effects of participation in sports and exercise on depression and anxiety have been studied under a variety of conditions. People from diverse popula-tions, including normal children and adults, psychiatric patients, and cardiac and other medically-ill patients have been studied. The exercise treatment programme has varied in length, frequency, intensity and type of exercise across studies. Further, a variety of outcome measures has been studied such as mood, personality, self-concept, and cognitive performance. This review is limited to studies that examine the effects of aerobic exercise on anxiety and/or depression and appeared in scientific, rather than popular, literature within the past 5 years. First, studies that provide evidence concerning the effects of *acute* exercise on depression and anxiety in clinical and normal populations are considered. Next, studies that provide evidence concerning the effects of *chronic* exercise, i.e. aerobic training, on anxiety and depression in clinical and normal populations are presented. Finally, directions for future research are described.

## ACUTE EFFECTS OF AEROBIC EXERCISE

### Clinical Populations

There are two contrasting views about the anxiolytic effects of acute exercise. Pitts and McClure[9] assert that exercise *provokes* anxiety attacks and anxiety symptoms. They postulate that anxiety neurotics feel anxious after exercise because physical exercise produces sensations such as arousal and muscle tension that are similar to, and likely to be confused with, symptoms of anxiety. Pitts[10] has suggested that the accumulation of lactic acid could be responsible for the subjective experience of anxiety associated with the stress-response. Since lactic acid is an exercise metabolite, exercising normal individuals could experience lactate-induced anxiety.

In contrast, Morgan[11] has suggested that exercise *reduces* anxiety through muscular relaxation. He conducted a series of studies to evaluate the effects of acute exercise on measures of anxiety. Subjects were required to exercise on a treadmill at 80% of their maximal aerobic power. Anxiety was measured by a well-known questionnaire called the State–Trait Anxiety Inventory (STAI). Whether the exerciser walked or ran, state anxiety was slightly increased early in the exercise session but decreased rapidly following exercise. This pattern of change was reported by both clinically anxious and normal subjects. Since lactate levels were significantly elevated, it appears that exercise had been sufficiently intense to have produced lactate-induced anxiety. Morgan concluded that subjective anxiety was reduced with exercise. A similar conclusion was reached by Orwin[12] who summarized his experience with patients suffering from agoraphobia. He used running as treatment in eight phobics and found that a single session of exercise actually reduced levels of subjective anxiety.

Taken together, these studies suggest that aerobic exercise is associated with a reduction in state anxiety. However, other studies in this area are needed to identify the individuals who are most likely to benefit from exercise, and to define the kinds of exercise most likely to reduce trait anxiety. Recent investigations on the effects of acute aerobic exercise on depression in clinical populations are lacking.

## Normal Populations

Several studies have examined the effect of acute aerobic exercise on mood in normal adults. For example, Lichtman and Poser[13] examined mood states in 64 adults who were enrolled in either a physical exercise class (45 min of jogging and other physical activities) or a hobby class. Change in mood was assessed by the Nowlis Mood Scale (a 14-factor shortened version of the Mood Adjective Checklist) and the Profile of Mood States (POMS). As indicated by the Nowlis Mood Scale, the exercise group felt significantly less depressed, less fatigued, less serious and more pleasant after they had exercised. The results of the POMS showed that the exercise group felt significantly less anxious, depressed, angry and fatigued after they had exercised. In contrast, the hobby group showed no significant changes on any of the factors of the Nowlis Mood Scale after participation in their class. Examination of their scores on the POMS revealed significant decreases on anxiety and depression subscales, but no significant changes on the other four subscales.

Berger and Owen[14] showed that another type of aerobic exercise, swimming, produces favourable changes in mood. These investigators used the POMS to assess change in mood in two groups of students who participated either in a swimming class or in a lecture class. The swimmers reported significantly less tension, depression, anger, confusion and more vigour after exercise than before. Individuals in the lecture-class control group did not report any significant changes in mood.

The results of these two studies suggest that exercise may be associated with beneficial psychological effects for the exerciser. However, subjects were not randomly assigned to conditions, and a number of factors other than exercise may have been responsible for the observed changes in mood. Other methodological aspects of these two studies such as the sole reliance on self-report instruments, particularly with a pretest–post-test design, make it difficult to draw any definitive conclusions. For example, self-reports may be biased by subjects' concern about evaluation, expectations about the effects of treatment, or desire to help the experimenter. When subjects are measured twice with the same instrument, the desire to appear consistent across time of measurement may be confounded with treatment effects.

This last potential source of error is evident in a study reported by Thaxton[15]. Thaxton examined the effects of acute exercise on depression in habitual runners using a randomized Solomon four-group design. This design consists of two replications of the same experiment, one with pretest and the other without. For the purposes of Thaxton's research, consistent findings in both replications would have led to greater confidence that exercise and not other factors such as the measurement procedure itself produced changes in mood. On the day of the experiment, two groups ran and two groups did not. Pretests were given to one of the running groups and one of the non-running groups. Mood was assessed by the POMS. Comparison across the non-pretested groups showed that the non-running group reported significantly higher depression scores than those who ran. If pretested subjects were not affected by the measurement procedure, a similar pattern should be observed. However, depression scores of the two pretested groups were similar whether they ran or did not. This pattern of results suggests that the observed effect of exercise may have been confounded with the effect of the measurement procedure. Thus, studies that rely on a pretest–post-test design or that rely exclusively on self-report should be viewed with caution.

Bahrke and Morgan[16] attempted to demonstrate the anxiolytic effect of aerobic exercise by comparing exercise with another anxiolytic intervention, i.e. meditation. 75 men were randomly assigned to 20 min of exercise at 70% maximum aerobic power, to non-cultic meditation, or to quiet rest in a sound-filtered room. All three conditions reduced state anxiety. The investigators concluded that something common to all three treatments, such as 'diversion', accounted for anxiety reduction and that 'time-out' or simple rest breaks may be as effective in reducing anxiety as aerobic exercise.

Direct comparisons between different kinds of interventions are difficult, however. Interventions may differ on a number of relevant dimensions, including intensity, degree of attention and social stimulation, and mode of action. Moreover, comparable results may be achieved via different mechanisms. Future research should attempt to identify which individuals could profit most from which interventions.

# CHRONIC EFFECTS OF AEROBIC EXERCISE TRAINING

## Clinical Populations

Interest in the use of an extended exercise programme in clinical populations has generally focused on two specific groups, psychiatric patients and patients with coronary heart disease (CHD). Many clinicians are optimistic about the therapeutic efficacy of an exercise programme in clinically depressed patients. However, because most previous research studies have used small samples, inadequate designs and no comparison groups, no definitive conclusions about the effectiveness of exercise are possible. For example, Blue[17] reported his experience with two clinically depressed individuals. These patients showed no response to more than 8 weeks of treatment with antidepressant medication and psychotherapy. After 3 weeks of an aerobic running programme, however, both individuals experienced a reduction in depression. Obviously, the small sample size, lack of control group and other methodological shortcomings make it difficult to interpret the results. If an appropriate control group was not readily available for this study, use of a multiple baseline cross-over design could have provided more direct evidence that the exercise *per se* was responsible for the clinical improvement.

Hartz *et al.*[18] used this alternative design. Seven clinically depressed outpatients proceeded through four phases of treatment over a 6 week period that included two segments of supervised aerobic conditioning and two segments of baseline or withdrawal. Daily measures of depression were obtained using the Depression Adjective Checklist (DAC) and Zung Self-rating Depression Inventory. Aerobic conditioning was measured by total exercise time and by 1 min pulse recovery after exercise. Examination of depression scores in the seven patients did not reveal a significant decrease in depression. However, *post hoc* analysis of subjects who showed significant improvements in mood revealed that the two subjects who experienced positive changes in their mood happened to be the only subjects who increased their aerobic conditioning. The five subjects who showed no change in conditioning showed no change in depression. These results imply that cardiovascular training, i.e. reduction in heart rates at submaximal workloads, may be necessary for exercise to relieve depression.

Most research has a number of potential sources of error variance that may lead to spurious conclusions. Repeated testing, i.e. daily assessments of depression as used by Hartz[18], is one example of a source of bias that may affect the results. Another potential source of bias is the 'special attention' associated with the treatment condition. Special attention refers to the fact that the treatment group may receive non-specific attention over and above the treatment that the control group does not receive. Thus, the experimental group differs from the control group not only because it receives a particular treatment, but also because it receives social attention and interaction that may be beneficial in and of itself.

Two potential sources of error, special attention and subject's expectation, were addressed in a study by Doyne *et al.*[19]. Four outpatients who were diagnosed as having a major depressive illness participated in both exercise (bicycle ergometry) and assertiveness training. It was assumed that assertiveness training would elicit expectations for change similar to those that exercise would elicit, and that subjects would experience similar amounts of attention in each condition. Assertiveness training also served as an attention-placebo baseline condition. One pair of subjects participated in the exercise condition until a training effect was achieved, and then participated in the attention-placebo condition. The other pair of subjects experienced the assertiveness training, followed by exercise training. A reduction in the percentage of 'depressed' adjectives, as measured by the DACL, was noted during the exercise treatment phase relative to the percentage endorsed during the attention-placebo baseline. Increases in the percentage of 'happy' adjectives endorsed on the DACL were also noted. The gains that appeared during treatment were maintained at a 3 month follow-up evaluation. In an inpatient study of depressed patients, Conroy et al.[20] reported that exercise produced significant reductions in depression. 17 patients volunteered to participate in a 6 week exercise pro-gramme. Nine patients participated in a minimum of three exercise sessions each week and reported a marked decrease in their depression. However, no other evidence of psychological benefits, such as feelings of self-acceptance or reductions in anxiety or anger, were found. The eight patients who participated in only one exercise session each week showed no significant changes on the psychological measures. Since the sample consisted of self-selected individuals and contained relatively few subjects, it is difficult to generalize the results to other psychiatric inpatients.

The efficacy of aerobic exercise as a treatment for depression was compared with other forms of therapy in depressed individuals by Greist et al.[21]. Patients were randomly assigned to time-limited, ten-session psychotherapy, time-unlimited psychotherapy, or to individual running with a running leader. Patients initially met with their running leader three times per week for 30–45 min and progressed from walking to running. Results indicated that the running treatment was as effective in alleviating depressive symptoms and complaints as either of the other two treatments.

Hilyer et al.[22] attempted to evaluate the use of exercise therapy in a special population. 60 institutionalized male juvenile delinquents were randomly assigned either to a 20 week physical fitness programme delivered by counsellors or to a control group. Other than meeting 3 days a week for 1½ hours, the routines of the experimental and control groups were similar. At the time of post-testing, between-group comparisons revealed that the exercise group reported less state anxiety as assessed by STAI, and less tension, less anger and more vigour assessed by POMS than the control group. No significant differences were found for depression assessed by Beck Depression Inventory. Within-group comparison of pre- and post-test scores revealed that the exercise group significantly reduced state and trait anxiety, depression, anger, fatigue and confusion. In contrast, the control group significantly increased state and trait anxiety, tension, depression, anger, fatigue, confusion and decreased vigour. This study again demonstrates some of the difficulties of conducting human research. Since the control group knew about the purpose of study, their responses may reflect the knowledge that they were in the no-treatment group, i.e. a deprivation effect. Furthermore, the differential degree of attention provided to subjects by counsellors confounds the exercise treatment.

In a series of investigations, the effects of exercise on depression were examined in a group of patients with coronary heart disease (CHD). Stern and Cleary[23] found improvement in depression in CHD patients who participated in a low-intensity exercise programme. This 6 week exercise programme was the prerandomization phase of The National Exercise and Heart Disease Project (NEHDP) and was of low intensity to acclimatize subjects to exercise. Comparison of pre- and postexercise measures revealed that after exercise, the number of depressed men and the mean scores on the MMPI depression sub-scale were reduced significantly. In these same individuals, however, the number of anxious men and the mean anxiety score as measured by Taylor Manifest Anxiety Scale actually increased significantly.

The results of the randomized phase of the 2 year NEHDP exercise programme[24] did not replicate the results of the preliminary phase. 651 men were randomly assigned to either a supervised exercise training programme or to a control group. Changes on three scales obtained from the MMPI, Depression, Taylor Manifest Anxiety and Katz Adjustment, were assessed at 6 months, at 1 year, and at 2 years. No significant changes in psychological functioning were found in either the exercise or the control group.

In another study[25] of post-MI patients, 106 individuals with significant physical and psychological impairment, more favourable results for exercise therapy were observed. The purpose of the study was to compare rehabilitation effectiveness of exercise therapy and group counselling. Criteria for subject selection involved either achievement of a mean work load of less than seven METs on treadmill testing and/or psychological ratings of significant anxiety and/or depression. Subjects were randomly assigned to an exercise, counselling or control group. Exercise training consisted of 1 hour sessions three times a week over 12 weeks. Group counselling consisted of 1 hour sessions once a week over 12 weeks. Decreases in anxiety and depression were reported in the exercise group, only reductions in depression was reported in the counselling group, and no change was reported by the control group.

Prosser et al.[26] examined the effects of exercise on anxiety and morale in a group of CHD male patients. 15 patients were randomly assigned to an exercise group and participated in a 3 month exercise programme that met twice weekly for 45 min. Eight patients were randomly assigned to a control group. While both groups improved in morale, the morale of exercise patients was significantly higher than the morale of patients in the control group. Further, the reduction in anxiety experienced by the exercise group was significantly greater than that experienced by the control group.

The results of these studies suggest that exercise therapy may be beneficial, particularly for patients with emotional or physical impairments. However, the precise mechanisms by which these benefits are achieved need to be clarified.


Normal Populations

A number of studies have examined the use of aerobic exercise in normal adults. The results of these studies generally show that the exercise group has lower scores of anxiety and depression after participation in an exercise programme than the no-exercise control group. However, many studies have employed a non-equivalent group design with the problems and potential confounds, e.g. expectancy effect, special attention, etc., that were described earlier. Improvement in mood is an expected effect of an exercise programme, and may even be one reason why participants elect to enter an exercise programme. In contrast, no changes are expected in volunteers who serve as a comparison group and who do nothing but complete tests on two different occasions.

In a study by Young[27], the effect of an 8 week exercise programme was assessed in 16 young or middle-aged men and women. A significant decrease in mean anxiety scores was found in young but not middle-aged subjects. No significant change was found on depression for any group. No control or comparison group was included in the design, however.

Blumenthal *et al.*[28] examined the effects of an aerobic conditioning programme on 16 deconditioned middle-aged adults. While a control group matched for age and sex maintained their sedentary lifestyle, the exercise group participated in a 10 week conditioning programme which met three times a week for 45 min. Exercise intensity was prescribed to produce an increased heart rate equal to 70–85% of the maximum heart rate achieved on each subject's initial treadmill test. Improved psychological functioning, including less state and trait anxiety assessed by the STAI, and less tension, depression and fatigue, and more vigour measured by the POMS was found for the exercise group but not for the control group. These results support the conclusion that exercise training can induce significant psychological benefits among healthy participants. However, since subjects were not randomly assigned to conditions, self-selection, expectancy or social attention factors could have been responsible for the observed changes in mood.

The effects of a 14 week conditioning programme on anxiety and physiological phenomena in young adults were assessed by McGlynn *et al.*[29]. The treatment consisted of an hour of exercise twice a week. All subjects were sedentary volunteers and were between 18 and 26 years old. The exercise group included 15 individuals from an aerobic exercise class, and the control group included 15 individuals from a health science class. Anxiety was measured by STAI. Physiological measures included an assessment of muscle tension determined by EMG activity and systolic blood pressure determined by standard sphygmomanometry. After the 14 week programme, the exercise group showed a significant decrease in state and trait anxiety while the control group showed no significant decrease in either state or trait anxiety. Another purpose of the study was to examine the effects of a conditioning programme during a stress situation. Subjects were asked to solve 15 anagrams, 12 of which had no solutions. After stress, the exercise group showed a significant increase in state anxiety and muscle tension, but no significant change of systolic blood pressure. The control group showed a significant increase in state anxiety, muscle tension and systolic blood pressure. While these results did not show that conditioning provided an antianxiety effect by self-report, the results of the blood pressure measure suggest that exercise may offer some beneficial psychophysiological effects. Thus, exercise training may attenuate the physiological concomitants of anxiety and depression. For a more detailed discussion of the effects of aerobic conditioning on the stress response the interested reader should see the recent review by Blumenthal and McCubbin[30].

Confirmation that exercise produces physiological benefits was reported in another study designed to investigate the relationship between exercise and stress. Lobitz et al.[31] were interested in examining the effects that stress would have on a physically fit person and recruited normal adults who experienced daily stress. The purpose of the study was to assess the relative effectiveness to withstand the pressure of stress by comparing different treatment programmes. 18 subjects were randomly assigned to one of three conditions: a 7 week aerobic exercise programme, a 7 week anxiety management training programme, or to a control group. State and trait anxiety were assessed by the STAI, and heart rate, blood pressure and blood chemistry were also assessed. Subjects in both treatment groups reported a significant reduction in state anxiety. Only subjects in the anxiety management training group reported a significant reduction in trait anxiety. These findings led investigators to conclude that both aerobic exercise programmes and anxiety management training were effective as stress prevention programmes. The physiological changes showed that the exercise group had significant decreases in heart rate, increases in high-density lipoprotein cholesterol and reductions in systolic blood pressure. These physiological results suggest that an aerobic exercise programme produces beneficial effects that other stress-prevention interventions may not provide.

The effects of exercise in 38 elderly adults were reported by Bennette et al.[32]. Subjects were randomly assigned either to an exercise programme that met twice a week for 45 min sessions for 8 weeks or to a control group. No significant reduction in depression as assessed by the Zung Depression Scale was found in either group. Further analysis revealed that a significant reduction in depression scores occurred in 11 individuals who were clinically depressed at the outset of the study. This finding is consistent with the idea that success of exercise therapy for depression may be limited to clinically depressed individuals.

While the results of these studies show that physical exercise programmes are associated with positive psychological changes in clinical and normal populations, and that those individuals who are less fit or who are in the most distress may profit most from exercise, methodological problems still plague researchers in the field so that it is not certain that exercise training itself induces improvements in mood.

## RESEARCH DIRECTIONS

The hypothesis that physical fitness reduces depression and/or anxiety has not been unequivocally demonstrated, primarily because of methodological limitations of previous research. Many studies provide suggestive evidence that aerobic exercise can provide psychological, as well as physical benefits to an exerciser. To advance our understanding in this area, however, future research should incorporate better techniques for identifying mechanisms responsible for change.

Methodological limitations of past research include examination of small self-selected samples, attrition of sample during the study, reliance only on self-report measures, inadequate description of characteristics of treatment (such as intensity, duration and mode of activity) and inadequate attention to characteristics of subjects (such as physical or mental status at the outset of the study). Attention to three methodological issues in particular is essential if we are to increase our understanding of the effects of aerobic exercise on mental health. Future studies should use a randomized experimental design, precisely characterize important subject factors such as level of physical health and mental health, and employ multiple assessment procedures including self-ratings, observer-ratings and psychophysiological response measures.

Although a number of investigators have examined the relationship between aerobic exercise and mood, the use of good research design has been limited. Only a handful of studies have used a randomized group design from which it is possible to make causal attribution to treatment for changes that were observed on the response measures. Many studies have used a non-equivalent group design so that a number of alternative explanations for the findings are possible. With the use of randomized experimental designs, a more precise understanding of the relationship between exercise and mood is possible.

The results of several studies suggest that use of heterogeneous samples may mask the effects of exercise on mood. Attention to individual differences is necessary to clearly identify populations most likely to benefit from aerobic exercise. Specifying what individuals do which kind of exercise for how long needs to be addressed, as well as evaluating whether other alternative interventions such as psychotherapy or pharmacological therapy may be as effective as exercise.

Other issues that require attention include identifying the mechanisms by which exercise effects psychological processes, ascertaining the factors that promote or deter adherence to exercise programmes, and identifying any harmful effects of exercise. For example, the role of endogenous opioids has recently received a great deal of attention as being one physiological mechanism by which exercisers feel better. A number of studies have demonstrated that $\beta$-endorphin and $\beta$-lipotrophin increase in response to acute exercise and chronic exercise training programmes, and elevated serum $\beta$-endorphin concentrations have been associated with improved mood and reduced pain perceptions[33-35]. By and large, no studies have reported the concurrent increase in endorphins and psychological well-being, however. In fact, studies of naloxone infusion find no difference in mood[36], indicating that mood changes may not be endorphin-mediated. Most of the current techniques for assessing opioid peptides are relatively crude, and further advances in the area of neurobiology will help to clarify this mind–body relationship.

If aerobic exercise is effective in improving mood, it must be practised on a regular basis. However, the problem of patient compliance cannot be underestimated. Since the drop-out rates from exercise programmes often exceed 50%, it is clear that many individuals find it difficult to adhere to an exercise programme[37]. Strategies for identifying patient drop-outs and improving compliance are currently being investigated[38]. The preliminary studies on the modification of exercise behaviour indicate that various interventions, including stimulus control, positive reinforcement and self-control procedures can improve exercise adherence. Few studies have focused on the maintenance side of exercise adoption, however, and more research in the area is essential.

Excessive involvement in jogging or running programmes has been described as a positive addiction[39]. However, when commitment to exercise assumes higher priority than commitments to work, family or interpersonal relations, a variety of problems may arise. Some researchers have gone so far as to suggest that compulsive exercise may be comparable to anorexia nervosa[40]. This issue remains a controversial one[41], and further research is needed to evaluate whether over-exercise can be too much of a good thing.

## ACKNOWLEDGEMENTS

The preparation of this chapter has been partially supported by a grant from the National Institute of Mental Health (Grant No. T32MH14660) to Duke University Center for the Study of Aging and Adult Development and by a New Investigator Award to Dr James Blumenthal from the National Heart, Lung, and Blood Institute (HL26609).

## References

1. Pate, R. R. (1983). A new definition of youth fitness. *Phys. Sportsmed.*, **11**, 77–83
2. Covert, B. (1977). *Fit or Fat?* (Boston: Houghton Mifflin Company)
3. *American College of Sports Medicine: Guidelines for graded exercise testing and exercise prescription.* (1980). 2nd Edn. (Philadelphia: Lea and Febiger)
4. Weissman, M. M., Myers, J. K. and Harding, P. S. (1978). Psychiatric disorders in a U.S. urban community: 1975–1976. *Am. J. Psychiatry*, **135**, 459–62
5. Gallant, D. M. (1976). Preface. In Gallant, D. M. and Simpson, G. M. (eds.) *Depression: Behavioral, Biochemical, Diagnostic and Treatment Concepts.* (New York: Spectrum Publications)
6. Petrick, J. and Holmes, T. H. (1977). Life changes and onset of illness. *Med. Clin. North Am.*, **61**, 825–38
7. MacKay, C. and Cox, T. (1978). Stress at work. In Cox, T. (ed.) *Stress.* pp.147–73. (Baltimore: University Park Press)
8. Spielberger, C. D. (1966). Theory and research on anxiety. In Spielberger, C. D. (ed.) *Anxiety and Behavior.* pp. 12–19. (New York: Academic Press)
9. Pitts, F. N., Jr. and McClure, J. N., Jr. (1967). Lactate metabolism in anxiety neurosis. *N. Engl. J. Med.*, **277**, 1329–36
10. Pitts, F. M., Jr. (1969). The biochemistry of anxiety. *Sci. Am.*, **220**, 69–75
11. Morgan, W. P. (1981). Psychological benefits of physical activity. In Nagle, F. J. and Montoye, H. J. (eds.) *Exercise in Health and Disease.* pp. 299–314. (Springfield, Ill.: Charles C. Thomas)
12. Orwin, A. (1981). 'The running treatment': A preliminary communication on a new use for an old therapy (physical activity) in the agoraphobic syndrome. In Sacks, M. H. and Sachs, M. L. (eds.) *Psychology of Running.* pp. 32–9. (Champaign, Ill.: Kinetics Publishers, Inc.)
13. Lichtman, S. and Poser, E. G. (1983). The effects of exercise on mood and cognitive functioning. *J. Psychosom. Res.*, **27**, 43–52
14. Berger, B. G. and Owen, D. R. (1983). Mood alteration with swimming – swimmers really do 'feel better'. *Psychosom. Med.*, **45**, 425–33

15. Thaxton, L. (1982). Physiological and psychological effects of short-term exercise addiction on habitual runners. *J. Sport Psychol.*, **4**, 73–80
16. Bahrke, M. S. and Morgan, W. P. (1981). Anxiety reduction following exercise and meditation. In Sacks, M. H. and Sachs, M. L. (eds.) *Psychology of Running.* pp. 57–66. (Champaign, Ill.: Kinetics Publishers, Inc.)
17. Blue, F. R. (1979). Aerobic running as a treatment for moderate depression. *Percept. Mot. Skills*, **48**, 228
18. Hartz, G. W., Wallace, W. L. and Cayton, T. G. (1982). Effect of aerobic conditioning upon mood in clinically depressed men and women: a preliminary investigation. *Percept. Mot. Skills*, **3**, 1217–18
19. Doyne, E. J., Chambless, D. L. and Beutler, L. E. (1983). Aerobic exercise as a treatment for depression in women. *Behav. Ther.*, **14**, 434–40
20. Conroy, R. W., Smith, K. and Felthous, A. R. (1982). The value of exercise on a psychiatric hospital unit. *Hosp. Commun. Psychiatr.*, **33**, 641–5
21. Greist, J. H., Klein, M. H., Eischens, R. R. and Faris, J. T. (1978). Running out of depression. *Phys. Sportsmed.*, **6**, 49–51, 54, 56
22. Hilyer, J. C., Wilson, D. G., Dillon, C., Carol, L., Jenkins, C., Spencer, W. A., Meadows, M. E. and Brookes, W. (1982). Physical fitness training and counseling as treatment for youthful offenders. *J. Counsel. Psychol.*, **29**, 292–303
23. Stern, M. J. and Cleary, P. (1981). The National Exercise and Heart Disease Project: psychosocial changes observed during a low-level exercise program. *Arch. Intern. Med.*, **141**, 1463–7
24. Stern, M. J. and Cleary, P. (1982). The National Exercise and Heart Disease Project: long-term psychosocial outcome. *Arch. Intern. Med.*, **142**, 1093–7
25. Stern, M. J., Gorman, P. A. and Kaslow, L. (1983). The group counseling vs. exercise therapy study. A controlled intervention with subjects following myocardial infarction. *Arch. Intern. Med.*, **143**, 1719–25
26. Prosser, G., Carson, P., Phillips, R., Gelson, A., Buck, N., Tucker, H., Neophytou, M., Lloyd, M. and Simpson, T. (1981). Morale in coronary patients following an exercise programme. *J. Psychosom. Res.*, **25**, 587–93
27. Young, R. J. (1979). The effect of regular exercise on cognitive functioning and personality. *Br. J. Sports Med.*, **13**, 110–17
28. Blumenthal, J. A., Williams, R. S., Needels, T. L. and Wallace, A. G. (1982). Psychological changes accompany aerobic exercise in healthy middle-aged adults. *Psychosom. Med.*, **44**, 529–35
29. McGlynn, G. H., Franklin, B., Lauro, G. and McGlynn, I. K. (1983). The effect of aerobic conditioning and induced stress on state–trait anxiety, blood pressure, and muscle tension. *J. Sports Med.*, **23**, 341–50
30. Blumenthal, J. A. and McCubbin, J. (1985). Exercise training as stress management. In Baum, A. and Singer, J. (eds.) *Handbook of Psychology and Health.* (New York: Lawrence Erlbaum Associates)
31. Lobitz, W. C., Brammell, H. L., Stoll, S. and Niccoli, A. (1983). Physical exercise and anxiety management training for cardiac stress management in a nonpatient population. *J. Cardiac Rehabil.*, **3**, 683–8
32. Bennett, J., Carmack, M. A. and Gardner, V. J. (1982). The effect of a program of physical exercise on depression in older adults. *Physical Educator*, **39**, 21–4
33. Berk, L. S., Tan, S. A., Anderson, C. L. and Reiss, G. (1981). $\beta$-EP response to exercise in athletes and non-athletes. *Med. Sci. Sports and Exercise*, **13**, 134
34. Bortz, W. M., Angevin, P., Mefford, I. N., Boarder, M. B., Noyce, N. and Barchas, J. D. (1981). Catecholamine, dopemine and endorphin levels during extreme exercise. *N. Engl. J. Med.*, **305**, 466–7
35. Colt, E. W., Wardlaw, S. L. and Frantz, A. G. (1981). The effect of running on plasma $\beta$-endorphin. *Life Sci.*, **28**, 1637–40
36. Markoff, R. A., Ryan, P. and Young, T. (1982). Endorphins and mood changes in long-distance running. *Med. Sci. Sports and Exercise*, **14**, 11–15
37. Dishman, R. K. (1982). Compliance/adherence in health-related exercise. *Health Psychol.*, **1**, 237–67
38. Martin, J. E. and Dubbert, P. M. (1982). Exercise applications and promotion in behavioural medicine: Current status and future directions, *J. Counsel. Clin. Psychol.*, **50**, 1004–17

39. Glasser, W. (1976). *Positive Addiction*. (New York: Harper and Row)
40. Yates, A., Leehey, K. and Shisslak, C. M. (1983). Running – an analogue of anorexia. *N. Engl. J. Med.*, **308**, 251–5
41. Blumenthal, J. A., O'Toole, L. C. and Chang, J. L. (1984). Is running an analogue of anorexia nervosa? An empirical study of obligatory running and anorexia nervosa. *J. Am. Med. Assoc.*, **252**, 520–3

# SECTION 3

# SOCIAL AND
APPLIED STUDIES

# 11

# Individual differences in non-verbal communication

## Peter E. Bull

---

### INTRODUCTION

Communication is concerned with the sharing of information; if we are to talk of non-verbal communication, it needs to be shown that information can be both transmitted and received through non-verbal behaviour, a process referred to as encoding and decoding through a socially shared signal system[1]. The focus of this chapter is on individual differences in non-verbal communication; they may be of importance with regard to both encoding and decoding, and need to be considered from both points of view. Communication can also be regarded as a skill; Argyle and Kendon[2], in a highly influential paper, argued that social interaction can be seen as a kind of motor skill, involving the same kinds of processes as driving a car or playing a game of tennis. For example, good timing is essential both for the successful tennis player and for the accomplished diplomat; again, the skilled perception of relevant information is important both for the motorist as he negotiates the traffic and for the successful bargainer as he makes a judgement of the most he can achieve from his negotiations. In this chapter, it is intended to discuss individual differences in non-verbal communication in the context of the social skills model, with particular reference to whether individual differences in the encoding and decoding of non-verbal cues can be regarded as reflecting different levels of skill in communication.

With regard to encoding, there may be individual differences concerning the extent to which people transmit information through non-verbal cues: some people may transmit a great deal of information through non-verbal cues, others relatively little. Non-verbal cues may also encode information about individual differences; for example, it is widely believed that non-verbal cues encode significant information about the personalities of others, that information about people's personality traits is in some sense encoded in their non-verbal behaviour. This would suggest that individual differences in encoding are important not only in that people may differ in the extent to which they transmit information through non-verbal cues, but also the non-verbal cues they do employ may encode significant information about what kind of person they are.

231

To what extent these individual differences in encoding reflect different levels of communication skill constitutes one main theme of this chapter.

Individual differences in decoding non-verbal cues constitute a second important theoretical issue. A number of studies have been carried out to investigate whether groups differ in their decoding ability, whether, for example, women are superior to men in this respect, or whether psychiatric patients are disadvantaged in comparison to the normal population. The importance of these studies with regard to the communicative status of non-verbal behaviour is that although non-verbal cues may encode information about, say, emotion, speech or individual differences, such information may not always be accurately decoded; if certain groups of people fail to decode non-verbal cues appropriately, then the significance of those cues as a form of communication may be limited to certain sectors of the population. In that sense the significance of non-verbal cues as a system of communication is dependent upon the decoding skills of the message receiver. Hence, individual differences in decoding will constitute the second main theme of this chapter; they will be discussed with reference to differences in age, culture, personality, psychopathology and sex, and with reference to what extent those individual differences in decoding can be seen as reflecting different levels of communication skill. The theoretical significance of these studies of decoding is that there may be individual differences in the extent to which non-verbal cues function as a system of communication; the importance of individual differences in both encoding and decoding non-verbal cues will form the central theme of this chapter.


## STUDIES OF ENCODING

### Individual Differences in Expressiveness

Individual differences in the extent to which people transmit information through non-verbal cues may in fact be seen as a personality trait, in that some people are highly expressive, others less so. Jones[3] claimed to find two personality types, which he labelled internalizers and externalizers. Internalizers show high galvanic skin responsiveness, but their outward behaviour is restrained and they are judged to be calm and poised in their social relationships. Externalizers show little galvanic skin responsiveness, but they tend to be talkative and animated, and display a great deal of motor activity. Jones' observations were based on a series of experiments with a group of adolescents, having first selected the 20% who were most reactive and the 20% least reactive in their galvanic skin responses. These two groups were then instructed to classify a series of words and phrases in terms of their emotional significance, while their galvanic skin response to those words and phrases was measured; the results showed the patterns of internalizer and externalizer behaviour described above.

Jones' work appears consistent with the belief that overt expression reduces the strength of emotion. The most famous exponent of this view is Freud[4], who maintained that verbal, bodily and physiological responses are alternative

232

channels for releasing emotional energy; if one channel is blocked, the response through the others should increase in intensity. Consistent with this hypothesis, a number of studies have shown significant negative correlations between overt facial expressions of emotion and physiological responsiveness. Typically, such studies have involved exposing an encoder to an emotionally arousing event while a decoder judges from his expression what event he is observing; the encoder's heart rate or skin conductance are both continuously monitored during the stimulus presentation[5, 6]. The results of these studies consistently indicate that decoders are most accurate with the least physiologically aroused encoders and least accurate with the most physiologically aroused encoders. One problem with these designs is that the assessment of overt expression is dependent on the measure of decoding accuracy and on the assumption that this reflects expressiveness. More recently, however, studies have included direct observations of the amount of facial expressiveness and have still found significant negative correlations with physiological arousal[7, 8].

Such studies suggest that differences in expressiveness can be seen as a personality trait. Other studies have shown that there are significant sex differences in expressiveness. Hall[9] was able to find 26 studies in which comparisons were made of sex differences in encoding through facial expression, body movement or content-free speech. In these studies, groups of judges ranging from 2 to 200 in number were asked to make judgements from either posed or spontaneous non-verbal expressions; if the judges were able to accurately identify the non-verbal expression, then the sender was regarded as a 'good' encoder. In the case of posed expressions, the task of the decoders was to judge the expression in terms of its meaning (emotional or otherwise), or degree of friendliness, or honesty; the criterion of 'good' encoding was whether that judgement concurred with the poser's intentions. In the studies of spontaneous expressions, the experimenters surreptitiously recorded the encoders' faces on film or videotape while they were viewing emotionally arousing incidents (on slides, videotape or in person); the criterion of 'good' encoding was whether the decoders could guess the particular incident viewed by the encoder. Of the 26 studies reviewed by Hall, nine showed a significant gender difference and eight of these showed that women were better encoders, a proportion which is significantly greater than the 50% which would be expected by chance. To make the studies statistically comparable, the size of effect was calculated in terms of standard deviation units $(d)$; $d$ is the difference between the mean of the two groups divided by their common standard deviation[10]. The mean effect size for visual studies was 0.88 standard deviation unit, while the mean effect size for vocal studies was only 0.01 standard deviation unit, a difference which is marginally significant ($p = 0.067$). Hence, it appears that female non-verbal encoding advantage is essentially confined to visual cues.

Differences in encoding can also be related to psychopathology. Winkelmayer, Exline, Gottheil and Paredes[11] arranged for normal and schizophrenic American women, closely matched for age and educational level, to relate three personal experiences, one which evoked happiness, another which evoked anger and another which evoked sorrow. A film was made of these accounts which was shown without sound to male American, British and Mexican students, who were asked to identify the emotion being described. The results showed a significant statistical interaction between diagnostic category and nationality of the judges, with American and British judges performing significantly better at guessing the emotions encoded by the group of normal women. This finding that schizophrenic women were relatively poorer at encoding information about emotion provides some support for the traditional description of schizophrenia as characterized by 'flattened affect'[12]. Flattened affect refers to a relative impoverishment of emotional expressiveness, a concept which is highly similar to that of poor encoding demonstrated in this study.

There are also cross-cultural differences in encoding. Shimoda, Argyle and Bitti[13] asked English, Italian and Japanese students to pose expressions in front of a camera for eight emotions (surprised, depressed, sad, disgusted, happy, anxious, angry, afraid) and for four interpersonal attitudes (superior, submissive, friendly and hostile). The results showed that the Japanese expressed emotions and attitudes significantly less clearly than the other two cultures, since the subjects from all three cultures (including the Japanese) did significantly worse when judging Japanese expressions.

Differences in encoding can thus be related to personality, sex, psychopathology and culture. Hall[9], in her review of sex differences in encoding, talks of 'good' encoders, with the implication that people whose expressions can be judged more easily are more skilled at encoding. But this begs the question as to what constitutes 'good' encoding. In certain circumstances, it may be inadvisable to show one's feelings, for example, for a subordinate to show anger to a person of superior status. 'Good' encoding in those circumstances might lead to rapid dismissal! The fact that Japanese expressions are difficult to judge even for the Japanese[13] probably reflects Japanese norms governing the display of emotions in public, such that 'good' encoding in Japanese culture may be maintaining a smiling demeanour and concealing signs of hostility or distress. Similarly, sex differences in encoding may reflect social norms regarding the behaviour considered appropriate for each sex; a man who displays his feelings too easily might be considered weak or effeminate, whereas a women who rarely shows her feelings might be considered hard or cold. Certainly, encoding may be regarded as a skill, but what constitutes good encoding cannot be divorced from cultural norms or situational context. Moreover, the person who is good at expressing his feelings when appropriate may be less able to conceal his feelings when necessary (and vice versa); indeed, work on the externalizer/internalizer dimension suggests that expressiveness is a personality trait and the study of Winkelmayer *et al.* on schizophrenia suggests this can also be related to psychopathology[11]. The person who is skilled at displaying a 'poker face' during a tense bargaining situation may not be the person who is good at expressing affection for a loved one or expressing sympathy for someone in distress. Hence, skill in encoding must be considered an interaction in which the personality of the encoder and the situation and culture in which he finds himself all play a role; it is simply not possible to make general statements about 'good' encoding independently of these factors.

## Encoding Information about Individual Differences

Individual differences in encoding are important not only in that people may differ in the extent to which they transmit information through non-verbal cues, but also the non-verbal cues which they do employ may encode significant information about individual differences. The implications of those individual differences in encoding for the concept of communication skill depends very much upon what information is conveyed about individual differences. For example, it is widely believed that non-verbal cues encode information about the personalities of others, that information about people's personality traits is in some sense encoded in their non-verbal behaviour. In a review of a number of studies investigating the relationship between personality traits and the encoding of non-verbal behaviour, Bull found little evidence to support this view; even where studies have shown significant correlations between a particular personality trait and particular non-verbal cues, the results often do not replicate[14]. Bull argued that the belief that non-verbal behaviour encodes significant information about personality may be an example of a decoding error, in which people mistakenly attribute significance to non-verbal behaviour which it does not in fact possess. This view has implications more for skill in decoding than for skill in encoding; it would suggest that one attribute of the skilled decoder is that he does not jump to sweeping conclusions about someone's personality on the basis of their non-verbal behaviour alone.

There are, however, a number of consistent and reliable sex differences in the encoding of non-verbal behaviour. For example, Exline[15] reviewed a number of studies which showed that women gaze more than men at other people, irrespective of their sex. Another commonly reported finding is that women smile more than men, again irrespective of the sex of their conversational partner[16]. Women appear to adopt closer interpersonal distances with each other than do men[17]. There also appear to be certain kinds of body movement which are sex-typed. Rekers, Amaro-Plotkin and Low[18] found that gestures considered to be effeminate used by gender-disturbed boys were in fact predominantly used by girls in a study of normal children. These gestures were what they called the limp wrist, flutters (a rapid succession of up and down movements of the forearm and/or upper arm while the wrist remains relaxed) and walking with a flexed elbow (where the angle between the upper arm and forearm is between 0° and 135°). In another study with a larger sample of American children (aged 4–5, 7–8 and 10–11 years), Rekers and Rudy[19] replicated these findings and in addition found that girls, irrespective of age, made significantly greater use of what they called a hand clasp (touching the hands together in front of the body) and palming (touching the palm to the back, front or sides of the head and above the level of the ears).

The significance of these sex differences in the encoding of non-verbal behaviour for the concept of communication skill depends very much upon the meaning which is attached to those differences. Frieze and Ramsey[20] argue that the non-verbal behaviours used by women are those which are associated with low status and so help to perpetuate the inferior position of women in society. Drawing upon ethological studies of animal behaviour, they argue that smiling is used as an appeasement signal against aggression, that smaller interpersonal distances are related to an inferior position in a dominance hierarchy and that lower status is also associated with increased gazing at others, since a responsiveness to the needs and behaviour of more dominant members of a group is necessary for survival. The main alternative explanation to this is that women are socialized to be more accommodating to others[21] and that they prefer warm, intimate relationships; the non-verbal behaviours which women use can be seen as encoding a more accommodating attitude, in that their clearer encoding makes their messages easier to understand and their greater use of gaze, smiling and closer interpersonal distances can be seen as encoding a more receptive, affiliative attitude to others. Of course these explanations are not necessarily mutually exclusive; being more accommodating to others could be seen as adopting a more submissive role in respect of others and hence adopting an inferior position in society.

These different concepts of the significance of feminine non-verbal behaviour reflect different views of the position of women in society and there is no obvious way of deciding between them. What can be said is that there are clear and reliable sex differences in the encoding of non-verbal behaviour; it is also proposed that such behaviours constitute a code for communicating information about masculinity and femininity. This can be demonstrated from the fact that people can make quite subtle judgements about the sex-role attitudes of others on the basis of their non-verbal behaviour alone. For example, Lippa[22] had videotapes made of men and women as they role played being junior high school maths teachers. These encoders also completed the Bem Sex Role Inventory[23], according to which it is possible to identify any person of either sex as possessing either masculine qualities, feminine qualities or as androgynous, with the latter possessing masculine and feminine traits in roughly equal proportions. The videotapes were rated by decoders on a number of rating scales, including masculinity and femininity. The results showed that when the decoders saw videotapes of the body only, their judgements of masculinity and femininity correlated significantly with those dimensions as measured by the questionnaire, thus demonstrating that information about sex-role attitudes can be communicated through bodily cues alone.

With regard to the concept of communication skill, the non-verbal communication of masculinity and femininity poses a number of problems. From a radical feminist perspective, it could be argued that if a woman uses traditional feminine non-verbal behaviours, she is encoding a submissive attitude and hence colluding in the social inequality of women. But if she adopts more assertive non-verbal behaviours, she may meet with hostility and outright rejection, which makes it extremely difficult for her to realize her aims in society. In that sense her rejection of traditional feminine non-verbal behaviour could be seen as socially unskilled, but in another sense it could be argued that changes in traditional concepts of sex-role behaviour cannot be brought about without offending and antagonizing others, so that this is a price which has to be paid if those aims are to be realized. Whether or not her behaviour is seen as socially skilled can only be judged in terms of what she intends to achieve. By the same token, a homosexual who uses 'effeminate' forms of body movement could be seen as highly skilled if he is successful in attracting prospective partners of the same sex – if that is his aim. A heterosexual male who makes use of the same behaviours and conspicuously fails to attract members of the opposite sex could be seen as highly unskilled – if his aim is to attract members of the opposite sex. The point here is that judgements about whether behaviour is skilled or unskilled can only be made in the context of the aims and intentions of the encoder; if the behaviour assists the encoder in achieving his aims, then it can be seen as skilled, but if it hinders him in achieving his aims, it must be regarded as unskilled.

The encoding of non-verbal behaviour is also systematically related to psychopathology. People suffering from anxiety make greater use of non-signalling hand movements (e.g. stroking oneself, hand tremors), use shorter glances and smile less frequently; observers can also decode differences in the self-reported degree of anxiety on the basis of non-verbal behaviour alone[24], thus demonstrating that anxiety can be communicated through non-verbal behaviour. People suffering from depression show a lack of eye contact, downward angling of the head, a drooping mouth and a lack of hand movement[25]; observers can also identify depressed patients on the basis of their non-verbal behaviour alone[26], thus demonstrating that depression, too, can be communicated through non-verbal behaviour. Autistic children show marked gaze aversion[27], which has been interpreted as a form of communication serving to maintain the isolation of the autistic child[28]. The belief that people suffering from schizophrenia show marked gaze aversion has not been supported by more carefully controlled studies; instead, schizophrenics apparently avert their gaze only when talking about their own personal problems[29]. Studies of psychopathy and delinquency are less clear-cut, but it appears that violent offenders and delinquent adolescents have abnormally large personal space preferences which are possibly modified by the effects of institutionalization[30–32].

The implications of these findings for the concept of communication skill can be considered not only with regard to the encoding of non-verbal behaviour by psychiatric patients but also with regard to the way in which that behaviour is decoded by psychiatrists and clinical staff. A major implication of the social skills model of social interaction is that if social behaviour is seen as a skill, then it is possible for people to improve their social effectiveness through appropriate training procedures. It has been argued[33] that certain psychiatric difficulties can be seen as a consequence of a lack of social skill leading to rejection and social isolation, resulting in turn in disturbed mental states and that this can be alleviated through the use of appropriate social skills training. According to this view, it could be argued that abnormal forms of encoding used by psychiatric patients constitute part of their problem; the implication of this is that therapeutic intervention should focus on changing that behaviour into more socially acceptable forms which will in turn change the reactions of others towards them and consequently alleviate their distress. For example, a number of studies have been carried out intended to modify the gaze patterns of schizophrenic patients[34]. But if we accept Rutter's conclusion that schizophrenic patients only avert their gaze when talking about personal matters which embarrass them[29], teaching them to look more at others is not necessarily going to make them feel less embarrassed, indeed it may have the reverse effect. Similarly, the kinds of behaviours which encode depression (lack of eye contact, downward angling of the head, drooping mouth, lack of hand movement) can be seen as a way of communicating a desire to reduce social contact; training people not to use these behaviours, even if it did have the effect of increasing their amount of social contact, is not necessarily going to reduce the feeling of depression – indeed, it might exacerbate it, as the social skills trainer teaches them only how to hide their feelings. Trower, Bryant and Argyle[33] acknowledge this problem by making a distinction between pathological conditions where the social skills failure is the primary problem and pathological conditions where abnormalities of social behaviour can be seen as the consequence of a deeper emotional disturbance. The critical question, however, is in how many cases can the social skills failure be seen as the primary problem; if in most cases abnormalities in social behaviour are a consequence of severe emotional distress, then training people to adopt more conventional forms of social behaviour is not going to deal with the underlying problem. Bull claims that a fundamental distinction needs to be drawn between posed and spontaneous forms of encoding on the grounds that the non-verbal expression of emotion has both innate and learned components and that these cannot be regarded as interchangeable[35]. If abnormalities in the encoding of non-verbal behaviour are regarded as expressive of emotional distress, then training psychiatric patients to change their encoding of non-verbal behaviour is simply training them to conceal their feelings; concealing one's feelings may be socially advantageous in certain circumstances, but is not going to deal with the problems underlying that emotional distress. It may well be the case that training in encoding should focus on changing the behaviour which leads to the emotional distress; but there has as yet been little attention to this possibility in the social skills training literature.

However, this does not mean that abnormalities in encoding are unimportant for the concept of communication skill; what is proposed here is that their significance lies not in providing the basis for attempts to directly change the symptoms of the patient through some form of social skills training but rather in developing the decoding skills of psychiatrists and clinical staff. If the encoding of non-verbal behaviour is systematically related to psychopathology, then sensitivity to such cues provides a useful diagnostic tool for the clinician. Moreover, a number of studies have indicated that as patients recover, there are associated changes in non-verbal behaviour, which may provide a useful guide to the patients' improvement. For example, Hinchcliffe, Lancashire and Roberts[36] conducted a standardized interview with patients suffering from depression and with patients who had recovered from depression (matched for age, sex and social class) and found that the recovered patients spent significantly more time gazing at the interviewer than did those still suffering from depression. Similarly, Ekman and Friesen (p. 215[37]) describe an unpublished study by Kiritz, in which hand movements of American female psychiatric inpatients suffering from psychotic depression, neurotic depression and schizophrenia were observed at hospital admission and discharge. The patients suffering from psychotic depression at admission showed the fewest number of illustrators (hand movements which follow the rhythm and content of speech), but there was a significant increase in their use of illustrators from the admission to the discharge interview. Fisch, Frey and Hirsbrunner[38] observed the movement patterns of depressed patients (both male and female) 4 days after admission and 3 days before discharge and found significant differences along three dimensions of movement. The recovered patients were more mobile (defined as the number of body parts in motion), their movements were more complex (defined as the degree to which the various parts of the body are simultaneously involved in movement) and they showed a greater level of dynamic activation (defined as the swiftness with which movement shifts to a different level of activation).

Abnormalities in encoding non-verbal behaviour may even be useful guides as to what therapy to employ. This was suggested in a recent study by Ranelli and Miller[39] in which they found that depressed women who responded to drug therapy (amitryptyline) could be distinguished from non-responders on the basis of their non-verbal behaviour observed in an interview which took place prior to their receiving any medication. Whereas responders used long speech pauses and long durations of head aversion, non-responders showed a high frequency of self-adaptors (movements which satisfy self or bodily needs), posture shifts, pauses and a low frequency of smiles. Thus, non-verbal behaviour may be of value to the clinician, not only as an aid to diagnosis and as an indicator of recovery, but also as a guide to the responsiveness of the patient to different forms of therapy.

Hence, the argument proposed here is that abnormalities in encoding non-verbal behaviour do have significant implications for the concept of communication skill, not in directly attempting to change the symptomatic behaviour of psychiatric patients but in facilitating the decoding skills of the clinician. If abnormalities in encoding non-verbal behaviour are taken as reflecting underlying emotional distress, then attempting directly to change those behaviours is not going to alleviate that distress; in effect, it is simply training people to conceal their feelings. Perhaps training in encoding should concentrate on modifying the behaviour which influences emotional distress, but there has been scarce attention to this issue in the social skills training literature. What the evidence does suggest, however, is that non-verbal cues can provide important guides to the diagnosis of a patient's condition, to whether there is any improvement and even to the responsiveness of the patient to different forms of therapy. Telling a person to smile more, to gaze more, not to drop their head or to use more hand gestures is not going to make them happy; but the presence or absence of these non-verbal behaviours may be useful cues to the clinician in whether to diagnose depression, in what treatment to recommend and in his assessment of whether recovery has taken place.

## STUDIES OF DECODING

Individual differences in decoding constitute a second important theoretical issue. If people differ in their ability to decode non-verbal cues, then the significance of those cues as a form of communication will vary according to those decoding skills. For example, subtle non-verbal cues of disapproval will be wasted on an insensitive individual who is relatively impervious to such communication and a more explicitly verbal approach may be required! An extensive series of studies of individual differences in decoding have been carried out using a test called the Profile of Non-verbal Sensitivity (PONS)[40], in which a number of scenes are posed by a young American woman. The information available to the decoder includes both bodily cues (pictures of the face and body from the neck to the knees) and speech, especially processed by electronic filtering or randomized splicing to disguise the actual words spoken but to retain vocal information, such as pitch and amplitude. The decoders are given two alternate descriptions for each film clip (e.g. nagging a child/expressing jealous anger) and are asked to state which is correct. The criterion of accuracy is based on a combination of what message the encoder intended to send and what message the researchers, the encoder and a panel of judges decided the encoder had in fact sent; the items which achieved the highest level of agreement were included in the final test. Results using the PONS show a number of significant effects due to age, sex, culture and psychopathology. Thus, when the PONS was administered to Americans of differing ages, accuracy was shown to increase in a linear fashion between the ages of 8 and 25. Cross-cultural studies show that non-American samples perform significantly better than chance but significantly worse than Americans (the encoder is of course American). Psychiatric patients perform significantly worse on the PONS than non-psychiatric groups and also seem unable to benefit from practice with the PONS. Women perform significantly better than men on the PONS and this sex difference also occurs even with children.

At first sight, these findings would seem readily explainable in terms of individual differences in decoding skill. Adults with their greater social experience are more skilled at decoding non-verbal cues than children. Americans not surprisingly are better than non-Americans at decoding non-verbal cues from a member of their own culture. The inferior performance of psychiatric patients in decoding non-verbal cues is consistent with the view put forward by Argyle[41] that a lack of social perceptiveness may be a causal factor in mental illness. The superiority of women in decoding non-verbal cues lends some support to the folk wisdom of female intuition, that women are more perceptive than men about other people.

Nevertheless, the fact that all these findings are based on a test of non-verbal perceptiveness which relies on posed expressions should lead us to regard this conclusion with caution. As was discussed above, I have argued elsewhere[35] that a fundamental distinction needs to be drawn between posed and spontaneous forms of encoding on the grounds that the non-verbal expression of emotion has both innate and learned components and that these cannot simply be regarded as interchangeable. This point is highlighted in a study by La Russo[42], who investigated the non-verbal perceptiveness of patients suffering from paranoid schizophrenia and found that whereas their performance with posed expressions was significantly inferior to a control group with no history of psychiatric disorder, their performance with spontaneous expressions was actually significantly better than the control group. Such a finding demonstrates that there are important differences between spontaneous and posed expressions and that to base our study of individual differences in decoding non-verbal cues on posed expressions alone may result in a profoundly distorted view of their significance.

The LaRusso finding is also important with regard to the extent to which decoding non-verbal cues can be regarded as a social skill. One might naively assume that the more socially skilled people are, the better they will be at decoding non-verbal cues. But the finding that patients suffering from paranoid schizophrenia were actually significantly better at decoding spontaneous expressions than a control group with no previous history of psychiatric disorder might suggest that in certain circumstances it may actually be socially disadvantageous to know too much. A heightened social perceptiveness of the feelings concealed behind the social mask may impair social effectiveness, not enhance it. Similarly, it suggests that there may be different kinds of decoding skill, such that the person who is skilled in decoding what another person intends to communicate is not necessarily the same person who is skilled at decoding what a person unintentionally communicates, picturesquely referred to by Ekman and Friesen[43] as 'non-verbal leakage'.

A similar idea is to be found in the work of Rosenthal and DePaulo[21] on sex differences in the decoding of non-verbal cues. They have proposed that women are socialized to be more accommodating towards others. The accommodating person, they argue, wants to understand what others are trying to communicate; consequently, the accommodating person decodes more accurately. But Rosenthal and DePaulo also argue that skill at decoding non-verbal cues may be detrimental to satisfactory social relationships under certain circumstances, especially if the encoder unwittingly conveys information that he actually does not wish to communicate. Consequently, Rosenthal and DePaulo argue that if women's superiority in decoding non-verbal cues is due to a desire to be accommodating, they will not show such an advantage in respect of unintentional communications.

Rosenthal and DePaulo tested this hypothesis in three different ways. In one set of ten studies, they showed American adults, college students and high school students scenes of visual cues with very brief exposures, arguing that very brief signals may be less controllable by the encoder and hence carry more unintended messages. To do this, they administered a special version of the PONS using scenes of visual cues with median exposure lengths of only 250 ms. These studies showed no significant advantage for women, irrespective of age.

In a second set of studies, Rosenthal and DePaulo rank ordered non-verbal cues according to the degree to which they considered they might give off unintended information. They argued that the face gives the most information and is best controlled by the encoder. From studies of deception carried out by Ekman and Friesen[43, 44], they argued that less attention is paid to the body which may reveal more unintended information. Tone of voice, they maintained, is less controllable than cues from the face or body and hence may give information about deception or stress. Very brief exposures of the face or body may offer further unintended cues which may be more difficult to control. Finally, they maintained that discrepant messages may be the most difficult to control, because they involve simultaneous communication in two different channels which may involve problems of co-ordination. These measures of sensitivity to non-verbal cues were administered to American high school and college students, the results showing that female advantage decreased significantly with cues which were hypothesized to be more difficult to control. A re-analysis of previous studies where a comparison was possible between these different types of information showed that female decoding superiority decreases with a change from face to body to tone of voice.

Finally, in a third series of studies, Rosenthal and DePaulo arranged for American male and female college students to be videotaped while describing a person they liked, one they disliked, one about whom they were ambivalent, one to whom they were indifferent, a person they really liked as though they disliked him or her and a person they really disliked as though they liked him or her. Thus, the first two encodings were of clear affects, the second two of mixed affects and the final two of deceptive affects. Each of the encoders also acted as a decoder and their ratings of the other encoders showed that women were significantly more accurate than men for the perception of liking and disliking, but that their advantage decreased significantly and linearly with the transition from ordinary to ambivalent to deceptive cues; this would again be consistent with the accommodation hypothesis.

Subsequently, one study has examined this accommodation hypothesis from a developmental perspective, using both a cross-sectional and a longitudinal design[45]. In the cross-sectional study, they compared American pre-high school students, high school students and college students; in the longitudinal study, their subjects were American children between 11 and 14 years old. The task involved comparing performance on the PONS over four types of non-verbal cue (face, body, tone of voice and discrepant cues) ranked from the most controllable to the least controllable channel. The results of the cross-sectional study showed a significant interaction, whereby as age increased, females lost more of their advantage for the more leaky channels but gained in advantage for the less leaky channels. The results of the longitudinal study supported those of the cross-sectional study – with increasing age, females lost more of their advantage in the more leaky channels. Hence, the results are consistent with a socialization interpretation that as females grow older, they learn to be more non-verbally courteous or accommodating in the sense that they become better at perceiving what others want them to know. Alternatively, it may be the case that women do not actually become less perceptive of unintentional than intentional cues, but simply learn that it is more courteous not to openly acknowledge such information, although they may still privately be aware of its significance. It is in fact difficult to test this alternative explanation, since if women are socialized to be more accommodating, this may well extend to taking psychological tests of non-verbal perceptiveness, such that in this situation as in any other they are reluctant to acknowledge awareness of unintentional non-verbal cues.

Whichever explanation is valid, an important feature both of the work of Rosenthal and his associates and of LaRusso's work[42] on paranoid schizophrenia is that there may be different types of skill in decoding non-verbal cues: the person who is skilled at decoding what the encoder intends to communicate may not necessarily be skilled at decoding spontaneous or unintentional communications. Moreover, different decoding skills may be appropriate in different situational contexts. For example, what constitutes 'good' decoding for a detective in the police may be the ability to detect from his suspect's unintentional non-verbal communication whether the suspect is telling the truth. But for the social hostess information about deception may be positively harmful, if she wishes to be popular and attractive to her guests; it may be more socially advantageous to accept the image which people project of themselves and accommodate to it rather than to pick up the cues to deception. A total inability to accept the pretensions and deceptions of society might even be a contributory factor in the development of paranoid schizophrenia. 'Good' decoding like 'good' encoding cannot be divorced from cultural norms or situational context or from the aims and aspirations of each individual; to ignore the social context in which decoding takes place is to ignore the very factors which are essential to evaluating skill in communication.

## CONCLUSIONS

In this chapter, individual differences in non-verbal communication have been discussed with regard to the concept of communication skill. It has been argued that there are consistent and reliable individual differences in decoding non-verbal cues, which can certainly be regarded as reflecting different levels of social skill. Nevertheless, there may be different types of skill in decoding, such that the person who is good at decoding what the encoder intends to communicate may not necessarily be the same person who is good at decoding spontaneous or unintentional communications. There are also systematic individual differences in encoding: non-verbal cues encode information about individual differences such as sex-role attitudes or psychopathology, while individuals also differ in expressiveness, in the degree to which they encode information through non-verbal cues. Encoding too can be regarded as a skill, but what constitutes good encoding cannot be divorced from cultural norms or situational context or indeed from the aims and aspirations of each particular individual. In fact, in a very real sense the concept of communication skill is underpinned by individual differences, since behaviour which may be highly appropriate and skilful for one individual may be totally inappropriate and unskilful for another; it all depends upon what each individual intends to achieve. Any comprehensive theory of non-verbal communication must be able to encompass individual differences; similarly, individual differences are central to the concept of communication skill. To demonstrate the interrelationship of these factors has been the purpose of this chapter.

## References

1. Wiener, M., Devoe, S., Robinson, S. and Geller, J. (1972). Non-verbal behaviour and non-verbal communication. *Psychol. Rev.*, **79**, 185–214
2. Argyle, M. and Kendon, A. (1967). The experimental analysis of social performance. In Berkowitz, L. (ed.) *Advances in Experimental Social Psychology*, Vol. 3, pp. 55–98. (New York: Academic Press)

3.  Jones, H. E. (1960). The longitudinal method in the study of personality. In Iscoe, I. and Stevenson, H. W. (eds.) *Personality Development in Children.* pp. 3–27. (Chicago: University of Chicago Press)

4.  Freud, S. (1946/1921). Instincts and their vicissitudes. In *Collected Papers.* Vol. 4. (London: Hogarth Press, 1946; originally published, 1921)

5.  Lanzetta, J. T. and Kleck, R. E. (1970). Encoding and decoding of non-verbal affect in humans. *J. Pers. Soc. Psychol.,* **16**, 12–19

6.  Buck, R. W., Savin, V. J., Miller, R. E. and Caul, W. F. (1972). Communication of affect through facial expressions in humans. *J. Pers. Soc. Psychol.,* **23**, 362–71

7.  Buck, R. W. (1977). Non-verbal communication of affect in pre-school children: relationships with personality and skin conductance. *J. Pers. Soc. Psychol.,* **35**, 225–36

8.  Notarius, C. I. and Levenson, R. W. (1979). Expressive tendencies and physiological response to stress. *J. Pers. Soc. Psychol.,* **37**, 1204–10

9.  Hall, J. A. (1979). Gender, gender roles and non-verbal communication skills. In Rosenthal, R. (ed.) *Skill in Non-verbal Communication: Individual Differences,* pp. 32–67. (Cambridge, Massachusetts: Oelgeschlager, Gunn and Hain)

10. Cohen, J. (1977). *Statistical Power Analysis for the Behavioural Sciences.* Rev. Edn. (New York: Academic Press)

11. Winkelmayer, R., Exline, R. V., Gottheil, E. and Paredes, A. (1978). The relative accuracy of U.S., British and Mexican raters in judging the emotional displays of schizophrenic and normal U.S. women. *J. Clin. Psychol.,* **34**, 600–8

12. Bleuler, E. (1950). *Dementia Praecox or the Group of Schizophrenias.* Trans. Tinkin, J. (New York: International Universities Press)

13. Shimoda, K., Argyle, M. and Bitti, P. R. (1978). The intercultural recognition of emotional expression by three national racial groups: English, Italian and Japanese. *Eur. J. Soc. P-sychol.,* **8**, 169–79

14. Bull, P. (1983). *Body Movement and Interpersonal Communication.* pp. 79–87. (Chichester: Wiley)

15. Exline, R. V. (1972). Visual interaction: the glances of power and preference. In *Nebraska Symposium on Motivation.* pp. 163–206. (Lincoln: University of Nebraska Press)

16. Duncan, S. and Fiske, D. W. (1977). *Face-to-face Interaction: Research, Methods and Theory.* (Hillsdale, NJ: Lawrence Erlbaum)

17. Giesen, M. and McClaren, H. A. (1976). Discussion, distance and sex: changes in impressions and attraction during small group interaction. *Sociometry,* **39**, 60–70

18. Rekers, G., Amaro-Plotkin, H. D. and Low, B. P. (1977). Sex-typed mannerisms in normal boys and girls as a function of sex and age. *Child Dev.,* **48**, 275–8

19. Rekers, G. A. and Rudy, J. P. (1978). Differentiation of childhood body gestures. *Percept. Mot. Skill,* **46**, 839–45

20. Frieze, I. H. and Ramsey, S. J. (1976). Non-verbal maintenance of traditional sex roles. *J. Soc. Issue.,* **32**, 133–41

21. Rosenthal, R. and DePaulo, B. M. (1979). Sex differences in accommodation in non-verbal communication. In Rosenthal, R. (ed.) *Skill in Non-verbal Communication: Individual Differences.* pp. 68–103. (Cambridge, Massachusetts: Oelgeschlager, Gunn and Hain)

22. Lippa, R. (1978). The naive perception of masculinity–femininity on the basis of expressive cues. *J. Res. Pers.,* **12**, 1–14

23. Bem, S. (1974). The measurement of psychological androgyny. *J. Consult. Clin. Psychol.,* **42**, 155–62

24. Waxer, P. H. (1977). Non-verbal cues for anxiety: an examination of emotional leakage. *J. Abnorm. Psychol,,* **86**, 306–14

25. Waxer, P. H. (1976). Non-verbal cues for depth of depression: set versus no set. *J. Consult. Clin. Psychol.,* **44**, 493

26. Waxer, P. H. (1974). Non-verbal cues for depression. *J. Abnorm. Psychol.,* **88**, 319–22

27. Hutt, C. and Ounsted, C. (1970). Gaze aversion and its significance in childhood autism. In Hutt, S. J. and Hutt, C. (eds.) *Behaviour Studies in Psychiatry.* pp. 103–20. (Exeter: Pergamon)

28. Clancy, H. and McBride, G. (1969). The autistic process and its treatment. *J. Child Psychol. Psychiatry,* **10**, 233–44

29. Rutter, D. R. (1978). Visual interaction in schizophrenic patients: the timing of looks. *Br. J. Soc. Clin. Psychol.*, **17**, 281–2
30. Kinzel, A. F. (1970). Body-buffer zone in violent prisoners. *Am. J. Psychiatry*, **127**, 59–64
31. Newman, R. C. and Pollack, D. (1973). Proxemics in deviant adolescents. *J. Consult. Clin. Psychol.*, **40**, 6–8
32. Beck, S. J. and Ollendick, T. H. (1976). Personal space, sex of experimenter, and locus of control in normal and delinquent adolescents. *Psychol. Rep.*, **38**, 383–7
33. Trower, P., Bryant, B. and Argyle, M. (1978). *Social Skills and Mental Health*. (London: Methuen)
34. Edelstein, B. A. and Eisler, R. M. (1976). Effects of modelling and modelling with instructions and feedback on the behavioural components of social skills. *Behav Ther.*, **7**, 382–9
35. Bull, P. (1984). The communication of emotion. Presented at the *Annual Conference of the British Psychological Society*, March 30–April 2, University of Warwick
36. Hinchcliffe, M. K., Lancashire, M. and Roberts, F. J. (1971). A study of eye-contact changes in depressed and recovered psychiatric patients. *Br. J. Psychiatry*, **119**, 213–15
37. Ekman, P. and Friesen, W. V. (1974). Non-verbal behaviour and psychopathology. In Friedman, R. J. and Katz, M. M. (eds.) *The Psychology of Depression: Contemporary Theory and Research*. pp. 203–32. (New York: Wiley)
38. Fisch, H.-U., Frey, S. and Hirsbrunner, H.-P. (1981). Analyzing non-verbal behaviour in depression. *J. Abnorm. Psychol.*, **92**, 307–18
39. Ranelli, C. J. and Miller, R. E. (1981). Behavioural predictors of amitriptyline response in depression. *Am. J. Psychiatry*, **138**, 30–4
40. Rosenthal, R., Hall, J. A., DiMatteo, M. R., Rogers, P. L. and Archer, D. (1979). *Sensitivity to Non-verbal Communication: The PONS Test*. (Baltimore: Johns Hopkins University Press)
41. Argyle, M. (1969). *Social Interaction*. (London: Methuen)
42. LaRusso, L. (1978). Sensitivity of paranoid patients to non-verbal cues. *J. Abnorm. Psychol.*, **87**, 463–71
43. Ekman, P. and Friesen, W. V. (1969). Non-verbal leakage and clues to deception. *Psychiatry*, **32**, 88–106
44. Ekman, P. and Friesen, W. V. (1974). Detecting deception from the body or face. *J. Pers. Soc. Psychol.*, **29**, 288–98
45. Blanck, P. D., Rosenthal, R., Snodgrass, S. E., DePaulo, B. M. and Zuckerman, M. (1981). Sex differences in eavesdropping on non-verbal cues: developmental changes. *J. Pers. Soc. Psychol.*, **41**, 391–6

# 12
## Movement and the personal style

*James J. Conley*

## INTRODUCTION

The experimenter measures the *what* of the product, but not the *how*. What is measured is the content of the response. The content is, of course, revealing, but so, too, are the expressive movements that go to waste. Emphasizing the *Geist*, psychologists are blind to the *Seele* as reflected in postures, handwriting, eye movements, voice, and even doodles[1].

Gordon Allport advocated a stylistic analysis that would integrate individual differences in movement with other aspects of the personality. Although this stylistic analysis had a very exciting beginning, it was never followed through. In 1933, Allport and Philip Vernon published an ambitious study relating personality theory and expressive movement[2]. Neither of the authors returned to empirical studies of movement, however, and their psychological colleagues did not actively pursue their discoveries. *Studies in Expressive Movement* became one of those classics that is admired but not emulated. As such, it represents one of the great missed opportunities of twentieth century psychology.

Individual differences in movement have, of course, been the object of many studies. Although out of favour for many years, there are signs that an analysis of individual differences in movement is once again coming into vogue[3,4]. The great majority of the studies relating personality and movement relate to temperamental aspects of personality such as neuroticism, social extraversion and impulse control. While these temperamental relationships are quite important, the analysis of personal styles is an even more appropriate vehicle for the study of certain aspects of human movement. The personal style is independent of the major dimensions of temperament and represents a different domain of personality phenomena[5].

History is an unfinished book and missed opportunities are often taken up in later times when conditions are more favourable. The study of human movement as an expression of personal style is a perspective that seems ripe for development. In the last two decades, there has been rapid progress in scientific studies of movement as well as some important innovations in personality

247

psychology (in particular, the restoration of a somatic basis for personality differences, the maturation of longitudinal studies, and the growing appreciation of the importance of data aggregation). An integration of personality studies and movement studies at both the theoretical and empirical levels may now be possible.

This chapter returns to the original work of Allport and Vernon on personal styles and expressive movement and examines the theory and the data they developed. Allport and Vernon left the analyses of both personal styles and expressive movement in a rather undeveloped condition and the relationships between movement and the other aspects of personal style were only roughly sketched. This chapter clarifies the general theory of personal styles, summarizes and reinterprets the work of Allport and Vernon on expressive movement, and suggests a number of new directions for research that would link individual differences in movement with a fascinating array of stylistic differences in other domains of human experience and behaviour.

## THE THEORY OF PERSONAL STYLES

The analysis of personal styles is derived from Dilthey's theory of worldviews[6]. Dilthey distinguished the worldviews of naturalism, objective idealism, and the idealism of freedom. Dilthey believed that the worldview acted as 'the foundation for a full valuation of life and for a comprehension of the world'. Spranger extended Dilthey's analysis into a theory of lifestyles or dominant personal values[7]. He identified six major styles: theoretical, economic, aesthetic, social, political, and religious. According to Spranger, these six represent ideal types of evaluative perspectives which are brought to bear in all aspects of perception and judgement. Allport and Vernon developed the Study of Values as a measure of Spranger's six styles. Later studies demonstrated that the types measured by the Study of Values can be adequately summarized by two dimensions[5,8]. The subjective–objective dimension contrasts the aesthetic with the economic and political values. The critical–acceptant dimension contrasts the theoretical and religious values. (The measurement of the social value presented such serious problems of reliability and validity that Allport recommended that this scale not be used in regular research[9].) These two dimensions are very similar to the ideational–professional and challenger–upholder dimensions identified by Helson in her study of the styles employed in literary criticism[10].

The subjective–objective and critical–acceptant dimensions define the four quadrants of personal styles: objective–acceptant, objective–critical, subjective–critical and subjective–acceptant. The effects of these personal styles permeate many areas of experience and behaviour, including personal preferences, types of fantasies, political and social attitudes, and vocational interests[11,12]. Figures 12.1 and 12.2 depict the patterns of occupational interest and personal preferences associated with the various personal styles. The data are drawn from the Kelly Longitudinal Study. The objective–acceptant style is rather conventional in nature. It is associated with religious and familial

248

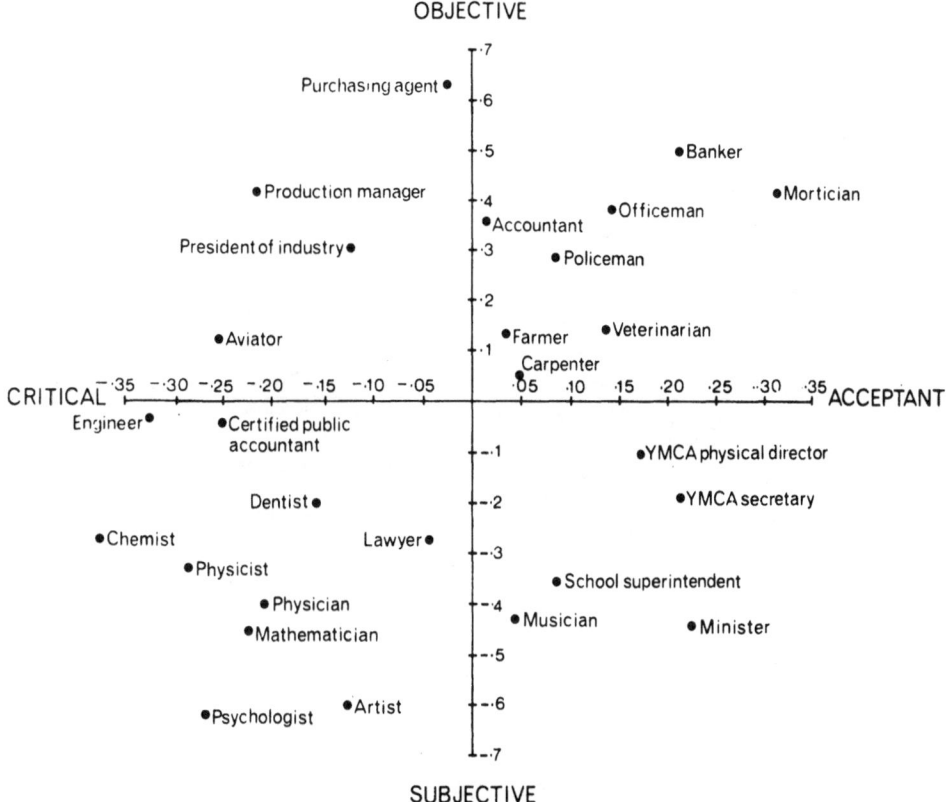

*Figure 12.1 Pearson product–moment correlations between scales of the Strong Vocational Interest Blank and the subjective–objective and critical–acceptant dimensions derived from the Allport–Vernon Study of Values*

preferences and interests in such occupations as banker, mortician, office worker, accountant, and policeman. The objective–critical style is related to strongminded preferences and interests in such occupations as production manager, president of an industrial concern and aviator. The subjective–critical style is associated with unconventional and culturally sophisticated preferences and interests in scientific, academic and artistic occupations. Lastly, the subjective–acceptant style is related to sensitive and compassionate preferences and interests in public service occupations.

An individual's personal style tends to be quite consistent over long periods of time. In the data of the Kelly Longitudinal Study the stability correlations of the dimensions of personal style were approximately 0.6 for a period of 19 years and 0.4 for a period of 45 years[5]. Given the pervasive influence of personal styles and their relative stability, it is reasonable to expect that they might be manifested on a physical level in movements as well as on the cognitive and emotional levels. Such an extension of the theory of personal styles requires the

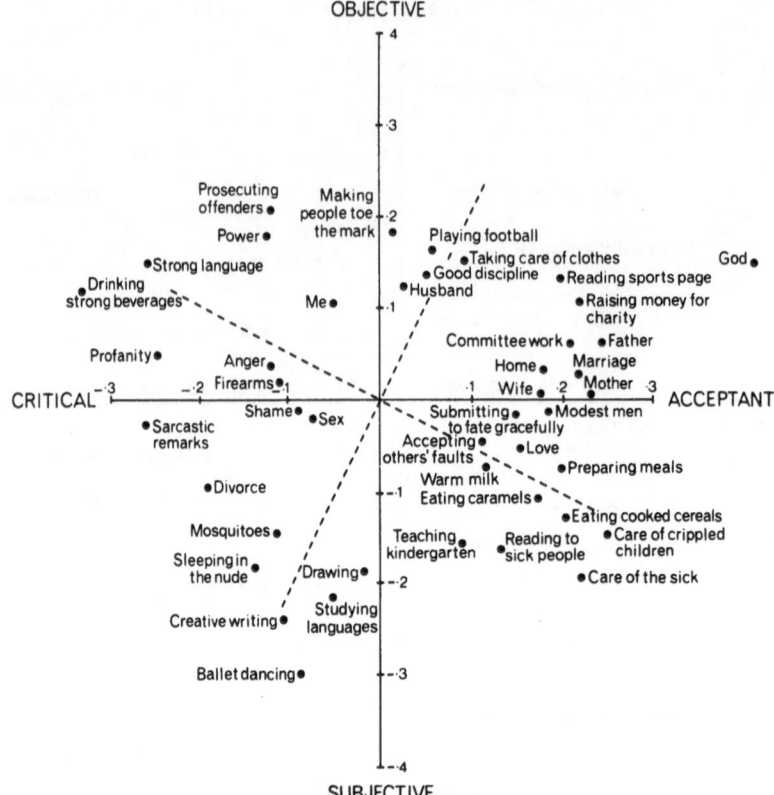

*Figure 12.2   Pearson product–moment correlations of evaluations of items from the Krout Personal Preference Inventory and the Semantic Differential with the subjective-objective and critical-acceptant dimensions derived from the Allport–Vernon Study of Values*

identification of the important parameters of movement so that they can be related to other aspects of the personal style. These parameters were identified by Allport and Vernon in their *Studies in Expressive Movement*.

## ALLPORT AND VERNON ON EXPRESSIVE MOVEMENT

Allport and Vernon summarized their interest in expressive movement very suc-cir-ctly: 'Our study of expressive movement is concerned with *individual differences in the manner of performing adaptive acts, considered as dependent less upon external and temporary conditions than upon enduring qualities of personality*' (italics in the original). Allport and Vernon employed several measures of movement and the individual differences in these measures defined three major factors: areal, centrifugal and emphatic. The areal factor included measures of the total space covered in expressive movement. The authors

250

*Table 12.1   Characteristics associated with the quadrants described by the centrifugal and emphatic group factors*

| Emphatic | Centrifugal |
|---|---|
| Intensity of voice | Overestimation of distance away from body (using legs) |
| Few parallel lines drawn in fixed space | Overestimation of distances away from body (using hands) |
| Much movement while speaking | |
| Strong pressure of handwriting | Binet cubes spaced over large area |
| Overestimation of weights | Underestimation of weights |
| Strong finger pressure on stylus | |
| Strong tapping pressure | |
| Underestimation of distance between hands | |
| | |
| Centripetal | Unemphatic |
| Underestimation of distances away from body (using legs) | Lack of voice intensity |
| Underestimation of distances away from body (using hands) | Many parallel lines drawn in fixed space |
| | Little movement while speaking |
| Binet cubes spaced over small area | Weak pressure of handwriting |
| Overestimation of weights | Underestimation of weights |
| | Weak finger pressure on stylus |
| | Weak tapping pressure |
| | Overestimation of distances between hands |

describe it as an 'expansive' motor tendency. The centrifugal factor covered tasks that involved movement away from the body. It was interpreted as a 'general outward tendency' in expressive movement. The emphatic factor included tasks that measured pressure, intensity, forcefulness and 'strong control'. The centrifugal and emphatic factors are of most interest to us because of their probable relationship with the personal styles. Table 12.1 describes the variables most strongly related to these two factors. Only variables with loadings of 0.4 or higher are listed in the table. The associations among the various aspects of movement suggested to Allport and Vernon that they were held together by psychological similarities.

'The discovery of such motor factors or "traits" in our population of subjects suggests that psychological and not physical categories are fundamental in the study of movement. *Emphasis*, for example, partakes to be sure, of the physical movements of pressure, but it involves other tendencies, such as the disposition to fill only a small part of the space at one's disposal in writing.'

Allport and Vernon did not commit themselves to a specific theory linking the factors of movement with personality measures, repeatedly arguing that such was 'beyond the scope of this inquiry'. It seems clear, however, that the centrifugal type of movement corresponds with the objective–acceptant personal style, the emphatic type of movement with the objective–critical style, the centripetal type of movement with the subjective–critical style and the subjective–acceptant type of movement with the unemphatic style. Table 12.2 gives the central portions of the descriptions provided by Allport and Vernon for

251

Table 12.2    *Allport and Vernon's case studies of psychomotor congruence*

| | |
|---|---|
| *Emphatic*<br>Subject no. 1<br>'Gives the impression of being vigorous, brisk but pleasant, efficient and "go-getting".' | *Centrifugal*<br>Subject no. 3<br>'This youth might be characterized in a single "reduced term", by saying that he habitually *oversteps*.' |
| *Centripetal*<br>Subject no. 2<br>'He is exceedingly animated, talkative, and given to gesticulation. His interests are almost exclusively aesthetic.' | *Unemphatic*<br>Subject no. 4<br>'The subject is in no way striking or gifted, not distinguished in appearance, manner or talent. He has an agreeable submissive nature.' |

the four case studies that they reported in substantial detail. This analysis of 'psychomotor congruence' is the closest Allport and Vernon come to relating the movement factors to personality characteristics. These four cases 'selected for their diversity' were, in fact, extreme examples of the quadrants portrayed in 12.1 and 12.2. The personological descriptions in Table 12.2 correspond nicely with the respective patterns of preferences and interests displayed in Figures 12.1 and 12.2. The only major disjunction involves Subject no. 3 who is seen as habitually 'overstepping' himself. This seems at first contrary to the conventional orientation of the objective–acceptant style. This subject, however, overstepped because of his ardent devotion to conventional goals for himself.

The objective–acceptant style is thus associated not only with conventional preferences/interests but with a centrifugal type of movement. This type of movement entails a certain awkwardness or lack of sophistication. There is a 'rawness' in the way the individual moves. The opposing style, the subjective–critical, is associated with unconventional and sophisticated preferences/interests as well as a type of movement involving small, 'refined' gestures and actions. The objective–critical style involves both strongminded and ambitious preferences/interests and a type of movement that is very forceful and definite. The opposite style, the subjective–acceptant, involves sensitive and compassionate preferences/interests and movement that is unemphatic and relaxed. These are the intuitive connections between types of expressive movement and other aspects of personal styles that underlie Allport and Vernon's discussion of their findings. These connections seem quite reasonable in light of the contemporary work on personal styles.

## OTHER STUDIES OF EXPRESSIVE MOVEMENT

Only two studies attempted to replicate the Allport and Vernon findings on expressive movement. One of these studies[13] used only a portion of the tests employed by Allport and Vernon. This study replicated the retest reliabilities of the original study but was unable to confirm or disconfirm the existence of the factors identified by Allport and Vernon. The other study[14] confirmed the existence of areal, centrifugal and emphatic factors with essentially the same pattern of loadings reported by Allport and Vernon.

An interesting but inconclusive line of research on expressive movement was carried out by Werner Wolff[15, 16] during the 1930s and 1940s. Wolff used a variety of matching techniques and demonstrated that people are able to link various aspects of individuals' external appearances and movements (face, profile, hands, voice, gait, handwriting, bodily rhythms) at levels far above chance expectations. As a demonstration of personality as a diffuse entity that 'penetrates the whole organism', Wolff's work is a *tour de force* and it can be used as a source for ideas about the kinds of phenomena that should be investigated in an individual differences analysis of movement. Unfortunately, Wolff resisted multivariate statistical analysis and never posited coherent structural theories of either expressive movement or the larger realm of personality. When Wolff moved on to other topics in the later 1940s, the personological study of expressive movement ceased to be a major concern in mainstream psychology. Especially in North America, the field of personality psychology was moving in very different directions after the Second World War. Expressive movement and personal styles were lost in enthusiasm for self-report inventories, social psychological experimentation and research on the authoritarian personality.

## MOVEMENT IN RELATION TO OTHER ASPECTS OF PERSONAL STYLE

Personal styles have been described in many different ways by various observers and an extraordinary array of correlates have accumulated over the years. Two recent stylistic paradigms are openness to experience[17] and Type A behaviour[18]. Openness to experience is essentially the subjective–critical style and as such is associated with the centripetal type of movement. Type A behaviour is essentially the objective–critical style and as such is associated with the emphatic type of movement. Voice quality is an especially strong correlate of the latter style. The loudness and tension in the voice were leading markers for the emphatic movement type in the Allport and Vernon study. A study conducted a few years later found that listeners could distinguish the subjective–objective personal style of target individuals on the basis of their voice quality[19]. A recent study found that voice volume and duration of vocalization were highly correlated with the Type A behaviour pattern[20]. The tension and emphasis of this type are thus manifested in the voice as well as in movement of the major muscles.

The Allport–Vernon Study of Values can serve as a key that relates many aspects of behaviour and experience to the types of movement. Especially important in this regard is some of the work of the 'New Look' psychologists. The scales of the Allport–Vernon Study of Values were shown to be related to the recognition thresholds of words[21–23]. For instance, persons with high scores on the political scale had low recognition thresholds for words such as 'govern', 'famous' and 'compete', while persons with high scores on the theoretical scale had low recognition thresholds for words such as 'verify', 'science' and 'logical'. Despite the replication of these findings, these studies have been neglected for almost 30 years. They are quite important to the theory of personal style both as an assessment methodology and as an avenue for explanatory research. In other experimental psychological studies, the scales of the Allport-Vernon Study of Values have been related to the concept span, facility of associations and graphological characteristics[24-27]. Personal styles have substantial relationships with individual differences in perceptual and memory processes. This opens up the possibility of relating them to individual differences in movement.

## THE STUDY OF MOVEMENT IN A REVITALIZED PERSONALITY PSYCHOLOGY

During the 1960s and the early 1970s, personality psychology (particularly in North America) underwent a severe crisis of confidence. Looking back on this period, we can identify five major factors that contributed to the confused and demoralized state of the field.

(1) Reliance on self-report measures. Although self-report is part of a general personality assessment, excessive reliance on this technique led to the vexed issues of response biases, implicit personality theories and self-concept interpretations of personality data.

(2) Univariate miniparadigms. The field was fractured into a multitude of literatures on individual dimensions or aspects of personality. Many of these were redundant and/or poorly conceptualized.

(3) Overuse of social explanation and social psychological experimental techniques. A generation of personality psychologists was trained to look only for social causes of personality differences and to assess these differences far from natural settings.

(4) Non-temporal research designs. Although personality was assumed to be temporally stable and to exert a formative influence over time, few powerful demonstrations of these phenomena were available.

(5) Use of inadequate samples of indicators. Self-report scales, behavioural observations and performance measures were usually correlated on a one-to-one basis and the resulting correlational patterns were vitiated and confusing.

Fortunately, recent years have seen shifts toward multimethod assessment and data aggregation, the maturation of several important longitudinal studies, the revival of temperamental and behaviour genetic perspectives, and an emerging consensus on the overall structure of personality. There has been a gradual revitalization of the entire field and the study of individual differences in movement has an important role to play in this exciting period. Movement studies can help to restore the naturalistic and somatic bases of personality psychology and they represent an important addition to multimethod assessment. The discovery of properly aggregated movement correlates of personality constructs will constitute a powerful argument for the validity and importance of the constructs.

Movement studies are much more sophisticated today than they were in the 1930s. There have been impressive advances in measurement, recording and simulation techniques. If these techniques can now be applied to a stylistic analysis of individual differences, the promise of the Allport and Vernon study can begin to be fulfilled. Charting the relationships among types of movement and other aspects of the personal style has the potential of bringing together movement studies and personality psychology at a time when both fields are in very exciting stages of development.

## References

1. Allport, G. W. (1961). *Pattern and Growth in Personality*. (New York: Holt, Rinehart and Winston)
2. Allport, G. W. and Vernon, P. E. (1933). *Studies in Expressive Movement*. (New York: Macmillan)
3. Tucker, L. A. (1983). Obesity, exercise, semato type, and psychological well-being: a factor analytic study. *J. Hum. Movement Stud.*, 9, 125–33
4. Tucker, L. A. (1984). Trait psychology and performance: a credulous viewpoint. *J. Hum. Movement Stud.*, 10, 53–62
5. Conley, J. J. (1984). Personal styles: their structure and longitudinal stability across the adult life span. Unpublished manuscript, Wesleyan University
6. Dilthey, W. (1957). In Kluback, W. and Weinbaum, M. (eds.) *Philosophy of Existence*. (New York: Bookman)
7. Spranger, E. (1928). *Types of Men*. (Halle, Germany: Max Niemeyer Verlag)
8. Stewart, L. H. (1964). Change in personality test scores during college. *J. Counsel. Psychol.*, 11, 211–20
9. Cantril, H. and Allport, G. W. (1933). Recent applications of the Study of Values. *J. Abnorm. Soc. Psychol.*, 28, 259–73
10. Helson, R. (1982). Critics and their texts: an approach to Jung's theory of cognition and personality. *J. Pers. Soc. Psychol.*, 43, 409–18
11. Conley, J. J. (1985). Personal styles as formative influences in adulthood and aging. Unpublished manuscript, Wesleyan University
12. Conley, J. J. and Fox, A. E. (1985). Personal styles as an integrative structural theory of the nontemperamental domain of personality. Unpublished manuscript, Wesleyan University
13. Eisenberg, P. A. (1937). A further study in expressive movement. *Character Pers.*, 5, 396–401
14. Carlson, W. S. (1938). Further studies in expressive movement. *Psychol. Rec.*, 2, 310–16
15. Wolff, W. (1943). *The Expression of Personality: Experimental Depth Psychology*. (New York: Harper)
16. Wolff, W. (1947). *The Personality of the Preschool Child*. (New York: Grune & Stratton)
17. Macrae, R. R. and Costa, P. T. (1985). Openness to experience. In Hogan, R. and Jones, W. H. (eds.) *Perspectives in Personality: Theory, Measurement and Interpersonal Dynamics*. (Greenwich, CT: JAI Press)
18. Friedman, M. and Rosenman, R. H. (1974). *Type A Behavior and Your Heart*. (New York: Alfred A. Knopf)
19. Fay, P. J. and Middleton, W. C. (1940). Judgment of Spranger personality types from the voice as transmitted over a public address system. *Character Pers.*, 8, 144–55
20. Howland, E. W. and Seigman, A. W. (1982). Toward an automated measurement of the Type A behavior pattern. *J. Behav. Med.*, 5, 37–54.

21. Postman, L., Bruner, J. S. and McGinnies, E. (1948). Personal values as selective factors in perception. *J. Abnorm. Soc. Psychol.*, **43**, 142–54
22. Postman, L. and Schneider, B. H. (1951). Personal values, visual recognition, and recall. *Psychol. Rev.*, **58**, 271–84
23. Haigh, G. O. and Fiske, D. W. (1952). Corroboration of personal values as selective factors in perception. *J. Abnorm. Soc. Psychol.*, **47**, 394–8.
24. Mayzner, M. S. and Tressett, M. E. (1955). Concept span as a composite function of personal values, anxiety and rigidity. *J. Pers.*, **24**, 20–33
25. Cantril, H. (1932). General and specific attitudes. *Psychol. Monogr.*, **17**, Whole No. 192
26. Dunn, S., Bliss, J. and Siipola, E. (1958). Effects of impulsivity, introversion, and individual values upon association under free conditions. *J. Pers.*, **26**, 61–76
27. Cantril, H. and Rand, H. A. (1935). An additional study of the determination of personal interests by psychological and graphological methods. *Character Pers.*, **3**, 72–8

# 13

## The value of traits in sport

### *Bruce D. Kirkcaldy*

---

## INTRODUCTION

The abundance of studies performed in sport psychology research bears witness to the appeal of the topic. On closer examination, however, it becomes obvious that its appearance is distorted by a profusion of incoherent and undifferentiated results. Consequently, a schism between the advocates and opponents of trait theory has arisen which resembles that observed between personality theorists and experimental psychologists[1]. A large part of the literature on personality and sport is characterized by studies of an 'unacceptably low scientific standard'[2]. The deficiencies include secondary source errors, failure to consider response distortion, inferior statistical analysis, implementation of diverse (often unreliable) measuring instruments, neglect of moderator variables, lack of operationalization of concepts and atheoretical enquiry.

## GENERAL FINDINGS

Despite some inconsistencies, a certain degree of generalization can be tentatively proposed[1, 2]. For instance, extraversion–introversion (E) emerges as a trait associated with an *interest* in sport participation. This extraverted temperament is common to both male and female athletes[3]. There is no indication that E is able to distinguish elite from average athletes[4-6]. Introverted athletes are inclined to gravitate towards individual as opposed to team-oriented physical activities, although the evidence here is less convincing: it seems that introverts select particular variations of a sport, e.g. long-distance running rather than sprinting or other power disciplines[7, 8], in addition to adopting a different playing strategy to extraverts, the latter sacrificing accuracy for greater speed[9, 10].

The implication of E with sport fits in well with the description of the extravert as active and vigorous, relishing the demands of strenuous activity and exercise. They are impulsive and pursue varied interests as a means of satiating their *stimulus hunger*. They prefer being with others rather than alone, enjoying participation in parties and other social gatherings.

Toughmindedness appears to provide the *propulsion* necessary for success in competitive sport[2, 6, 11]. The primary constituents of this higher order trait include aggressiveness, achievement motivation, assertiveness, masculinity, sensation-seeking, manipulation and dogmatism[12]. These are attributes which appear congruent with competitive sport. The scale represents the antithesis of rigid, rule-bound behaviour and there is evidence that an excess of tough-mindedness may be debilitating for certain types of sport. In team sports it may be an undesirable trait since it implies uncooperativeness, which may explain why its obverse, 'social conformity' (lie-scale), is occasionally found to be high in disciplined group sports[13, 14]. Male and female athletes display elevated toughmindedness scores compared to the population norm, but a sex difference persists (sportsmen having markedly higher scores[6]) so that 'sex differences in aggressiveness appear to be part of a wider pattern of sex differences in the propensity to engage in competitive social interaction[15]'.

Emotionally less stable persons tend to avoid competitive situations[16]. Outstanding athletes are characterized by a less neurotic profile[1-3, 17]. This emotional stability provides a certain degree of *immunity* to the stress of competition (a feature shared with toughmindedness). Emotionality declines with age so that younger athletes will appear less stable in relation to veteran athletes. Offensive players are frequently amongst the most emotional of all athletes. There is some indication that outstanding sportswomen are more stable than their male counterparts.[6]

The personality dimension emotionality comprises the traits anxiety, depressiveness, obsessiveness, dependence, inferiority feelings, hypochon-driasis and guilt[12]. Persons high on this higher order trait are inclined to worry about the possibility of failure, a concern which is likely to distract them from the task-relevant aspects of their performance.

Trait-sceptical Position

Mummendey[18] has emphasized the diametrically divergent conclusions which characterize studies in the area of sport and personality as evidence that traits have little relevance to sport. In so doing, he inadmissibly aggregates a vast array of studies with a disregard to the *quality* of research. He employs a method of dichotomizing studies in terms of those favourable and those opposing trait relevancy in sport. Such absolute distinctions are meaningless since, 'If one good, carefully designed research study based on reasonable theoretical predictions gives a consistency of 0.80, this is not negated because another scruffy, poorly designed study based on no theoretical foundations gives a consistency of 0.0![19]' Sack[20] performs an equally meaningless evaluation of the literature in that he continually collapses results across scales, 'in a total of 27 investigations, on average 12% of the scales produced statistically significant differences.' It ought to be clear that secondary analyses can be self-defeating exercises, contaminated by *errors of selection* and cumulative errors of transmission. A critical stance is necessary when examining secondary sources and this means examining the reliability and validity of the tests used, nature of the sample employed, theoretical framework, etc.

## METHODOLOGICAL AND STATISTICAL ISSUES

### Response Distortion

There are many personality inventories which do not include a lie-scale (L) (incorporated to assess response distortion) such as forms A and B of Cattell's 16PF which have frequently been implemented in sport studies. In instances where the scale has been available, there has been a tendency to neglect it. It is a valuable scale for determining the exclusion of those persons who are inclined to dissimulate, that is, respond deceptively.

There are some conditions in which individuals may feel motivated to present more positive self-images. This susceptibility to faking can be demonstrated when subjects are requested to produce desirable or undesirable responses. For instance, completion of a personality test in a positive direction produces lower neuroticism (N) scores. The fact that this does not occur under ordinary conditions of testing supports the notion that people are generally honest in their completion of such questionnaires. This is augmented by the finding that the major dimensions E and N do not change significantly when persons are allowed to fill in the inventory in anonymity. Furthermore, when ratings are obtained from relatives, colleagues and friends, these are in good agreement with the profile description obtained on the basis of the test[21].

Nitsch and Allmer[22] criticized the use of traditional trait questionnaires in sport since the items which are deemed to measure neuroticism incorporate subjective reports such as 'frequent sweating', 'accelerated heart rate', etc., responses which are typical for the situational demands commonly confronted by the athlete. If this was indeed the case, the athlete ought to exhibit an emotionally less stable profile. This is not so. One of the most consistent findings is that of emotional stability amongst athletes.

Mummendey has claimed that inconsistencies are the rule in sport personality studies. Furthermore, he felt that scales of E and N are saturated with items which serve excellently as Social Desirability questions. Content analyses of these items reveal that they relate to predominantly illness-oriented concepts such as tremor, sickness and sleepiness, symptoms which are not consistent with the idea of 'sport as healthy'. As a result, athletes will adopt an 'impression management strategy', displaying the stable extravert profile beneficial for selection. It is surprising that athletes should modify their responses in the direction of a hypothetical norm when Mummendey's initial contention was that there did not exist any coherent differences on the basis of his secondary analysis[23]. Furthermore, it is interesting that both critics of trait research in sport themselves arrive at divergent conclusions as to the athletic profile!

In the same discussion article, Simons suggested that there will be a strong desire to obtain recognition and therefore produce a more positive self-image in such situations as competitive sport so it is not surprising that '. . . successful athletes will be inclined to display higher scores on social conformity (EPI)'. In contradiction, he claims that desirable responding may equally well be coupled with deflated L-scores since honesty and willingness to admit small weaknesses are themselves positive characteristics. In a study involving 192 Olympic athletes compared to 500 male non-athletes[2], the sportsmen in addition to having low N and high E and P scores were characterized by *low* L-scores. In a large sample of West German athletes[6], there was no evidence of dissimulation as indexed by the intercorrelation between N and L-scales. Furthermore, the correlation between E and L was towards the lower end of the scale[24] indicating a distinct lack of response distortion. The scales P (psychoticism, alternatively labelled toughmindedness) and L were, however, significantly negatively correlated, so that the elevated P scores typical of athletes would have been even higher after correction.

## Size of Effect

It has been claimed that even when consistent differences are found between athletes and non-athletes, successful and less successful, individual and team-oriented athletes, etc., the magnitudes of these effects are too small for adequately describing, explaining or predicting behaviour. Kroll[25] had considered that researchers using traditional trait inventories have been fishing for minnows with a nomological net designed for whales. An equally sceptical evaluation of the implementation of broad, enduring behaviour dispositional concepts which produce personality coefficients rarely exceeding $+0.30$ has been expressed by Fisher[26], so that '. . . to embark on a research strategy knowing you are so limited is tantamount to committing experimenter suicide.' The fact that individuals adapt their behaviour according to the specific demands of the situation is used as evidence against the trait model of personality.

A distinction must be made between a statistically *significant* finding (referring to a relatively rare event, which in itself does not imply a large or meaningful effect) and the *strength of association*[27]. Equivalent levels of significance may correspond to quite different magnitudes of experimental effect. If a sufficiently large sample is used, small differences, which may be trivial for predictive purposes, may nevertheless yield significant results. One of several indices which can be used for estimating the magnitude of an experimental effect is Hay's *omega squared ratio*. It is the proportion of the total variance which is accounted for by the independent variables.

Simons[23], unconvinced that differences observed in the personality profiles of athletes and non-athletes were of any practical value, estimated omega squared for the data from Eysenck, Nias and Cox's study[2] which had reported highly significant results on all three major personality dimensions. The traits accounted for a negligible proportion of the total variance (P, 6%; E, 4%; N, 1%). The higher order personality traits P, E and N are, however, independent so that the additive effects of all three will be in excess of 10%.

In a study reported by Sack[23] involving 364 track and field athletes, including 120 of the best young West German athletes, the group was found to be significantly less depressive and less excitable, enthusiastic, calm and self-reliant compared to non-athletes. The percentage of the variance attributable to personality variables was between 0 and 8%, a finding which appears damaging to the adoption of a trait model of personality in sport. On this occasion, a reduced version of the Freiburg Personality Inventory had been used (eight scales incorporating seven items per scale) in which the scales were interrelated. Furthermore, the abbreviated version did not contain a scale for assessing dissimulation. Another weakness in this instrument was the absence of a higher order scale corresponding to toughmindedness (which is present in the original FPI). His estimate of omega squared cannot, therefore, be taken as a serious challenge to the trait model.

The omega squared ratio is popularly used as an index of 'transituational generality' of individual differences, that is the stability of behaviour across a variety of situations. Although it does *technically* represent the percentage total variation, it fails to index the theoretical property of consistency. Omega squared cannot be interpreted unambiguously in terms of its magnitude alone. It is susceptible to variations in the heterogeneity of the sample. By suitable selection of personality traits and situations any set of results can be obtained. *Coefficients of generalizability* are the estimates which carry inferential weight in apportioning variance[28].

Consider several athletes competing in a number of races ranging from 100 metre sprint to 400 metres. If the assumption is made that the trait running speed is perfectly reliable across situations, athletes will retain their rank order of finishing all races. The variations observed in finishing time (dependent variable) among runners (individual differences) will be small relative to that observed between events (situational factors). The proportion of the total variance accountable for by individual differences will be negligible in those instances where runners of roughly equal ability are selected to participate over a wide range of distances. On the other hand, by limiting the events to a narrow range and choosing runners of diverse ability, individual differences will emerge as significantly more influential than situational factors[29].

Rosenthal and Rubin[30] have discussed the *problem of interpretation* of various effect size estimators. There is a widespread tendency to underestimate the importance of effects simply because they are associated with low values of $r^2$. For instance, a correlation coefficient of 0.32 which corresponds to a coefficient of determination ($r^2$) of only 0.10 is the equivalent of improving selection rates from 34 to 66%! The binomial effect size display is considered an appropriate index of the magnitude of experimental effect.

The 0.30 Barrier

Behavioural inconsistency appears commonplace in contradiction to what would be expected on the basis of broad, stable response dispositions (traits). Low reliability is reported when *single* instances of behaviour have been correlated with the same behaviour on another occasion: the magnitude of the correlation coefficient rarely exceeds 0.30, representing 10% variance. It is a popular misconception to assume that trait theorists believe that traits can be accurately inferred from single items of behaviour (which, like items on an inventory, are characterized by low reliability and low generalizability[31]), nor for that matter, can single items of behaviour be predicted using such limited and unreliable sampling.

*Aggregation* of data is a suitable method for reducing the error of measurement thus raising the temporal reliability. In a study in which daily self-reports of positive and negative emotional experiences were kept over a period of 24–34 days, the mean correlation between two days was found to be less than 0.20 (a value consistent with that reported by critics of trait theory[9]). Stability coefficients in excess of 0.80 were demonstrated, however, when the mean was calculated over a large number of observations (all the even days matched with all the odd days)[29]. This increment in reliability allowed for more coherent patterns to emerge between objective behavioural measures, personality questionnaire scores and rating data.

Aggregation is frequently implemented in sport competition, e.g. scoring in gymnastics, dancing and ice-skating, where it serves to reduce the error variance due to an unrepresentativeness between evaluators. The concept of a national rank-listing of athletes based on their level of performance in a variety of tournaments (aggregation over situations), e.g. tennis, provides a more reliable, hence predictive index of a player's ability than observing his or her success in any one competition.

Sources of Variance in S–R Inventories

Several S–R inventories have been constructed by sport psychologists, enabling a three-way analysis of variance to be performed to determine the percentage of total variance attributable to situations, persons, modes of response and their interactions. The inventory incorporates a number of anxiety-eliciting sport-related situations[32] such as, 'One week before an important game the coach told you that it was going to be your job to control the high scoring player of your opposition'; and 'You have just committed a foul with the score tied at 90–90 and only 2 seconds remaining in the game. Your action may have cost your team the game.' In addition, there are several modes of response – 'emotion disrupts actions', 'mouth gets dry', 'feel exhilarated and thrilled', 'becomes immobilized' – the athlete being required to respond on a five-point scale as to the degree of response for each particular mode. Modes of response usually account for a considerable part of the variance, followed by situations. The contribution of variance from persons is often substantially lower than the other two main effects. There are reasons which suggest that a *two-way* analysis of variance is more appropriate. The use of *modes of response* as a separate factor in the statistical analysis has been criticized[33]. Persons respond *through* a mode and not *to* a mode. As such, its inclusion serves to inflate the total pool of variation. Furthermore, there is evidence that modes of response represent a coalescence of two types of emotional expression, an *anxiety* class, e.g. 'need to urinate' – and a *pleasurable anticipation* category, e.g. 'enjoy the challenge'. The relative proportion of variance cannot be accurately assessed using mean squares; instead each *component of variance* must be compared with the sum of all the components in the analysis in order to obtain an accurate estimate. Finally, one of the weaknesses of the S–R inventory is that the situations are not only qualitatively different, they vary in the level of threat elicited. By increasing the range of threat across situations, its relative size (component of variance) can be raised.

There are a number of *theoretical limitations* associated with using an analysis of variance design to estimate the relative importance of persons, situations, response modes and their interactions. One of these has already been examined (the difficulty in representative sampling of persons, situations and modes of response). Persons and situations cannot be treated independently of each other – individuals select situations on the basis of their needs[34], e.g. toughminded persons seek competitive situations, whereas neurotics prefer to avoid social interaction, etc.

This effect operates both prior to a situation, e.g. the decision of a person to participate in physical activity as opposed to inactivity, and during the situation itself, e.g. the manner in which the individual behaves in the sport setting – assertive, restrained, confident, etc. This 'structural affinity'[35] between dispositional needs and situational characters is frequently ignored in laboratory studies in which persons are assigned to particular situations.

Social situations imply that other people constitute a part of the context in which an individual finds him- or herself; the outcome is determined by *relative* rather than absolute attributes[36]. In selecting a team leader it is the *more* assertive member (from those available) who will be appointed. The allocation of players to specific positions within a team will also depend on the extent that an individual demonstrates a supremacy relative to the others on those skills necessary for the task.

The situations can themselves be modified or 're-defined' by the constituent members. Of course, people vary in their ability to evoke responses in others and some situations are more difficult to influence than others[37]. A coach may be able to threaten or intimidate an athlete; he may be able to offer him guidance and reassurance in stressful situations. There is evidence that extraverted athletes cope with states of anxiety, anger, apathy and depression by implementation of *socially-oriented regulatory techniques*[38]. They deal with defeat by seeking social support (stress attenuation mediated through social interaction). In instances of failure, introverted athletes are inclined to feel threatened by the group situation, preferring isolation and not affiliation.

Moderator Variables

It is unjustified to assume that consistency at the intervening variable (trait) level necessarily means overt behavioural consistency[39]. A trait will have an indirect relationship with behavioural responses due to a confounding by other moderator variables (other personality traits, mediating variables and situational factors). These moderator variables influence the effect that a variable may have on another. The traditional research design (classic experimental- and control-group set-up) fails to take account of the complexity of behaviour, neglecting interactions caused through moderator variables.

The belief that interactionism provides an alternative to resolving the person–situation controversy is based on a semantic misconception. Trait theorists have emphasized the sensitivity/dependency of personality variables towards situational components[19] and the labels of the traits themselves (sociability, activity, sensation-seeking, suggestibility) explicitly refer to the conditions necessary for evoking trait-expresion. This is best illustrated with a few examples from sport.

Essing and Eberspaecher[40] found that the situational variable, 'class of competition' partially moderates the relationship between popularity and leadership in football. Those football teams participating at local club level exhibited a high positive correlation between popularity and leadership choice. The correlation coefficient was lowest for national teams and intermediate for regional clubs. Furthermore, popularity and competency were highly correlated for local club sportsmen and progressively lower for national team players. A trait such as sociability seems of considerable value in facilitating group interaction and fulfilling socioemotional needs at lower levels of competition, but is replaced by task-related competency demands in professional sport. The function of a leader in professional sport serves a different purpose to that of the amateur sportsman. If we fail to appreciate the effect of a moderating variable such as class of competition, coherent results can be annihilated by 'averaging' inappropriately.

In a series of studies[41] performed with parachutists (including 33 experienced parachutists with at least 100 jumps and an equal number of novices with less than five jumps), subjective anxiety and aversive feelings were registered on the ten-point scale on 14 occasions prior to a jump. The novice parachutists displayed a peak in tension (avoidance tendency) at the 'ready' signal. Fear decreases after this decision to jump has been made but remains fairly high at the moment of jumping. The experienced jumper is relatively high on subjective, that is, felt anxiety a week before the event and the level of anxiety increases on the night before the jump, reaching a maximum on the morning of the jump. From this stage on up to the point of free-fall, anxiety gradually decreases (and rises again on landing). Both groups of parachutists displayed an increase in anxiety followed by a drop prior to the jump; the temporal shift in trend, however, indicates that the decision to jump is taken earlier by experienced jumpers. Physiological measures of heart rate, respiratory rate and skin resistance revealed discordant results for the veteran parachutists. All three physiological variables increased up to the phase of intermediate altitude, whereas self-reported anxiety had long ceased to rise. The novices did not display this lack of correspondence; for them both subjective and physiological anxiety seemed coupled, with a dramatic increment in activity at maximum altitude. The feeling of anxiety appears very much a function of situational variables and the more experienced athlete seems better able to cope with impending fear, orienting attention to the external task demands involved in successful performance.

A frequently ignored moderating variable is age. A group of male marathoners were compared to a group of joggers on the primary traits of the

16PF[42]. The marathoners were more reserved (A –), intelligent (B), less happy-go-lucky (F –), more tender-minded (I), imaginative (M), less forthright (N), less apprehensive (O –), more self-sufficient ($Q^2$) and controlled ($Q^3$). The authors attempted to elucidate these findings. They interpret the data as providing evidence for specific traits as prerequisites for the arduous, persevering training involved in marathon running. The samples differed in age by some 14 years (mean age of marathoners $34.4 \pm 1.4$ and joggers $20.6 \pm 0.6$ years). Age had been found to be positively correlated with the primary traits I, M, N and $Q^2$ and negatively correlated with A. These are all traits which are closely related to the higher order factor toughmindedness (P). The statistical regression observed with age has also been demonstrated by Eysenck and Eysenck[21] (Figure 13.1).

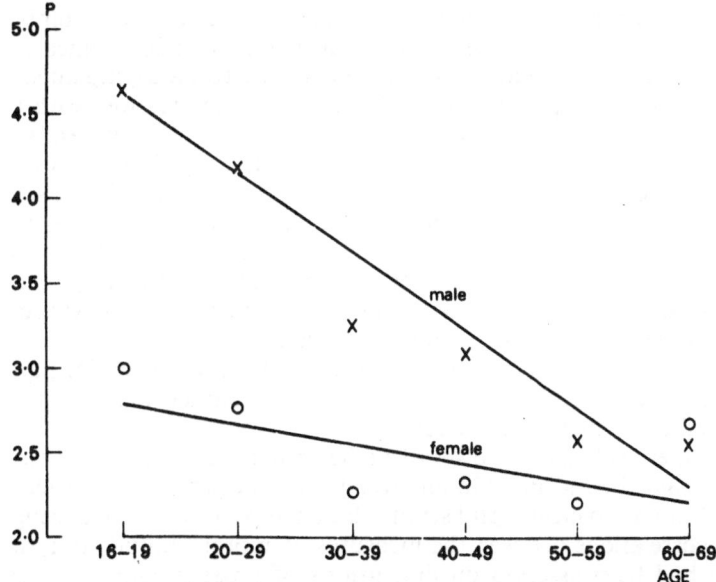

*Figure 13.1    Age regression of male and female P scores (reprinted with kind permission from Eysenck, H. J. and Eysenck, S. B. G.[21])*

The marked decrement in P with increasing age is even more pronounced in males! Any differences observed in personality profile between marathoners and joggers cannot be attributed to the 'structuring' effects of physical activity or trait gravitation (people search for situations which fulfil a need compatible with their personalities). It is necessary to control for the effects of age prior to interpretation of data.

For this reason, studies which contrast athletes and non-athletes, or athletes on the basis of their sport discipline, must consider whether a predominance of veteran athletes, e.g. in sailing, shooting and fencing, outweigh younger athletes. If for instance, modern pentathalon athletes are compared with gymnasts – the latter being characteristically younger – trait differences could not be attributable to the criterion 'multiple–single sport disciplines'.

## Higher Order Factoring

The majority of studies in sport personality research have used multiphasic tests such as the California Psychological Inventory, Edwards Personal Preference Schedule and Cattell 16PF. There is a statistical problem which arises whenever large variable sets are involved. Significant results will occur by chance when more than 20 variables are being considered; at least one of these will be expected to be statistically significant at the 0.05 probability level on the basis of chance effects of sampling, thus increasing the likelihood of making a type 1 error (rejecting the null hypothesis when it is true).

It has been demonstrated that the components of multitraits tests are themselves interrelated tending to cluster together in the form of second order traits. For instance, anxiety as a major determinant of temperament combines the primary traits of excitability associated with sympathetic dominance as well as a cycloid dispositional factor (moodiness) related to parasympathetic dominance, and a trust–suspicious element[43]. This corresponds well with findings that the 16PF primaries of C − (emotional instability), H − (shy, restrained and threat-sensitive), L + (suspecting and irritable), O + (guilt-proneness, apprehensive and insecure) and $Q_4$ + (tense and frustrated) coalesce in the secondary trait anxiety. The major contribution to predictive variance comes from the secondary rather than primary trait level[44]. Moreover, there have also been difficulties in replicating these primary source traits. Frequently, items which have been assigned to a particular scale are found to load heavily on other factors with item heterogeneity on several scales[2].

If indeed the two superfactors, E and N, contribute the major part of the valid variance in predicting a criterion, statistical artifacts may result if evaluation is limited to first order factors.

The greater explanatory power of higher order factors is well illustrated in a study discussed by Kane[45]. In an attempt to link personality structure with physical abilities, no meaningful set of relationships were revealed using simple bivariate correlations between the measures of motor aptitude (physical performance had been assessed on dimensions of *gross physical strength*, e.g. endurance, dynamic and explosive strength, *body strength*, e.g. muscularity and linearity, and *sports' participation*) and the personality variables (16 *primary traits*) (Figure 13.2). Successive factoring produced a more parsimonious

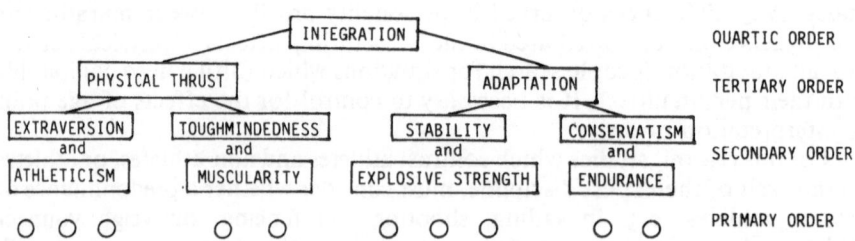

*Figure 13.2   A hierarchical structure of the relationship between motor aptitudes and personality (redrawn from Kane,[45])*

pattern. The five primary traits which cluster together as the second order factor extraversion were significantly associated with general athletic ability, the latter being a conglomerate of speed, strength and power. Similarly, the other second order factors were more predictive as well as having greater face validity than the univariate solution. The third order factors (*physical thrust* and *anxious radicalism*) were more difficult to explain in functional terms. The hierarchical factor ordering cumulated in the extraction of a fourth factor which combines these complexes with principal loadings on athleticism and extraversion. For female athletes it was stability rather than extraversion which was related to the physical vector. A high degree of sport participation is significantly associated with the variables dominance (E), low tension ($Q_4 -$) and group dependence ($Q_2 -$) accounting for 20% of the variance (for both men and women).

The transition from simple bivariate correlations through multiple to canonical correlations revealed that multivariate analyses are better able to filter out the structural relationship between personality and sport performance. This is demonstrated by the link toughminded, stable extraversion with general athletic ability. (Multivariate analysis uses an alpha level which is not affected by the number of dependent variables involved, and therefore prevents inflated group differences which may occur due to intercorrelations between the dependent variables).

At the very least, higher order factors serve to package information more meaningfully. Consider a study[14] performed on three groups of 'sensation-seeking athletes' including 30 of the best 300 drivers during the period 1966–71 (17 professionals and nine World Class Grand Prix drivers), 43 outstanding US male parachutists all having had a minimum of 1000 free-falls, and 50 football players from National football leagues. The three types of athlete were remarkably similar relative to the average – they were more intelligent, happy-go-lucky, toughminded, forthright and less rule-bound.

These traits bear some similarity with the secondary trait toughmindedness. The individual-oriented sportsmen, that is, the parachutists and drivers, differ with respect to a number of primary traits when compared to footballers. They were assertive, slightly more stable, more toughminded, more experimenting, more self-sufficient and more reserved than footballers. It is unfortunate that the authors restricted their level of statistical analysis to two-tailed *t*-tests for uncorrelated means. It is more preferable to use the more reliable descriptors of secondaries (individually oriented sportsmen emerging as introverted and more toughminded relative to team sportsmen).

Eysenck, Nias and Cox[2] have warned against drawing hasty conclusions on the basis of multivariate analyses without first *cross-checking* the validity of the findings on another sample. Although these more sophisticated statistical analyses are informative, they are inclined to capitalize on chance error which may occur when the sample is small relative to the number of variables involved.

Contextual and Temporal Proximity

Personality *types* are broad traits with strong predictive qualities for aggregates of behaviour. Narrow traits are, however, usually better predictors of specific behavioural responses, due to the contextual proximity between predictor and criterion variable. It has been demonstrated[46] how a general personality factor such as 'reducing–augmenting'* is a relatively good predictor of trait constituents (sensation-seeking and risk-taking) but not significantly related to habitual or specific responses: the specific response of pinball playing was, however, associated with the more proximal response pattern (gambling) (Figure 13.3). It is clear that correlation coefficients are attenuated in instances where predictors are selected remote from the behaviour studied.

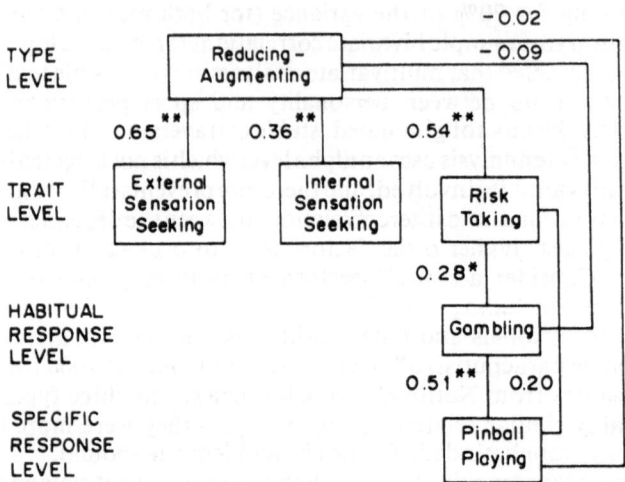

Figure 13.3   Hierarchical structure of sensation-seeking and pinball playing. *p < 0.05; **p < 0.01 (reprinted with kind permission from Barnes, G. E. (1984). Person. Indiv. Diff. Vol. 5, pp. 361–3. (Pergamon Press Ltd.))

States frequently yield the best predictors of behaviour. Morgan[1] presents a series of studies using a combination of trait and state inventories to determine which aspects of personality distinguish elite, successful athletes across several sports – running, wrestling and rowing – from less successful ones. The champion athlete was significantly lower on trait anxiety, tension and depression and high on mental vigour. Furthermore, he was inclined to score lower on state anxiety, fatigue, confusion, neuroticism and conformity (lie-scale) and high on extraversion and somatic perception.

*My attention has been drawn to the fact that Barnes *et al.*'s use of terms 'sensation-seeking' and 'augmenting–reducing' refers to the Vardo scale which is simply an arousing-seeking questionnaire, where high scorers are rather arbitrarily termed 'reducers'. Buchsbaum and Zuckerman have employed the augmenting–reducing scale in reference to the cortical evoked potential where they found that augmenters are the *high* sensation-seekers not the low ones. Reducers emerge as low sensation-seekers. By failing to distinguish between Vardo and Petrie (KFA which does not relate to either Vardo or SS scales) and Buchsbaum's defined augmenting-reducing, there is a tendency to perpetuate the error.

The profile of mood states for successful competitors was characterized by an 'iceberg profile' which refers to its graphical configuration. This was consistent for all disciplines (figure 13.4).

## The "Iceberg" Profile

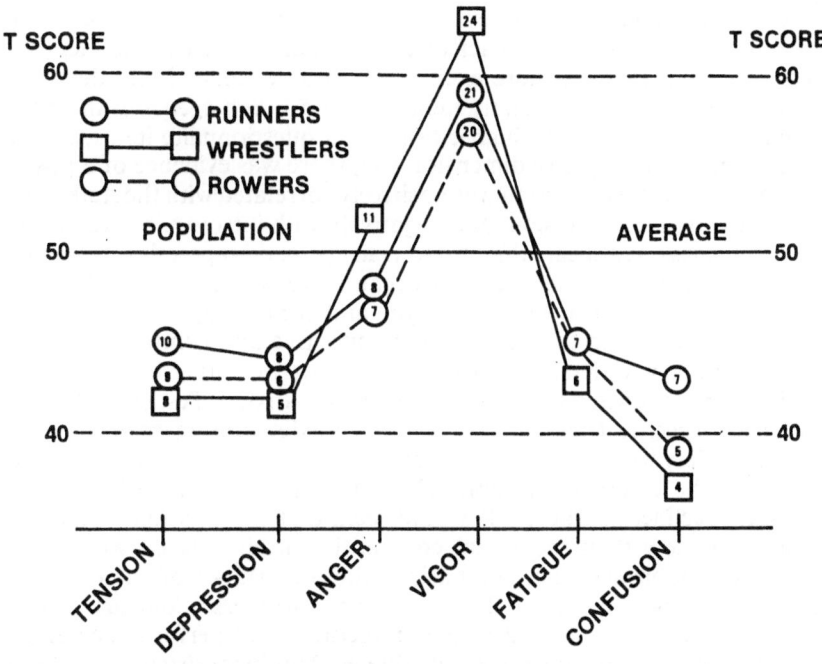

PROFILE OF MOOD STATES (POMS)

*Figure 13.4  Profile of mood states (POMS) summaries for elite wrestlers, distance runners and rowers (reprinted with kind permission from Morgan, W. P. (1980). Res. Q. Exercise Sport, **51**, 65 AAHPERD)*

The effectiveness of states in predicting sports' performance is due to the temporal proximity (inventories are administered shortly prior to competition) of these measures with the coping behaviour. States are transient moods, representing responses in delimited periods of time. There are theoretical problems associated with their use[31]; they are likely to be contaminated by *trait elements* (identical precompetitive anxiety state scores between athletes may signify quite different emotional reactivity, for one athlete it may be a decrease in resting anxiety level, for another it may be an increase); *temporal incongruency* (states are self-reports based in the present whereas traits are memories of previous states); and states suffer from the same limitations as other single measures, that is, they are of *low reliability* (this refers solely to temporal stability, but not necessarily to internal consistency of measures) and high *situational specificity*. Traits have been described as the aggregate of states[47].

In an attempt to relate state and trait concepts[48], 149 persons were administered a multidimensional state scale (EWL) in which 162 adjectives of momentary feeling (reducible to 15 state scales) were responded to. The first two factors extracted using principal component analysis (orthogonal rotation for the derived solution) resembled E and N. A profile analysis of high and low trait (EPQ) neuroticism scorers revealed that the neurotics' response style (state descriptions) appeared less differentiated than stables (low neurotics). They were less concentrated, more deactivated and numb, introverted, less self-assured, less good-spirited, more excitable, sensitive, fearful and depressed. The state inventories contain many items which are *homogeneous* in content and semantically similar to the higher order trait questionnaire items. In addition to a higher order negative dimension (N), there was evidence of a positive trait factor (E). Trait extraversion was positively correlated with the states good-spirited, activation, extraversion, and negatively with introversion, fearfulness and depressiveness. It appears that broad traits (E and N) permit prediction of the kind of states implemented in Morgan's study on successful athletes (tension, depression, anger, vigour, fatigue and confusion).

In a study[49] designed to examine precompetitive and competitive anxiety patterns in junior wrestlers, 464 of the athletes participating in the National Championships completed the Sport Competitive Anxiety Test (SCAT) which assesses sport-specific trait anxiety, and an anxiety rating scale. A linear increase in anxiety was observed across precompetitive measures, state anxiety increasing as the competition approaches but once the competition began, anxiety state declined markedly. It would seem that anticipation of the event elicits more anxiety than the actual competition itself. Placed winners had reported less trouble sleeping, emphasized the importance of the event, felt more confident and were older than non-placed winners. Contrary to other studies[41], no differences existed in precompetitive and performance anxiety between the successful and unsuccessful athletes. This inconsistency may be due to the *physical danger* in some high-risk sports, e.g. parachuting, compared to the *interpersonal threat* component which characterizes less dangerous pursuits, e.g. wrestling.

The wrestlers were divided into low and high trait anxious groups on the basis of their scores on the SCAT (Figure 13.5). Significant differences in state anxiety emerge 24 h, 1 h and 2 min prior to the event (a progressive divergence in anxiety ratings as the competition draws near) as well as when competing against the toughest opponent. The high trait anxious athletes expressed more anxiety when the threat was proximal. The lower anxious (SCAT) sportsmen rated themselves higher in ability, more confident in their predictions, considered that they would be highly placed, less worried, have less trouble in sleeping, and did not feel that nervousness would necessarily debilitate their performance. Multiple regression analysis revealed that *trait anxiety* and *importance to self to perform well* were influential factors in predicting competitive anxiety. It is clear that state anxiety is a function of both the level of *situational stress* (nearness to competitive event) and the athlete's *susceptibility*

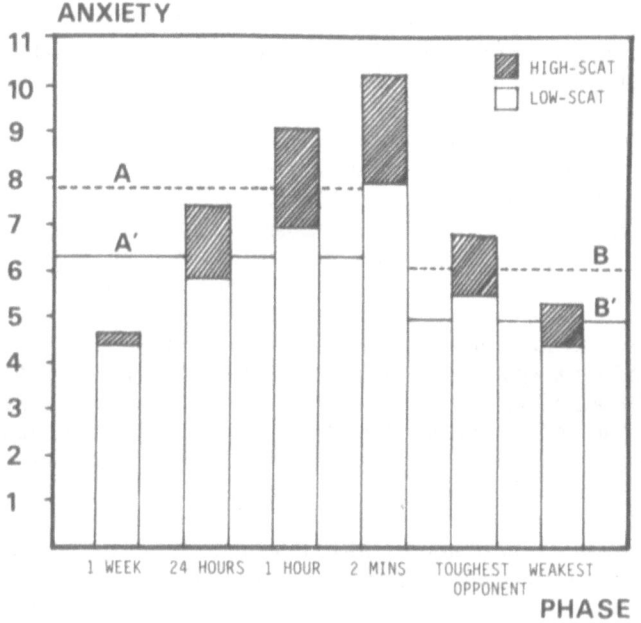

A and A' are mean pre-competitive anxiety for high and low SCAT-groups
B and B' are mean performance anxiety for high and low SCAT groups
respectively

*Figure 13.5  Anxiety ratings of high and low trait anxiety (SCAT) wrestler anxiety-responses (redrawn from Gould, Horn and Spreeman[49])*

*to anxiety* (trait anxiety). The sport competitive trait anxiety resembles a more narrowly defined trait and the state elements used are not far removed from a trait in that they are based on reports of how the wrestlers *typically* feel in certain situations thus relying more on memory components.

Schwenkmezger[50] examined the two components of anxiety, 'emotionality' (state anxiety inventory score) and 'worry' (intensity of task irrelevant cognitions) in a group of 35 National handball players in two situations, a practice game ('low importance') and a trial for selection ('high importance'). The sample was dichotomized into high and low anxious athletes on the trait anxiety scale and it was found that high trait anxious athletes were more likely to exhibit state anxiety in both situations on the emotionality dimension. In the non-threatening, practice game, the two groups did not differ significantly in the frequency of task irrelevant cognitions but differences did exist in the more stressful (trials) situation. The high trait anxious athlete does appear to engage in more performance-distracting cognitive deliberations.

The latter study suggests that even when broad anxiety traits are employed, used correctly, they are good predictors of competitive state anxiety but a trait such as anxiety will generally only gain expression when the situations are appropriate.

271

## Operationalization of Sport

The concept 'sport' is too global and undifferentiated for research purposes, and it is improbable that many general relationships will be disclosed between personality and sporting activities[2]. Overall contrasts between sportsmen are insufficient: there is a danger in aggregating inappropriately over heterogeneous groups. Consider the four distinct questions for which it would be meaningless to average results. Are there personality differences between sport-interested and uninterested persons? Do differences exist between sport participants and (passive) spectators? Do competitive athletes differ from non-competitive athletes? What characterizes the outstanding athlete? It is unlikely to expect *identical* traits to operate with equal potency at every selection level. Another important factor, in addition to the issue of *level of involvement* and achievement, is the *between sports* level of analysis. It has been claimed that it is important to isolate which *specific* traits are consistently associated with which specific sports and well documented that more reliable and valid indices of sport can be obtained by using *criterion analysis* of the sports themselves, e.g. team vs. individual, contact vs. non-contact, open-skills vs. closed skills, rigid rules vs. flexible rules, strategic vs. physical, etc. There is an endless array of categories, some obviously more important than others; for example, it would be expected that broad traits such as anxiety and sensation-seeking are probably implicated in sports involving high risks. By providing a theoretical explanation of sport, Zuckerman[51] was able to construct a paradigm for empirical testing of the theory. He used the criterion 'element of risk-taking' as a means of classifying sports, *high risk* sports included car-racing, hang-gliding, parachuting, skiing, mountaineering and scuba-diving, *moderate risk* sports included team sports such as rugby, football and handball which entail the occasional bone injury and low risk sports included running, gymnastics, tennis, etc. in which injuries of a serious nature are rare.

The multidimensional 'sensation-seeking' scale contains personality variables assumed *coherent* with the features inherent in risky sports. In a review of 12 studies, it was confirmed that the trait, sensation-seeking, was related to those sports involving novel sensations and risks and that this relationship was most pronounced in the more experienced participant. The high sensation-seeker was inclined to underestimate the risk involved and was more likely to be injured (as a result?). Low sensation-seekers preferred to avoid high risk activities; a small negative correlation had been reported between a narrow trait anxiety (fear of physical injury) and sensation-seeking.

Sensation-seeking appears to interact with trait anxiety producing approach or avoidance behaviour. The trait 'toughmindedness' has been shown to correlate with the two subscales of sensation-seeking, 'disinhibition' and 'boredom susceptibility'[52]. The socially undesirable aspects of toughminded behaviour may explain why they are under-represented in the more institutionalized sport disciplines requiring persistence and conformity with respect to training schedules.

Dowd and Innes[53] selected two open-skilled sports (demanding perception of external cues): volleyball and squash. The volleyball players tended to be less anxious and more forthright than squash players, traits which were assumed to facilitate performance on a team-oriented task (requiring social co-operation amongst players). Other traits gain expression as higher levels of competitive ability are reached, for example state volleyball players tended to be more intelligent, assertive and self-sufficient than squash players, traits which may well serve to draw the attention of selectors towards a talented player. This study suggests that between-sport comparisons are quite likely *confounded* by other factors such as *level of achievement*.

It is possible for relatively homogeneous groups to show considerable variation *within sports* e.g. variations in playing position within team sports, or differences in style or strategy of play in individual sports.

Kirkcaldy[3] differentiated team athletes according to their position within the team (defenders, midfield and attackers). Attackers were the most toughminded of all players and midfield the least, with defenders lying midway. This partially supports the view that there is a tendency to be physical amongst defensive (and offensive) players in sport. This has been referred to as the *era of the hard defence* in which 'young talent have no option but to acquaint themselves with the entire repertoire of fouls which had transformed their predecessors into world-class athletes'[54]. Extraversion was unrelated to playing position; offenders were significantly more emotionally unstable relative to other players. The most stable athletes were midfield and defensive players, midfield players were somewhat more conservative than offenders (Table 13.1). Separate

Table 13.1  Comparison of means (univariate t-test) for personality variables between classes (position of play) – male and female combined, L > 11 were removed from the analysis[3]

| Factor | Position | | No. | Mean | SD | Probability | | |
|--------|----------|---|-----|------|-----|---|---|---|
| | | | | | | O | M | P |
| Psychoticism | Offense | (O) | 70 | 6.60 | 2.77 | — | 0.02* | 0.39 |
| | Middle | (M) | 53 | 5.58 | 2.17 | | — | 0.34 |
| | Defense | (D) | 25 | 6.08 | 2.00 | | | — |
| Extraversion | Offense | (O) | 70 | 14.96 | 3.46 | — | 0.22 | 0.39 |
| | Middle | (M) | 53 | 14.23 | 3.87 | | — | 0.42 |
| | Defense | (D) | 25 | 14.96 | 3.46 | | | — |
| Neuroticism | Offense | (O) | 70 | 10.96 | 4.01 | — | 0.01** | 0.02* |
| | Middle | (M) | 53 | 8.83 | 4.86 | | — | 0.82 |
| | Defense | (D) | 25 | 8.56 | 5.28 | | | — |
| Lie-scale | Offense | (O) | 70 | 5.29 | 2.75 | — | 0.08 | 0.51 |
| | Middle | (M) | 53 | 6.13 | 2.54 | | — | 0.54 |
| | Defense | (D) | 25 | 5.72 | 3.08 | | | — |

discrimination analyses for each sex revealed that whilst N and P were powerful determinants in the function (between class comparison), this was the case for *males only*. It is probable that for sportsmen, the toughminded, sensation-seeking, emotional attacker has a very different function from the less extraverted, stable, tenderminded midfield player. The latter is more concerned with tactical planning and organization during the game ('constructional play'), whereas attackers must have a collection of well-rehearsed moves at their disposal. The *drive* quality of a relatively high N may well enhance less cognitively demanding performance.

Regarding this issue shooting sports have been studied across ten groups[9]. The prone rifle shooter allows for plenty of time for taking the shot which is executed in the lying flat position. The free-pistol shot shares the feature of allowing time to concentrate but he has to stand and thus exercise considerable control in minimizing extraneous movements. These two groups were significantly more introverted. The rapid-fire pistol event does not allow the period of concentration provided by the other two events for a series of shots must be fired successively at a series of targets and the shooter has to adapt rapidly to each newly exposed target. Such an event shares many of the explosive characteristics of short-distance events and so it is perhaps not too surprising that the rapid-fire pistol shooter emerges as the most extraverted of the groups. There was some indication that the *impulsivity* component of extraversion was the determining factor in relation to the number of factors involved.

Such differences within sports are consistent with what is theoretically predictable and replicable.

## CONCLUSION

The inability to replicate findings in sport personality research is insufficient reason to abandon a perfectly good theory. The rejection of a sound theory on the basis of unfavourable results constitutes a type 2 error, '. . . where the failure of the experiments in question to give positive results is due, not to defects of the theory, but to errors in the minor premises of the syllogism used to make the prediction, to assumptions about the tests used which are in fact erroneous, or to failure to take into account the whole theory to be tested, including the deductions about the parameter values contained in it[19].'

Consider the typical shot-gun approach which until recently prevailed in studies relating sport and personality. Any one of an array of multiphasic trait inventories was administered to whichever groups of athletes were available. The level of inquiry was frequently *atheoretical* with no hypothesis being derived on the basis of specific theories – the criteria were invalid and unreliable – researchers neglected specifying the parameters of testing (traits cannot be treated in isolation of situations and other moderator variables) and statistical analysis was inappropriate. To compare this secondary reviews have tended to ignore the issue of 'quality' of research.

It is unfortunate that sport psychologists have invested considerable effort in attempting to denounce trait theory by demonstrating a low level of cross-situational generalization of behaviour or concentrating on the pseudo-issue of the relative importance of people, situations and their interactions, an area saturated with methodological and statistical artifacts. It is based on a misunderstanding of what trait theorists propose. It is possible to demonstrate consistency at the intervening variable level but not at the behavioural level. Broad

274

nomothetic traits are unlikely to be accurate predictors of single instances of behaviour, the latter being unreliable and too narrow in scope (low generalizability). Narrow traits such as the Sport Competitive Anxiety Scale, in which situations relevant to sport are specified, are clearly more contextually proximal than broad traits. State measures will be superior predictors of behaviour when administered shortly before a competitive event (increased potency attributable to 'temporal proximity'). The 0.30 barrier can be broken through aggregation which serves to reduce the error of measurement of single observations. Traits can be considered as sampling behaviour over time for a class of situations.

A few higher order traits seem preferable to many, diverse primary traits, the latter adding little to predictive validity and themselves of low replicability. Multivariate statistical methods provide the most appropriate way of dealing with complex phenomena such as physical performance and sport. Researchers must, however, acquaint themselves with the *underlying assumptions* of these statistical techniques to ensure valid inferences.

The sceptics of trait theory must pose themselves several questions before discarding their nets. Thus returning to the figurative language of Kroll. Are we agreed over the identity of fishes? This relates to whether the criteria are valid and reliable. How can we catch them? This concerns the selection of appropriate measuring instruments which assess traits relevant to criteria. Where do we fish? The importance of describing situational parameters should not be underestimated. When do we fish most effectively? The temporal proximity determines the potency of measures. What emerges is a technician who will supplement his nets with others. The trait and state concepts should not be considered as if they were mutually exclusive. If we fail to take account of the constraints on a theory, we may well end up 'angling in polluted waters!'

## References

1. Morgan, W. P. (1980). The trait psychology controversy. *Res. Q.*, **51**, 50–76
2. Eysenck, H. J., Nias, D. K. B. and Cox, D. N. (1982). Sport and personality. *Adv. Behav. Res. Ther.*, **4**, 1–56
3. Kirkcaldy, B. D. (1982). Personality and sex differences related to positions in team sports. *Int. J. Sport Psychol.*, **13**, 141–53
4. Schmitz-Scherzer, R., Bierhoff-Alfermann, D. and Bierhoff, H. W. (1977). Sport, Freizeit und Persönlichkeitsmerkmale – ein Vergleich zwischen Sportlern and Nichtsportlern. In Schmitz-Scherzer, R. (ed.) *Aktuelle Beiträge zur Freizeitforschung*, **7**, 64–74. (Darmstadt: Steinkopff Verlag)
5. Knobloch, J. (1977). *Stress und Stressanfälligkeit – eine psychophysiologische Untersuchung an Sportlern and Nichtsportlern.* Unpublished doctoral dissertation, Freiburg University
6. Kirkcaldy, B. D. (1982). Personality profiles at various levels of athletic performance. *Pers. Individ. Diff.*, **3**, 321–6
7. Kane, J. E. (1968). Personality and physical ability. In Kenyon, G. (ed.) *Proceedings from the International Congress of Sports' Psychology.* pp. 131–41. (Washington: Athletic Institute)
8. Thomas, T. R., Zebas, C. J., Bahrke, M. S., Araujo, J. and Etheridge, G. L. (1983). Physiological and psychological correlates of success in track and field athletes. *Br. J. Sports Med.*, **17**, 102–9

9. Coleman, J. A. (1979). *Personality and stress in shooting sports.* Unpublished
10. Kruse, V. (1977). Persönlichkeitseigenschaften von Fussball and Tischtennisspielern. *Leistungssport*, 7, 231-6
11. Sage, G. H. (1972). An assessment of personality profiles between and within intercollegiate athletes from eight different sports. *Sportwissenchaft*, 2, 408-15
12. Eysenck, H. J. and Wilson, G. (1976). *Know Your Own Personality.* (Middlesex: Penguin)
13. Nation, J. R. and LeUnes, A. D. (1983). Personality characteristics of collegiate football players as determined by position, classification and red-shirt status. *J. Sports Behav.*, 6, 92-102
14. Johnsgard, K., Ogilvie, B. and Merritt, K. (1975). The stress-seekers: a psychological study of sport parachutists, racing drivers and football players. *J. Sports Med.*, 15, 158-69
15. Gray, J. E. (1973). Casual theories of personality and how to test them. In Royce, J. R. (ed.) *Multivariate Analysis and Psychological Theory.* pp. 409-63. (London: Academic Press)
16. Furnham, A. (1981). Personality and activity preference. *Br. J. Soc. Psychol.*, 20, 57-68
17. Kane, J. E. (1978). Persons, situations and performance. In Glencross, D. (ed.) *Psychology and Sport.*. pp. 120-43. (Australia: McGraw Hill)
18. Mummendey, H. D. (1983). Sportliche Aktivität und Persönlichkeit. *Sportwissenschaft*, 13, 9-23
19. Eysenck, H. J. (1981). General features of the model. In Eysenck, H. J. (ed.) *Models of Personality.* pp. 1-37. (Berlin: Springer Verlag)
20. Sack, H. G. (1982). Sport und Persönlichkeit. In Thomas, A. (ed.) *Sportpsychologie – ein Handbuch in Schlüsselbegriffen.* pp. 148-65. (Munich: Urban and Schwarzenberg)
21. Eysenck, H. J. and Eysenck, S. B. G. (1976). *Psychoticism as a Dimension of Personality.* (London: Hodder and Stoughton)
22. Nitsch, J. R. and Allmer, H. (1978). *Sportpsychologie – eine Standortbestimmung.* (Köln: bps)
23. Kirkcaldy, B. D., Mummendey, H. D., Eysenck, H. J., Sack, H. G. and Simons, H. (1984). Sportliche Aktivität und Persönlichkeit: Diskussion. *Sportwissenschaft*, 14, 73-92
24. Michaelis, W. and Eysenck, H. J. (1971). The determination of personality inventory factor patterns and intercorrelations by change in real-life motivation. *J. Genet. Psychol.*, 118, 223-34
25. Kroll, W. (1970). Current strategies and problems in personality assessment of athletes. In Smith, L. E. (ed.) *Psychology of Motor Learning.* pp. 349-67. (Chicago: Athletic Institute)
26. Fisher, A. C. (1984). New directions in sport personality research. In Weinberg, R. S. (ed.) *Psychological Foundations of Sport and Exercise.* (In press)
27. Plutchik, R. (1983). *Foundations of Experimental Research.* 3rd Edn. (New York: Harper and Row)
28. Golding, S. L. (1975). Flies in the ointment: methodological problems in the analysis of the percentage of variance due to persons and situations. *Psychol. Bull.*, 82, 278-88
29. Epstein, S. (1977). Traits are alive and well. In Magnusson, D. and Endler, N. S. (eds.) *Personality at the Crossroads: Current Issues in Interactional Psychology.* pp. 83-98. (Hillsdale: Lawrence Erlbaum Ass., Wiley)
30. Rosenthal, R. and Rubin, D. R. (1982). A simple, general purpose display of magnitude of experimental effect. *J. Educ. Psychol.*, 14, 166-9
31. Epstein, S. (1983). Aggregation and beyond: some basic issues on the prediction of behaviour. *J. Pers.*, 51, 360-92
32. Fisher, C. (1979). Multidimensional scaling of sport personality data: an individual differences approach. *J. Sport Psychol.*, 1, 76-86
33. Cartwright, D. (1975). Trait and other sources of variance in the S-R Inventory of Anxiousness. *J. Pers. Soc. Psychol.*, 32, 408-14
34. Bowers, K. (1973). Situationalism in psychology: an analysis and a critique. *Psychol. Rev.*, 80, 307-36
35. Sack, H. G. (1975). *Sportliche Betätigung und Persönlichkeit.* (Ahrensburg: Czwalina)
36. Argyle, M. (1976). Personality and social behaviour. In Harré, R. (ed.) *Personality.* (Oxford: Blackwell)
37. Wachtel, P. (1973). Psychodynamics, behaviour therapy, and the implacable experimenter: an inquiry into the consistency of personality. *J. Abnorm. Psychol.*, 82, 324-34
38. Eitel, W. (1980). *Naive Techniken der Selbstregulation im Leistungssport.* Unpublished Diploma Thesis. (Cologne: DSHS)

39. Eysenck, H. J. and Eysenck, M. W. (1980). Mischel and the concept of personality. *Br. J. Psychol.*, **71**, 191–204

40. Essing, W. and Eberspächer, H. (1974). Untersuchungen über Rollendifferenzierung in Sportgruppen. In Decker, W. and Lämmer, M. (eds.) *Jahrbuch der Deutschen Sporthochschule Köln 1973*. pp. 71–86. (Schorndorf: Karl Hofmann)

41. Epstein, S. (1977). Versuch einer Theorie der Angst. In Birbaumer, N. (ed.) *Psychophysiologie der Angst*. pp. 208–66. (Munich: Urban and Schwarzenberg)

42. Vailliant, P. M., Bennie, F. A. B. and Valiant, J. J. (1981). Do marathoners differ from joggers in personality profile: a sports psychology approach? *J. Sports Med. Phys. Fitness.*, **21**, 62–7

43. Royce, J. R. (1973). The conceptual framework for a multi-factor theory of individuality. In Royce, J. R. (ed.) *Multivariate Analysis and Psychological Theory*. pp. 305–407. (London: Academic Press)

44. Reynolds, C. H. and Nichols, R. C. (1977). Factor scales of the C.P.I.: Do they capture the valid variance? *Educ. Psychol. Meas.*, **37**, 907–15

45. Kane, J. E. (1982). Mental and personality correlates of motor abilities. In Geron, E. (ed.) *Handbook of Sport Psychology*, Vol. 1, pp. 98–107. (Tel Aviv: Wingate Institute)

46. Barnes, G. E. (1984). A brief note on two often ignored principles that tend to attenuate the magnitude of correlation. *Pers. Individ. Diff.*, **5**, 361–3

47. Zuckerman, M. (1979). Traits, states, situations and uncertainty. *J. Behav. Assessment*, **1**, 43–54

48. Kirkcaldy, B. D. (1984). The interrelationship between state and trait variables. *Pers. Individ. Diff.*, **5**, 141–49

49. Gould, D., Horn, T. and Spreeman, J. (1983). Competitive anxiety in junior elite athletes. *J. Sports Psychol.*, **5**, 58–71

50. Schwenkmezger, P. (1980). Untersuchung zur kognitiven Angsttheorie im sportmotorischen Bereich (state–trait-anxiety). *Z. Exp. Angew. Psychol.*, **27**, 607–30

51. Zuckerman, M. (1983). Sensation-seeking and sports. *Pers. Individ. Diff.*, **4**, 285–93

52. Furnham, A. (1984). Extraversion, sensation-seeking, stimulus screening and type A behaviour pattern – the relationship between various measures of arousal. *Pers. Individ. Diff.*, **5**, 133–40

53. Dowd, R. and Innes, J. M. (1981). Sport and personality: the effects of type of sport and level of competition. *Percept. Mot. Skills*, **53**, 381–9

54. Schmidt, H. G. (1982). Gewalt vom Sportlern. In Pilz, G. A. (ed.) *Sportliches Gewalt*. pp. 25–34. (Hamburg: Rowohlt)

# 14

# Personality and recreational behaviour

## *David K. B. Nias*

INTRODUCTION

In parallel with the many and well-known studies on intelligence and vocational interests, there have also been studies on recreational interests. At a time of increasing unemployment and early retirement, the use of leisure is becoming more and more of an issue in social psychology. This chapter outlines the beginnings of a systematic attempt to arrive at a greater understanding of how individuals choose their leisure time activity, and the effects it has on them. We start by describing the factorial studies made to arrive at a classification of recreational interests, and go on to see how these interests are related to personality, motivations and other possible causal factors.

CLASSIFICATION OF INTERESTS

The structure of different personality traits and of different cognitive abilities has been thoroughly investigated, resulting in the delineation of such well-known dimensions as emotionality, extraversion, spatial ability and verbal intelligence. Vocational interests have also been investigated, with the best known series of studies producing the *Strong Vocational Interest Blank*[1]. Early studies tended to include recreation along with vocational interests but, with the increasing relevance of leisure time, recreational interests are now being studied in their own right.

Typical of the early studies on interests generally is one by Sandall[2]. He subjectively classified some 500 specific interests into 28 categories and, on the basis of ratings from 429 school children, arrived at an eight-factor classificatory system using Thurstone's Centroid method. These factors were seen to be similar to those from other factorial studies, especially those from a large-scale study led by Guilford[3].

A limitation common to all these early studies was that only a few interests were analysed or, worse, that factor analysis was performed on *a priori* groups of items rather than on specific activities. This meant that the researcher was partially prejudging the issue by subjectively grouping activities thought to belong together, before conducting the factor analysis. In those days, researchers were restricted by the limited power of computers to analyse data in more detail. After reviewing the literature on interests generally, Eysenck[4] expressed the problem as follows: 'No large-scale study of . . . intercorrelations between items has yet been carried out, and there is little doubt in the writer's mind that only by such a study, using oblique and second-order factors if necessary, can a really firm foundation be laid for a proper system of classification of interests and values'. Responding to this need, Nias[5] carried out the first factor analysis of a large number of interest items that did not involve any prior subjective classification.

Table 14.1   Interest factors based on analysis of individual items

| School children | | Adults | |
|---|---|---|---|
| (1) Watching sport - TV sport, newspaper sport, etc. | 0.88 | (1) Sport when young - interest in sport when at school | 0.91 |
| (2) Children's entertainment - TV cartoons, comics | 0.97 | (2) Current affairs - TV documentaries, news | 0.95 |
| (3) Academic interests - English, TV news | 0.93 | (3) Romance - romantic films and magazines | |
| (4) Pop music - listening to and reading about pop | 0.83 | Social - talking to friends, holidays | 0.62 |
| (5) Sport - school games, athletics | 0.82 | (4) Crime and mystery - detective stories, thrillers | 0.79 |
| (6) Animals - looking after pets, animal books | 0.88 | (5) Sport - present participation in sports | 0.87 |
| (7) Art - model making, school art | 0.72 | (6) Films - adventure films, westerns | |
| (8) Romance - romantic films and stories | 0.78 | Romance - romantic films and magazines | 0.60 |
| (9) Crime and horror - TV horror films, detective stories | 0.97 | (7) Encouraging children - to join clubs and to mix socially | 0.92 |
| (10) Science - school chemistry, physics | 0.91 | (8) Academic - encouraging child in school work | |
| (11) War - TV war films, war stories | 0.88 | Music - listening and playing | 0.66 |
| (12) General interests - various home interests - sewing, cooking | 0.72 | (9) True stories - true and adventure stories | |
| | | Animals - looking after pets, TV animal programmes | -0.52 |
| | | (10) Home - gardening, work around the home | 0.83 |

Note: Factor similarity coefficients are given for males/females, showing that most of the factors are closely replicated across sex. Where the coefficient is low it has been necessary to give a different label for males/females. Based on Nias[5]

School subjects, hobbies, TV programmes, reading topics and sports, totalling some 80 items, were rated for degree of interest on a five-point scale by 1152 school children aged 12–16 years. A similar set of 70 interests (minus the school subjects and specific sports) were rated by the parents of the children (1270 adults). A principal components analysis with a Promax oblique rotation resulted in a set of 12 factors for the school children and ten factors for the adults. Table 14.1 lists these factors, together with examples of high loading items.

The main point to emerge was that the factors were concerned with specific rather than broad interest areas. For example, interest in watching sport constituted one of the factors for children but this was relatively independent of another factor concerned with active participation in sport; the correlation between the factors was 0.17 for boys and 0.24 for girls. Similarly, academic and scientific interests constituted separate and relatively independent factors. Because of this it did not prove possible, using second-order analyses, to arrive at a smaller number of more general but still meaningful factors. Rounds and Davis[6] also found 'circumscribed' factors when, for the first time, individual items (not groups of interests) were factored from the *Strong Vocational Interest Blank*.

*Table 14.2   Comparison of interest factors from early studies*

| Sandall's factors | Similar factors |
|---|---|
| (1)  Rural/Practical – crafts, pets, garden | Things v. people[11] <br> Outdoor work[3] |
| (2)  Sociable – dancing, acting, cinema | People[12] <br> Social activities[11] <br> Sociability[3] |
| (3)  Humanitarian – religion, charities, first aid | Working with people[1] <br> Social welfare [3, 13] <br> Anti-aggressive[14] |
| (4)  Entertainment – indoor games, amusements | Diversion[3] |
| (5)  Physical – athletics, games, sports | |
| (6)  Literate – writing, serious reading | Language[12] <br> Business[12] <br> Facts and figures[1] <br> Clerical and culture[3] |
| (7)  Aesthetic – art, music | Aesthetic[14] <br> Aesthetic appreciation[3] <br> Aesthetic expression[3] |
| (8)  Scientific/Mechanical – engineering, calculations | Scientific[12, 14] <br> Science[1] <br> Scientific v. display[13] <br> Mechanical[3] |

Note: Examples of the content of high-loading items are given for Sandall's factors. Based on Sandall[10]

Comparing the factors (Table 14.1) with those from earlier studies on recreational[7,8] and academic[9] interests reveals that the present study has produced more factors and ones of a more specific nature. Table 14.2 presents a summary of a table prepared by Sandall[10] for showing that his children's factors compare well with those from previous studies. Even though they tend to be more specific, most of the factors from Table 14.1 could be added to Sandall's table. This is reassuring in view of the different populations sampled, the different methods of analysis, and the different items selected for analysis. In particular, there was more of an emphasis in the present study on recreational rather than vocational interests.

Two other studies on classifying interests should be mentioned. Noting that previous studies were all limited to evidence from a single sample, Bishop[15] analysed data from four separate populations. His subjects were obtained from four stratified random samples, and were asked how frequently they participated in some 25 activities. Three clear factors emerged for each of the four communities, and were labelled:

(1) *Active-Diversionary* - concerned with action and movement (e.g. going swimming) rather than sedentary pursuits in familiar surroundings (e.g. watching TV);

(2) *Potency* - communion with nature by way of masculine activities seen as 'hard, tough, rugged and severe' (hunting, camping and fishing);

(3) *Status* - cultural or 'high brow' activities (plays, concerts and art).

In naming these factors, Bishop saw a parallel with Osgood's model of connotative meanings - Evaluative (the Status factor), Activity and Potency. Had Bishop analysed more than 25 items, however, and had he asked his subjects to rate their preferences (rather than just frequency of participation), he might well have obtained a larger set of more specific factors.

An extension to Bishop's study was carried out with school children by Witt[16]. This resulted in four factors, replicated across three samples, which he labelled: (1) *Sports*, (2) *Outdoor–Nature*, (3) *Social*, and (4) *Sophisticated*. The results represented a close replication of the study on adults. Only the Social factor had no direct parallel in the adult study, and Witt suggested that social participation in adults takes place in a more formalized context and so is represented on the other factors. Such a conclusion, however, may not be warranted since other studies (see Table 14.2) have revealed a Social factor for both children and adults.

The conclusion from these various factorial studies, especially the large-scale ones, seems to be that the dimensions of leisure are fairly specific. Few of the factors are general in the sense of combining activities from different domains. As a consequence, the nature of the factors obtained has depended very much on the nature of the items selected for analysis. This explains why highly specific factors (such as Animals, Crime and Horror, and War) can arise in a study (Table 14.1) where items on each of these topics are included. On the evidence of the specific factors obtained in the present study, it seems that the previous procedure of subjectively grouping apparently similar activities cannot be justified.

282

The conclusion that interest factors tend to be fairly specific contrasts with the conclusion from personality and intelligence research where broad, underlying, dimensions have been readily discovered. The aim with classifying recreational interests should perhaps now shift from attempting to arrive at a definitive set of dimensions, and instead move on to recognizing the specific nature of the factors that are obtained.

## PERSONALITY AND OTHER CORRELATES OF INTERESTS

In an attempt to help interpret the nature of the factors identified, most of the recent studies have included correlating the factors with demographic and other variables. At the same time this approach addresses the question of what type of person is attracted to the different interest areas, such as the 'sports type' v. the 'academic type'.

In the study by Nias[17, 18] loadings of over a dozen correlates on each of the factors (Table 14.1) were obtained using the Factor Extension method[19]. It was predicted that clear differences would emerge in the characterization of each factor. But in the event, the factors were relatively independent of such other variables as personality, intelligence, physique, family size, popularity, urban or rural home, and so on. Also few of the correlates that were statistically significant were replicated across sex. For example, in the case of extraversion several loadings were above 0.20 but only for one sex. For the school group, extraversion loaded most highly on the *Watching sport* factor for boys (0.26), *Pop music* for boys (0.27), and *Sport* for girls (0.43). For the adult group, extraversion was related to the *Social* factor for women (0.37), to the *Encouraging their children socially* factor for men (0.27), and negatively with the *Academic* factor for men (−0.20). The corresponding loadings for the opposite sex were in each case below 0.20. The impression thus emerged that, with few exceptions, it was not possible to define the type of person most likely to be attracted to a given interest area.

An example of an attempt to relate social class, not to choice of leisure activity but to *amount*, is provided by Willmott[20]. He interviewed people about their work and leisure and found that, apart from being more 'involved' in their work (e.g. thinking about it when at home), higher paid men were also more involved in their home life and participated in a wider range of leisure activities compared with the lower paid. The higher paid group had done more things in the past year, were more active in physical recreation, belonged to more clubs and associations, and were more likely to meet their domestic responsibilities (family, house and garden). This evidence suggests that involvement in one sphere of life is not necessarily at the expense of involvement in another. A limitation of this study is that only social class was assessed. The higher paid group may have been more active recreationally, not because of their social class, but because they differed in personality and other attributes. Only by assessing subjects for a range of attributes can alternative explanations of this sort be ruled out.

Furnham[21] looked at the link between values or lifestyle preferences and personality. After criticizing previous work as atheoretical ('giving Ss a number of apparently randomly selected scales and seeing simply how they relate to one another'), he gave reasons to expect differences in value preferences as a function of personality. In particular, the hypothesized need for arousal in extraverts, and the personal problems experienced by neurotics, should lead to characteristic preferences. 70 sixth form students, aged 16–18 years, were assessed for personality (with the *EPQ*) and asked to rank order a set of 18 values according to personal preference (with the *Rokeach Value Survey*). As predicted, extraverts tended to value a Comfortable life (a prosperous life) and an Exciting life (a stimulating, active life). Also the group scoring high on neuroticism tended to value Freedom (independence and free choice) and Inner harmony (freedom from inner conflict).

In arguing that Murray's needs are more appropriate than other personality models to a study of leisure interests, Allen[22] assessed 212 students with Jackson's *Personality Research Form-E*. The students rated their degree of interest in 51 leisure activities. Factor analysis revealed nine interest factors, and these in turn were related to the personality profiles by canonical analysis with a structure matrix. This analysis yielded four independent relationships between the personality needs and the leisure interests. Table 14.3 shows that the first represents a dominant, athletic type interested in physical competition, the second a cautious type with few interests, the third an educated, confident type, and the fourth an independent type with a liking for solitude. Although the analysis used by Allen tends to confound personality and interests (the four types representing a cross between the two domains), it does yield a pattern that is psychologically meaningful. On this evidence, his suggestion that a personality need model is appropriate to interests seems to be worth pursuing.

*Table 14.3 Personality needs related to leisure interests*

| Type | Personality needs | | Interest factors | |
|------|-------------------|------|------------------|------|
| (1) Athletic | Play | 0.51 | Sports | 0.60 |
| | Dominance | 0.36 | Outdoor–Activity | 0.43 |
| | Understanding | −0.60 | Cultural–Intellectual | −0.49 |
| | Harm avoidance | −0.49 | Hobby–Domestic | −0.22 |
| (2) Cautious | Harm avoidance | 0.70 | Social interaction | 0.22 |
| | Social recognition | 0.25 | Nature | −0.59 |
| | Sentience | −0.48 | Outdoor–Active | −0.56 |
| | Understanding | −0.41 | Mechanics | −0.42 |
| (3) Confident | Exhibition | 0.62 | Social interaction | 0.65 |
| | Dominance | 0.49 | Cultural–Intellectual | 0.41 |
| | Aggression | 0.46 | Hobby–Domestic | −0.43 |
| | Abasement | −0.34 | Swimming | −0.29 |
| (4) Independent | Autonomy | 0.52 | Mechanics | 0.40 |
| | Nurturance | −0.62 | Hobby–Domestic | −0.69 |
| | Affiliation | −0.57 | Social interaction | −0.47 |
| | Sentience | −0.56 | Sports | −0.24 |

Note: Examples of the highest loading items for each type are given. Based on Allen[22]

Howard[23] also correlated Murray's needs with leisure interest factors in a group of 139 high school students. Having replicated three of Witt's four factors, he found several of the need scores from Jackson's questionnaire to correlate up to 0.30 with these factors. The needs of aggression, impulsivity and play correlated around 0.23 with the Sports' factor, while order and nurturance produced negative correlations of a similar size. The needs of endurance, dominance and autonomy correlated around 0.18 with the Outdoor–Nature factor, with harm avoidance correlating negatively. Finally, the needs of exhibition and dominance correlated around 0.24 with what he labelled an Aesthetic–Sophisticate factor.

In conclusion, personality has been shown to be related to interest preferences, but at a rather low level. Perhaps because of the specific nature of interest factors, it is expecting too much for general personality dimensions to show anything other than tenuous relationships to them. A more fruitful approach might be to relate specific personality traits to the interest factors. With the different components of extraversion, we would be in a better position to define the sports type as opposed to the social type (both of which are related to general extraversion). Similarly, personality assessment based on Murray's need theory may help further in differentiating between the specific interest types.

## FAMILY INFLUENCE

Choice of leisure activities may, instead of reflecting personality or other attributes, be more a function of family or peer influence. In the study by Nias[5], because the adult sample consisted of the parents of the school children, it was possible to look at husband–wife similarities in interest preferences[24]. Although it was not possible to control for the degree to which these couples had similar interests before meeting, it may be worth looking at the nature of the interests they have in common after at least 12 years of marriage. Table 14.4 shows the interest preferences for which husbands and wives had the most and least degree

*Table 14.4   Interests for which couples were most and least similar*

|  | *Two highest correlations* | | *Two lowest correlations* | |
|---|---|---|---|---|
| Leisure | Going out for a drink | 0.34 | Cooking | 0.01 |
|  | Going to dances | 0.34 | Reading | −0.04 |
| TV | Variety shows | 0.29 | Adventure films | 0.07 |
|  | Pop music programmes | 0.37 | News | 0.07 |
| Reading | Pop music magazines | 0.31 | Newspaper news | −0.01 |
|  | Romance magazines | 0.22 | Adventure stories | 0.00 |
| Sport | Watching favourite sport | 0.40 | Sports ability at school | 0.03 |
|  | Watching with children | 0.47 | Watching aged 10–15 years | 0.04 |
| Encouraging | Music | 0.57 | Practical school subjects | 0.18 |
| children in: | Part-time jobs | 0.51 | Looking smart | 0.23 |

Note: Data are from 586 husband–wife pairs. Based on Nias[24]

of similarity. The average correlation between the 586 couples for 82 interest items was 0.18. This was higher than a correlation of 0.08 obtained for a set of 80 personality items answered by the same sample. There was no evidence of a general tendency for couples to have opposite or complementary interests, with the correlation of $-0.04$ for reading being the nearest to a significantly negative relationship.

The interest items showing the highest correlations between couples tended to be for activities they encouraged in their children, such as music and part-time jobs. These items are concerned with a common interest, i.e. their child. Other relatively high correlations were concerned with activities that couples can do together, such as going out for a drink, i.e. a joint interest. One of the highest correlations from the personality inventory was also of this nature, i.e. 'Do you like going out a lot?'. In contrast, the interest items with the lowest correlations between couples were concerned with more solitary activities, such as reading and cooking.

There is also evidence that type of leisure activity is related to marital satisfaction. Orthner[25] attempted to demonstrate the truth of the slogan, 'The family that plays together, stays together', with a sample of just over 200 couples. Those pursuing joint or shared leisure activities expressed a greater degree of marital satisfaction than did those pursuing parallel activities. Worst off were those pursuing individual activities. The results were most clear for those couples who had not been married for long.

Nias[5] also looked for parent–child similarities in interest preferences. The correlations between parents and their children, for the interests they had in common, were small but positive giving an average of 0.11 (which, because of the large sample size, was still significant). There was a slight tendency for the highest correlations to be between children and their same sex parent. The single highest correlation was between mother and daughter for playing a musical instrument (0.40); other high correlations included watching sports (especially for father and son), reading about sport, and watching cartoon films. Items at the other extreme gave an interesting contrast, with the lowest being between father and daughter for shopping ($-0.07$) and for going to dances ($-0.07$). Although these two negative correlations are of borderline significance, it is not difficult to think of reasons why fathers may lack enthusiasm for these activities if their daughters are too keen!

We thus have evidence for a small degree of similarity in the interests of married couples, and of parents and their children. If the similarity of couples is over and above what they had on first meeting, then this evidence together with that for parents and children is consistent with the hypothesis that choice of leisure time activity is partly determined by the family. As with personality, however, it must be stressed that the relationship is only slight, which leads to the general conclusion that a person's interests are determined by an interaction of many influences of which no single one is dominant and, of course, that interests are determined by factors other than those evaluated so far. Peer influence is almost certainly another determinant, but has yet to be studied in relation to interests. That such an approach is likely to be fruitful is suggested by studies on addiction, which show that the use of heroin and other drugs tends to start and spread among groups of friends[26].

## MOTIVATIONS

In considering the determinants of leisure activity, and noting that the usual personality and demographic correlates reveal only a slight relationship, it should be recognized that individuals may choose to pursue the same interest but for different reasons. Nias[5, 17] suggested that closer relationships would be obtained by relating personality and other variables 'not to interest areas, but to the motives people have for pursuing these interests'. A recent study has approached the issue in this way.

Instead of looking for the dimensions of leisure interests, Tinsley and Kass[27, 28] factor analysed the needs or motivations underlying leisure participation. Selecting the leisure activity (jogging, watching TV, etc.) with which they were most familiar, 417 students were asked to rate 'how true' each of 45 need-satisfiers (independence, activity, advancement, etc.) were regarding participation in that activity. These need items were then factor analysed giving some eight factors. The first was interpreted as being concerned with 'self-actualization' or fulfilment of proficiency, the second 'being with others', and so on. In order to see which need factors were perceived as being met by leisure activity, these eight factors were correlated with the ten leisure activities upon which they were based. This revealed a number of meaningful relationships. For example, jogging was found to represent the need for self-actualization and for autonomy, rather than the need for intellectual challenge.

Although it is relevant to enquire which needs are met by given leisure activities, it is difficult to know from this study the extent to which the students' answers reflected *their own* need satisfactions. It is possible that in rating 'how true' a need is concerning an activity, they were relying on *intellectual* rather than *personal* evaluation. In other words, to say that it is 'very true' that the need for self-actualization is met by jogging makes good sense, but does it really mean that the rater's need is met in this way? The evidence needs to be supplemented by showing that people high on the need for self-actualization are, indeed, more likely to participate in jogging than are people low on this need. Such evidence is available regarding participation in 'wilderness' weekends.

The *Personal Orientation Inventory* by Shostrom attempts to measure a person's degree of self-actualization or positive mental health. Items were selected from this scale by Young and Crandall[29] to see if wilderness users scored higher than did a random sample of the population. It was thought that the wilderness, involving an aesthetically pleasing and physically challenging environment, would help provide the chance for 'peak experiences' or moments of transcendence that are basic to the concept of self-actualization. In Illinois, it is necessary to apply for a permit to make use of the wilderness areas and it was thus possible to compare a group of 222 permit holders with a group of 503 randomly selected adults. As predicted, the wilderness users did obtain a significantly higher score on self-actualization. Not too much should be made of this result, however, since the reliability of the widely-used Shostrom scale is open to question[30].

The approach of assessing the needs that are met by involvement in different leisure activities, and supplementing this with evidence that people high on these needs are indeed more likely to participate in such activities, seems to be a useful line of attack. The work by Allen and Howard relating Murray's personality need theory to leisure activities, already described, lends further support to this recommendation[22, 23].

## HEREDITY

Discussions of the factors that determine leisure preferences almost always leave out the possible role of heredity. This topic, however, should perhaps be taken as the starting point in considering alternative theories on what it is that influences an individual's choice of leisure time activity. Presumably it is through the inheritance of personality traits, including needs, that heredity plays a part in influencing choice of leisure activity.

After an exhaustive review of the twin evidence, including his own large-scale surveys, Nichols[31] concluded that identical twin correlations are higher than fraternal twin correlations by about 0.20 for a variety of traits of ability, personality, and interests. For interests, the difference between weighted averages from intraclass correlations for identical and fraternal twins ranged from 0.22 for artistic interests to 0.11 for business or enterprising interests. Nichols was struck by the remarkable similarity of results for ability, personality and interests as well as for the more specific traits within the three domains. All this was interpreted as indicating that about half of the variation among people in a broad spectrum of psychological traits, including interests, is due to genetics. Essentially the same conclusion has emerged from our own work on the inheritance of traits of altruism, empathy, nurturance, aggressiveness and assertiveness[32].

## EFFECTS OF RECREATION

Numerous studies provide evidence on the effects that leisure activity can have on happiness, well-being and mental health. A few examples will suffice to illustrate the potential importance of leisure.

It has often been demonstrated that job satisfaction is related to overall happiness or self-rated quality of life. London and colleagues[33] extended this to include leisure. A nationally representative sample of 1297 adults rated the overall quality of their life by responding to the question: 'How do you feel about your life as a whole?' on a seven-point scale ranging from 1 (delighted) to 7 (terrible). The mean score obtained was 2.59 indicating some degree of happiness. They were also asked to rate how they felt about aspects of their work and leisure. Job and leisure satisfactions were found to be relatively independent, with both being related to overall quality of life. Table 14.5 presents the mean scores for the leisure items, together with an indication of how each was related to quality of life. The average person claimed to derive most satisfaction from activities involving the whole family (score of 2.19), and this item was the one most closely related to perceived quality of life (*beta* weight of 0.26).

288

*Table 14.5  Leisure satisfaction and perceived quality of life*

| Item | Mean | Beta weight |
|---|---|---|
| (1) The things you do and the times you have with your friends | 2.46 | 0.17 |
| (2) The things you and your family do together | 2.19 | 0.26 |
| (3) The people you see socially | 2.21 | −0.01 |
| (4) The organizations you belong to | 2.48 | 0.05 |
| (5) The sports and recreation facilities you yourself use, or would like to use – I mean things like parks, bowling alleys, beaches | 3.16 | 0.06 |
| (6) The entertainment you get from TV, radio, movies, and local events and places | 3.48 | 0.04 |

Note: Adults described their feelings about each item on a seven-point scale ranging from 1 (delighted) to 7 (terrible). The *beta* weights indicate the degree to which each item predicted 'quality of life'. Based on London, Crandall and Seals[33]

Another example of a study to identify the factors contributing to life satisfaction was carried out among women aged 65 years and over[34]. Leisure activity participation (time spent socializing with friends, gardening, going for walks, etc.) was closely associated with perceived life satisfaction (happiness, morale, etc.). The association was even higher than it was for income or health, which probably means that lack of money or health problems restricts participation in leisure activity which in turn detracts from overall happiness.

Direct evidence of an effect of leisure participation comes from a study by Griest and colleagues[35]. Moderately depressed neurotic outpatients were randomly assigned to behavioural or dynamic psychotherapy or to a graduated programme of walking–jogging–running. The jogging and behavioural psychotherapy groups appeared to improve as assessed by self-ratings of mood, with the improvement still apparent at follow-up over the next year. Also most of the patients had continued with their new found interest in jogging. The results of this study are based on too small a sample to be significant, but it does fit in with the observation that a range of activities (occupational therapy, relaxation classes, being interviewed, etc.) can act to reduce mood dysfunction on a daily basis (i.e. at least in the short term) in some depressed people.

A final area worth mentioning concerns the effects of competitive sport. Several researchers have suggested that competition can detract from the intrinsic value of sport[36]. For example, it has been demonstrated that children feel more anxious following a competitive task if the competition is with others rather than with themselves[37]. It is, however, also likely that some individuals derive satisfaction from the competitive nature of sport, and would not participate were it not for this rivalry. As in other areas, individual differences always exist to prove the rule.

## CONCLUSIONS

First, factor analysis indicates leisure activity preferences to be specific rather than general. This conclusion contrasts with the general dimensions found to underlie abilities and personality. Second, the genetic component to interest preferences has to be taken into account, and seems to be similar to that for abilities and personality. The genetic mechanism, probably acting via specific personality traits and needs, might explain why a closer relationship between personality and interests has been obtained for specific needs than for the major dimensions of personality. Third, the finding that parents express similar interests to their children, albeit only slightly, is consistent with the notion of a family influence on interest development.

The size of the correlations so far obtained between different leisure preferences, and between leisure preferences and their correlates, is not really high enough to justify individual assessment and guidance. At the moment the findings are of more relevance to group research and policy than to individuals. The correlations, in the sense of being prediction coefficients, are both smaller and fewer than are those for occupations[38]. The parallel to vocational guidance, involving the use of empirical tests linking an individual's profile to career choice, does not yet seem to be a practical proposition – although we are moving in that direction.

Improvements in research design may help to change this state of affairs. So far researchers have tended not to build on to previous research, with the result that different studies have not been properly integrated and the research has tended to be atheoretical. We have seen that many researchers have attempted to arrive at a classificatory system for interests, with different names being given to similar factors. These studies have involved different sets of items, different instructions to the subjects, and less than rigorous methods of analysis. Moreover, theoretical formulations have not been made and even basic questions, such as whether it matters if the subjects are not familiar with the activities being rated, have not been investigated.

Interviews with children and their parents often reveal that boredom is a major problem. In one large-scale survey, American children were found to have few hobbies or outside interests, spent most of their spare time watching TV, and complained of feeling bored[39]. This pattern was especially true for the more disadvantaged children. Since constructive leisure pursuits can enhance happiness (e.g. people often express surprise at the pleasure a new hobby or pastime can give them), and since for the unemployed leisure is a forced alternative to work, people should benefit from being educated and encouraged to make good use of their leisure. To this end, books on leisure counselling[40] are beginning to emerge, providing a practical application of the type of research reviewed in this chapter.

## References

1. Strong, E. K. (1943). *Vocational Interests of Men and Women*. (California: Stanford University Press)
2. Sandall, P. H. (1960). An analysis of the interests of secondary school pupils. PhD thesis, University of London.

3. Guilford, J. P., Christensen, P. R., Bond, N. A. and Sutton, M. A. (1954). A factor analysis study of human interests. *Psychol. Monogr.*, **68**, Whole No. 375
4. Eysenck, H. J. (1970). *The Structure of Human Personality*. 3rd Edn. (London: Methuen)
5. Nias, D. K. B. (1975). Personality and other factors determining the recreational interests of children and adults. PhD thesis, University of London
6. Rounds, J. B. and Davis, R. V. (1979). Factor analysis of *Strong Vocational Interest Blank* items. *J. Appl. Psychol.*, **64**, 132–43
7. Chisnall, B. (1942). The interests and personality traits of delinquent boys. *Br. J. Educ. Psychol.*, **12**, 76
8. Hammond, W. H. (1945). An analysis of youth centre interests. *Br. J. Educ. Psychol.*, **15**, 122–6
9. Stephenson, W. (1936). A new application of correlation to averages. *Br. J. Educ. Psychol.*, **6**, 43–57
10. Sandall, P. H. (1967). *Manual of Instructions of the Factorial Interest Blank*. (Slough: NFER)
11. Cottle, W. C. (1950). A factorial study of the Multiphasic, Strong, Kuder and Bell inventories using a population of adult males. *Psychometrika*, **15**, 25–47
12. Thurnstone, L. L. (1931). A multiple factor study of vocational interests. *Pers. J.*, **10**, 198–205
13. Vernon, P. E. (1949). Classifying high-grade occupational interests. *J. Abnorm. Soc. Psychol.*, **44**, 85–96
14. Brogden, H. E. (1952). The primary personal values measured by the Allport–Vernon test 'A Study of Values'. *Psychol. Monogr.*, **66**, Whole No. 348
15. Bishop, D. W. (1970). Stability of the factor structure of leisure behaviour: analyses of four communities. *J. Leisure Res.*, **2**, 160–70
16. Witt, P. A. (1971). Factor structure of leisure behavior for high school age youth in three communities. *J. Leisure Res.*, **3**, 213–19
17. Nias, D. K. B. (1977). The structuring of recreational interests. *Soc. Behav. Pers.*, **5**, 383–8
18. Nias, D. K. B. (1979). The classification and correlates of children's academic and recreational interests. *J. Child Psychol. Psychiatry*, **20**, 73–9
19. Gorsuch, R. L. (1974). *Factor Analysis*. (Philadelphia: Saunders)
20. Willmott, P. (1971). Family, work and leisure conflicts among male employees. *Hum. Relations*, **24**, 575–84
21. Furnham, A. (1984). Personality and values. *Pers. Individ. Diff.*, **5**, 483–5
22. Allen, L. R. (1982). The relationship between Murray's personality needs and leisure interests. *J. Leisure Res.*, **14**, 63–76
23. Howard, D. R. (1976). Multivariate relationships between leisure activities and personality. *Res. Q.*, **47**, 226–37
24. Nias, D. K. B. (1977). Husband–wife similarities. *Soc. Sci.*, **52**, 206–11
25. Orthner, D. K. (1975). Leisure activity patterns and marital satisfaction over the marital career. *J. Marriage Fam.*, **37**, 91–102
26. Hughes, P. H. and Crawford, G. A. (1972). A contagious disease model for researching and intervening in heroin epidemics. *Arch. Gen. Psychiatry*, **27**, 149–55
27. Tinsley, H. E. A. and Kass, R. A. (1978). Life activities and need satisfaction: a replication and extension. *J. Leisure Res.*, **10**, 191–202
28. Tinsley, H. E. A. and Kass, R. A. (1979). The latent structure of the need satisfying properties of leisure activities. *J. Leisure Res.*, **11**, 278–91
29. Young, R. A. and Crandall, R. (1984). Wilderness use and self-actualization. *J. Leisure Res.*, **16**, 149–60
30. Ray, J. J. (1984). A caution against use of the Shostrom *Personal Orientation Inventory*. *Pers. Individ. Diff*, **5**, 755
31. Nichols, R. C. (1979). *Heredity and Environment: Major Findings from Twin Studies of Ability, Personality and Interests*. (New York: IAAEE)
32. Rushton, J. P., Fulker, D. W., Neale, M. C., Nias, D. K. B. and Eysenck, H. J. (1985). Altruism and aggression: to what extent are individual differences inherited? *J. Pers. Soc. Psychol.*, in press
33. London, M., Crandall, R. and Seals, G. W. (1977). The contribution of job and leisure satisfaction to quality of life. *J. Appl. Psychol.*, **62**, 328–34
34. Riddick, C. C. and Daniel, S. N. (1984). The relative contribution of leisure activities and other factors to the mental health of older women. *J. Leisure Res.*, **16**, 136–48

35. Griest, J. H., Klein, M. H., Eischens, R. R., Faris, J., Gurman, A. S. and Morgan, W. P. (1979). Running as treatment for depression. *Compr. Psychiatry*, **20**, 41–54
36. Dickinson, J. (1976). *A Behavioural Analysis of Sport*. (London: Lepus Books)
37. Corbin, C. B., Barnett, M. A. and Matthews, K. A. (1979). The effects of direct and indirect competition on children's state anxiety. *J. Leisure Res.*, **4**, 271–7
38. Ghiselli, E. E. (1966). *The Validity of Occupational Aptitude Tests*. (New York: Wiley)
39. Loesch, L. C. and Wheeler, P. T. (1982). *Principles of Leisure Counseling*. (Minneapolis: Educational Media Corporation)
40. Medrich, E. A., Roizen, J., Rubin, V. and Buckley, S. (1982). *The Serious Business of Growing Up: A Study of Children's Lives Outside School*. (Berkeley: University of California Press)

# 15
## Sex differences in play

## *Marsha B. Liss*

---

## INTRODUCTION

Over the past 50 years much has been written about children's play with a concentration on sex roles or sex-differentiated activities. A great deal of this literature has focused primarily on what children choose to play with and the corresponding gender-identification measures as well as the role of parents, teachers and peers in influencing these decisions. An extensive discussion of these aspects can be found in Liss[1]. This chapter, however, will concentrate on *how* children play with these toys and the relationship of toy play to skill learning. The chapter will examine how the types of toys children choose affect their skill development in the area of movement and play.

First there will be a brief summary of the sex-differentiated areas of play typically found in most Western cultures from preschool (ages 3–5) through secondary school. Then attention will shift to the major areas in which investigators have examined the incorporation of skills into play. Following this will be a section on the amenability to change or modify sex-typed play and the implications of these changes for later development.

## SEX-DIFFERENTIATED ACTIVITIES

Surveys of what children prefer to play with are the oldest type of sex-linked play studies. Over 50 years ago pioneering researchers[2–4] examined with whom and with what children played. Each of these researchers found that boys played predominantly with boys and girls with girls. The types of inter-actions within the same-sex dyads and groups were similar for boys and girls beginning with *non-interactive* play (such as solitary functions) and then progressing first to *parallel* play and finally to *co-operative* play. Moreover, the researchers found that the boys and girls tended to play in different sections of the classrooms, findings which have been replicated in varying degrees to this day.

293

The most commonly cited female-traditional areas have been kitchen, dolls, sewing, dress-up, and singing/music, while those traditionally followed by boys have been transportation toys, blocks, guns and sports. In addition to the early investigations mentioned above, there have been periodic replications (e.g. 1960s[5, 6], 1970s[7–9], 1980s[10, 11]). The vast majority of these studies have centred on observations of the preschool classroom. However, there have been a few studies tracing sex-differentiated play interests to infancy[12] and the toddler period[13]. There have been relatively few studies in the social sciences focusing on sex-differentiated play in the older grade school or secondary school years; exceptions to this lack are the works of Liss and Etaugh[14] and Plumb and Cowan[15].

Liss and Etaugh[14] found that boys prefer to play with and request to receive sex-typed toys (such as balls and transportation toys) more than girls want female-traditional items (such as arts and crafts and dolls) with a maximum sex difference in the middle years. Moreover, they noted that there were more age than sex differences in their study. Plumb and Cowan[15] showed that boys greatly differentiated between male and female toys compared with girls' assessments. The cross-sectional work of Plumb and Cowan was based on adolescent subjects noting that 'tomboys' showed the fewest sex-typed choices as predicted. These tomboys are girls who do not prefer male-traditional activities, but rather, choose *both* male and female activities approaching destereotyping or androgyny. The age trend issue emerging from these studies has not been addressed extensively and is probably less reliable than the sex-typing issue.

A recent review of the literature on sex-related preferences[16] found strikingly *fewer* differences than similarities. Liss concluded that the literature has focused on the small number of differences perhaps due to the problems of statistical significance at the cost of overlooking or not reporting similarities. In addition, methodological considerations make many of the sex-differentiated play findings non-comparable or the results at least ambiguous. Lastly, the lack of consistency in recent studies of sex differences in play may reflect evolving societal notions of early sex roles which may become consistent or disappear altogether with time. The reader is advised to keep these qualifications in mind when reading the remainder of the chapter and original articles.


## HOW BOYS AND GIRLS PLAY

There are surprisingly few studies addressing how children play with similar materials. In this literature researchers examine not only how children play with their favourite items but how they handle the *same* play materials. The questions addressed here ask what skills boys and girls bring to their play and what they acquire in play. An underlying theme states that prior experience with the sex-differentiated toys given by parents, and activities encouraged by teachers, direct boys and girls to play and develop differently. This notion of play styles and the relationship to particular skills is best articulated by Block[17]. Block examined sex-differentiated play both on observation and theoretical levels developing a model of how one activity leads to the next. The most commonly cited distinction falls within activity levels and motor skills – between gross and fine motor skills, the former attributed to boys and the latter to girls.

## High Activity Level

The category of high activity includes such dimensions as gross motor skills and aggression. Gross motor skills have been associated with play by boys fostered by activities classified as traditionally masculine (transportation toys, sports highlighting contact sports and aggressive activities). One study examining play with transportation toys[18] looked at both absolute behaviours and rating of children at play. More than any other toy activity, truck play yielded more movement about the room (coded as activity level) and more actions termed as gadgetry. Males were furthermore labelled as more active by observers as well as more familiar with, enjoying more and playing correctly (or traditionally) with trucks compared with girls. The truck play movement scores were contributed primarily by males but the contrary was found for gadgetry (to be discussed further later in this chapter).

One highly microlevel analysis was performed by Halverson, Roberton and Langendorfer[19]. They found that early kindergarten arm-throwing movements by boys and girls were not significantly different from one another but over the course of the grade to secondary school years the sexes' abilities in this area diverged dramatically. Self-reports by the observed subjects indicate that boys engaged in more practice and use of this movement than girls did which then resulted in enhanced abilities usually associated with male sports.

*Aggressive* play has been called alternatively *rough-and-tumble* play or gross motor play. Often associated with males it is seen in adult sports activities such as football, ice hockey and the like. This type of play is characterized by frequent contacts with a goal of knocking down the other player, but without an explicit goal of inflicting harm on the playmate. Rough-and-tumble play differences are found in both human and primate young and are dominated by males[20]. Until recently most of the studies on this subject reported expanded or all-encompassing categories of active play within the category. For example, Langlois, Gottfried, and Seay[21] found that males were the recipients and instigators of aggression but did not distinguish aggressive play from active play from rough-and-tumble play. Likewise, according to the landmark cross-cultural work of Whiting and Edwards[22], males engage in more rough-and-tumble play defined as including aggression and unfortunately obscuring interpretation in this cross-cultural work.

However, DiPietro[23] broke down the category of rough-and-tumble play into several components and observed triads of preschoolers. She found that on all but two categories (out of a possible 12 dimensions) males were the aggressors as well as the recipients. These included wrestling, taking, activity level as well as more negative aspects such as physical assault (differentiated further into playful and aggressive). Girls, on the other hand, engaged in high activity behaviours but of a qualitatively different nature: girls tended to jump.

This is not surprising if one looks at the type of games young girls enjoy such as jump-rope and skipping. Girls also waited turns more than boys did. DiPietro further examined two sources contributing to this effect: the type of interactions with mothers (e.g. engaging in active play with their young and play with another identified only by gender) as well as biological predispositions to that effect. While no conclusive evidence for the latter is presented, evidence from the non-human primate literature is used as support.

Halliday and McNaughton[24] report measuring rough-and-tumble play along with choice of play-area and toy. While rough-and-tumble play occurred too infrequently to perform statistical tests of significance it is noteworthy that *only* males engaged in this behaviour. Likewise only males engaged in what Halliday and McNaughton called aggressive behaviour. Furthermore, Halliday and McNaughton found few other differences in what boys and girls do; girls engaged in more parallel play compared with boys' solitary play especially in climbing. It also appears that girls were more active physically with respect to climbing. This result, however, is qualified by teachers' proximity to the climbing equipment encouraging dominance by girls. See Liss[1] for discussions of influence of teacher presence. Aside from climbing results, other contentions regarding high energy level activities favouring boys were supported.

In the context of studying males with gender identity problems, Klein and Bates[25] measured a series of sex-differentiated movements during play. The first three were called *gender presentation movements* and refer to movements believed to be sex-typed and serve to enhance or inhibit play[26]: leg separation, pelvis roll and trunk–limb independence. The male correlates to these variables (legs at 10–15° angles, pelvis rolled back and trunk–limb independence) enhance rapid activity with larger more powerful movements. They also tested such variables as expensive movements, large space usage, erect posture, fluid movements and purposeful movements. Although their final study involved only boys they noted that highly masculine identified boys showed the foregoing behaviours while those with identity issues had patterns resembling those predicted for girls.

In a recent meta-analysis of aggression sex-differences[27], Hyde reports few discussions of sex differences in the play literature over the past few years. She further states that the conclusion reached by Maccoby and Jacklin in 1974[28] that there are sex differences in aggression is an illusory conclusion. Hyde says that there are fewer studies reporting such differences than there are those finding patterns of similarity between males and females. However, as noted earlier, the significant differences literature surpasses the similarities literature in part due to tendencies to report positive rather than negative results (rejections rather than failures to reject the null hypothesis).

Low Activity Level

The main dimension of low activity level, examined in the literature to date, has been fine motor skills. This opposite end of the activity continuum is associated with female play such as doll play, sewing and arts and crafts. In addition these types of female-preferred areas require fairly sedentary behaviours on the part of the participant; dolls are not generally thrown or chased, art work requires sitting, 'house' is not highly active in terms of space. These differences may contribute to the absence of gross motor and rough-and-tumble play of girls. Even in their reasonings there are signs of physical movement differences and conceptions of interactions between the sexes.

Using dolls as the medium, Liss[18] examined skills or behaviours generated by boys and girls in this type of play. Doll play generated more aggression as well as more nurturance on the part of both sexes compared to play with other toys. Females were, however, more nurturant than boys as well as displaying more positive affect in their comments. Girls were also rated as more talkative in doll play than in other types of play and more talkative in doll play than boys were. Girls were also rated as more active in doll play although it should be noted that their doll play was less active as defined earlier than boys' truck play. Females were more gentle in all forms of play but especially when playing with dolls. In contrast to the results for boys mentioned earlier, girls were more familiar, enjoyed and played more traditionally with dolls than boys did.

As discussed above, Liss[18] reported a most curious finding in the area of truck play as measured by ratings of gadgetry. While earlier work (see Maccoby and Jacklin[28]) would have labelled the gadgetry behaviour as masculine, results here point to the use of traditionally female skills as a strong component transferred to other play. That is, the fine motor skills and movements used in dressing and playing with dolls, sewing and other female traditional acts are then incorporated into play with the masculine toy of trucks. This finding of girls' truck play using the gadgetry behaviour is further evidence of the training of fine motor skills in traditionally female categories and the generalization of this skill to other activities.

Teacher Influences

Carpenter and Huston-Stein[29] have discussed a new notion with respect to method of play, called *structure*. Their series of studies (summarized in Carpenter[30]) show that boys and girls play in activities with different levels of structure and that girls favour the more structured areas. Their work involved observational methods of data collection and categorization of the types of activities. They further note that structure is related to teacher presence (such as that mentioned in discussing Halliday and McNaughton's work[24]) and differences in cognitive skills.

Another researcher with extensive work in the area of preschoolers' sex-typed behaviours in the classroom is Fagot. Through a series of studies[11, 31–33]. Fagot explored social play in preschool and the effects of teacher feedback on peer relationships and sex-typed play. She noted that teachers often direct children to sex-linked activities and that both peers and teacher give more positive feedback to sex-traditional children[32, 34]. Fagot's more recent work has shifted to examining the relationship of social play behaviours to cognitive and movement variables. An early effort in this area[31] positively correlated preschool participation in male traditional play activities with later interest in science and mathematics, especially for girls. In particular she has used a factor analytic approach to develop factors of play which outline skill development and sex differences[11]. For instance, males are more explorative in play, less verbal, more likely to hurt, shove and play with technical toys as well as being more active and acting more upon the environment than girls.

## Additional Variables

Another factor affecting children's sex-typed play which has received attention from a scant number of researchers is children's *clothing*. This represents a truly pragmatic consideration – some clothes are easier to play in than other clothes (skirts are not suitable for climbing, for instance). It is therefore no coincidence that Kaiser and Phinney[35] found that children recognize that traditional female clothes (skirts or dresses) are associated with female activities (not just with females *per se*) of a sedentary nature while boys' apparel and more androgynous female's clothes (trousers) are associated with male activities. The ease of play in climbing and running is clear and needs no further elaboration except to indicate that the way a child is dressed creates expectations for the child's behaviour and gives a clear message directing him/her to certain types of play.

Etaugh[36] points out that *group size* and *type of play* behaviour are related to gender. Boys' activities foster group play according to rules and high energy activities. The boys make contact within the context of play as in sports but not in intimate social interactions. Girls, on the other hand, play in smaller groups with less physical direct contact but with more proximity to one another and more verbal social skills.

## INTERVENTION STUDIES

Another important area for discussing sex-differentiated play refers to the studies aimed at modification or intervention. The general plan of such studies is to take children with highly sex-typed behaviours (play choices or styles) and modify or influence these behaviours. The most common paradigms are direct reinforcement and modelling techniques. Typically, the age groups involved have been preschool (ages 2–4) or kindergarten (ages 5–6) periods.

The intervention studies fall into three categories: (1) those whose aim is to affect changes in toy preferences or choices; (2) those whose aim is to increase cross-sex play; and (3) those whose aim is to train children in specific skills. Most of those studies have been laboratory studies but those performed in classrooms will be noted as they arise.

## Modelling Studies of Toy Preferences

Wolf[37] and Liss[8], for instance, showed male and female children single live or multiple videotaped models, respectively, playing with toys. While the subjects generally played with sex-typed toys, those who had seen same-sex models playing with opposite-sex traditional (or sex-non-traditional) toys chose to play with those toys at significantly increased rates compared to other children.

Critics of the generalizability of these studies have cited the strong presence of sex-typed behaviours in classrooms and peer playgroups as drawbacks to the programme's utility in destereotyping children. Liss and Doyle[38] addressed this type of criticism by pointing to the impact of peers as modifiers of modelling effects. As before, each subject viewed videotaped models at play and then was given the opportunity to play with a range of sex-typed and non-sex-typed toys. In contrast to earlier projects, two subjects each of whom had viewed the 'programme' separately were then brought to the playroom. The effect of the peer (also a subject) eliminated the expected modelling effect. Other studies of this genre have been performed with similar results: increased flexibility of toy choice if allowed to view and play alone, but lack of change of breadth of play from traditional behaviours if a peer is present. It is clear that to retain the flexibility all children need to know is that their peers are willing to play with non-traditional toys as well.

Reinforcement Studies of Cross-sex Play

The second group of studies is typified by a 1977 endeavour by Serbin, Tonick and Sternglanz[39]. This research differed from the above in two ways: setting (classroom vs. laboratory) and paradigm (direct reinforcement vs. modelling). Teachers verbally reinforced boys and girls for cross-sex play with respect to both type and gender of playmate. During the experimental phases boys and girls increased rates of cross-sex co-operative play. The importance and extent of this type of environmental control has been discussed by Fagot and Leinbach[11]. Fagot and Leinbach believe that teachers' and peers' response (*naturalistic* occurrence) or intervention (*planned*) can significantly develop wider ranges and experiences for boys and girls. However, they indicate that in most classrooms, teachers and peers are bound by traditional choices. This point is further elaborated by Bianchi and Bakeman[40, 41] who describe an open classroom (non-structured) with broadly encouraged experiences for boys and girls. Children in these special environments behave like the subjects in Serbin, Tonick and Sternglanz's experimental phase[39].

Development of Special Skills

The last type of activity in this section is represented by the work of Serbin and her colleagues[42-45]. They have demonstrated that specific skills (visual–spatial skills) can be developed and maintained. The importance of their work is the implication that visual–spatial skill differences between boys and girls are easily modifiable and may be derivatives of early play and reinforcement histories rather than innate differences between the sexes. As with the cross-sex play studies, these experiments have involved *reinforcement paradigms*. In addition, they have included training on tests such as the Children's Embedded Figures Test (CEFT) showing how skills transfer to the test settings. The basis for these tasks is the hypothesis that male-traditional toys promote the development of visual–spatial skills by use of eye–hand co-ordination and movements and transformations such as found in gross motor activities and block play, for example. Serbin's work casts doubt on Maccoby and Jacklin's claim[28] of male inherent dominance in visual–spatial skills.

## SUMMARY

In this chapter several questions regarding the issue of sex-differences in play have been addressed: What do boys and girls play with? Are there differences in boys' and girls' play behaviours such as fine and gross motor activities? Are there differences in preparation for play? Do children learn the same skills from male-traditional and female-traditional toys and do they transfer these skills to other toys? Are children's preferences, play behaviours and play-related skills predetermined by gender or are they subject to learning and subsequent modification?

In reviewing the answers suggested by the research discussed in this chapter, the reader may come to the conclusion that there is ongoing change in the area of sex differences in play. It will be important to continue to examine the changes in the literature itself within the decade. The most important lesson for movement, however, is that children learn *through* play and that exposure to a wide variety of sex-linked activities increases breadth.

## References

1. Liss, M. B. (1983). Learning gender-related skills through play. In Liss, M. B. (ed.) *Social and Cognitive Skills: Sex Roles and Children's Play*. pp. 147–66. (New York: Academic Press)
2. Benjamin, H. (1932). Age and sex differences in toy preferences of young children. *J. Genet. Psychol.*, **41**, 417–29
3. Bridges, K. M. B. (1927). Occupational interests of three-year old children. *J. Genet. Psychol.*, **34**, 415–23
4. Parten, M. B. (1932). Social participation among preschool children. *J. Abnorm. Soc. Psychol.*, **27**, 243–62
5. Clark, A. H., Wyon, S. M. and Richards, M. P. M. (1969). Free play in nursery school children. *J. Child Psychol. Psychiatry*, **10**, 205–16
6. Fagot, B. I. and Patterson, G. R. (1969). An *in vivo* analysis of reinforcing contingencies for sex-role behaviors in the preschool child. *Dev. Psychol.*, **1**, 563–8
7. Fagot, B. I. (1977). Consequences of moderate cross-gender behaviour in preschool children. *Child Dev.*, **48**, 902–7
8. Liss, M. B. (1979). Variables influencing modelling and sex-typed play. *Psychol. Rep.*, **44**, 1107–17
9. Smith, P. K. and Connolly, K. (1972). Patterns of play and social interaction in preschool children. In Jones, N. B. (ed.) *Ethological Studies of Child Behaviour*. (London: Cambridge University Press)

10. McLoyd, V. C. (1980). Verbally expressed modes of transformation in the fantasy play of black preschool children. *Child Dev.*, **51**, 1133-9
11. Fagot, B. I. and Leinbach, M. D. (1983). Play styles in early childhood: social consequences for boys and girls. In Liss, M. B. (ed.) *Social and Cognitive Skills: Sex Roles and Children's Play*. pp. 93-116. (New York: Academic Press)
12. Goldberg, S. and Lewis, M. (1969). Play behaviour in the year-old child. *Child Dev.*, **40**, 21-31
13. Fein, G., Johnson, D., Kosson, N., Stork, L. and Wasserman, L. (1975). Sex stereotypes and preferences in the toy choices of 20 month-old boys and girls. *Dev. Psychol.*, **11**, 527-8
14. Liss, M. B. and Etaugh, C. (1983). *Home, School and Playroom: Training Grounds for Adult Sex Roles*. (Anaheim, California: American Psychological Association)
15. Plumb, P. C. and Cowan, G. (1984). A developmental study of destereotyping and androgynous activity preferences of tomboys, nontomboys, and males. *Sex Roles*, **10**, 703-6
16. Liss, M. B. (1985). The play of boys and girls. In Fein, G. and Rivkin, M. (eds.) *The Play of Boys and Girls*. (Washington, DC: National Association for the Education of young children) (In Press)
17. Block, J. H. (1979). Socialization influences on personality development in males and females. In Parks, M. M. (ed.) *APA Master lecture series on issues of sex and gender in psychology*. (Washington, DC: American Psychological Association)
18. Liss, M. B. (1981). Patterns of toy play: an analysis of sex differences. *Sex Roles*, **7**, 1143-50
19. Halverson, L. E., Roberton, M. A. and Langendorfer, S. (1982). Development of the overarm throw: movement and ball velocity changes by seventh grade. *Res. Q. Exercise Sport*, **53**, 198-205
20. Hartup, W. W. (1974). Aggression in childhood: developmental perspectives. *Am. Psychol.*, **29**, 336-41
21. Langlois, H. J., Gottfried, N. W. and Seay, B. (1973). The influence of sex of peer on the social behaviour of preschool children. *Dev. Psychol.*, **8**, 93-8
22. Whiting, B. and Edwards, C. (1973). A cross-cultural analysis of sex differences in the behaviour of children aged three through eleven. *J. Soc. Psychol.*, **91**, 177-88
23. DiPietro, J. A. (1981). Rough-and-tumble play: a function of gender. *Dev. Psychol.*, **17**, 50-8
24. Halliday, J. and McNaughton, S. (1982). Sex differences in play at kindergarten. *N. Z. J. Educ. Stud.*, **17**, 161-70
25. Klein, A. R. and Bates, J. E. (1980). Gendertyping of game choices and qualities of boys' play behaviour. *J. Abnorm. Child Psychol.*, **8**, 201-12
26. Birdwhistell, R. L. (1970). *Kinesics and Context*. (Philadelphia: University of Pennsylvania Press)
27. Hyde, J. S. (1984). How large are gender differences in aggression? A developmental meta-analysis. *Dev. Psychol.*, **20**, 722-36
28. Maccoby, E. E. and Jacklin, C. N. (1974). *The Psychology of Sex Differences*. (Stanford, California: Stanford University Press)
29. Carpenter, C. J. and Huston-Stein, A. C. (1980). Activity structure and sex-typed behaviour in preschool children. *Child Dev.*, **51**, 862-73
30. Carpenter, C. J. (1983). Activity structure and play: implications for socialization. In Liss, M. B. (ed.) *Social and Cognitive Skills: Sex Roles and Children's Play*. pp. 117-95. (New York: Academic Press)
31. Fagot, B. I. and Littman, I. (1976). Relation of preschool sex typing to intellectual performance in elementary school. *Psychol. Rep.*, **39**, 699-704
32. Fagot, B. I. (1973). Influence of teacher behaviour in the preschool. *Dev. Psychol.*, **9**, 198-206
33. Fagot, B. I. (1978). Reinforcing contingencies for sex-role behaviours: effects of experience with children. *Child Dev.*, **49**, 30-6
34. Fagot, B. I. (1985). Peer and teacher reactions to boys' and girls' play styles. *Sex Roles*. (In Press)
35. Kaiser, S. B. and Phinney, J. S. (1983). Sex-typing of play activities by girls' clothing style: pants versus skirts. *Child Stud. J.*, **15**, 115-32

36. Etaugh, C. (1983). Introduction: the influences of environmental factors on sex differences in children's play. In Liss, M. B. (ed.) *Social and Cognitive Skills: Sex Roles and Children's Play*. pp. 1–19. (New York: Academic Press)
37. Wolf, T. M. (1973). Effects of live modelled sex-inappropriate play behaviour in a naturalistic setting. *Dev. Psychol.*, **9**, 120–3
38. Liss, M. B. and Doyle, T. (1982). *Sex-typing and Play: When Modelling Doesn't Work*. (Sacramento, California: Western Psychological Association)
39. Serbin, L. A., Tonick, I. J. and Sternglanz, S. H. (1977). Shaping cooperative cross-sex play. *Child Dev.*, **48**, 924–9
40. Bianchi, B. and Bakeman, R. (1978). Sex-typed affiliation preferences observed in pre-schoolers: traditional and open school differences. *Child Dev.*, **49**, 910–12
41. Bianchi, B. and Bakeman, R. (1983). Patterns of sex-typing in an open classroom. In Liss, M. B. (ed.) *Social and Cognitive Skills: Sex Roles and Children's Play*. pp. 219–33. (New York: Academic Press)
42. Connor, J. M., Schackman, M. and Serbin, L. A. (1978). Sex-related differences in response to practice on a visual–spatial test and generalization to a related test. *Child Dev.*, **49**, 24–9
43. Connor, J. M., Serbin, L. A. and Schackman, M. (1977). Sex differences on children's response to training on a visual–spatial test. *Dev. Psychol.*, **13**, 293–4
44. Serbin, L. A. and Connor, J. M. (1979). Sex-typing of children's play preferences and patterns of cognitive performance. *J. Genet. Psychol.*, **134**, 315–16
45. Sprafkin, C., Serbin, L. A., Denier, C. and Connor, J. M. (1983). Sex-differentiated play: Cognitive consequences and early interventions. In Liss, M. B. (ed.) *Social and Cognitive Skills: Sex Roles and Children's Play*. pp. 168–92. (New York: Academic Press)

# Index

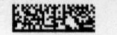